W0080623

Fundamentals of
DENTAL RADIOLOGY

Fourth Edition

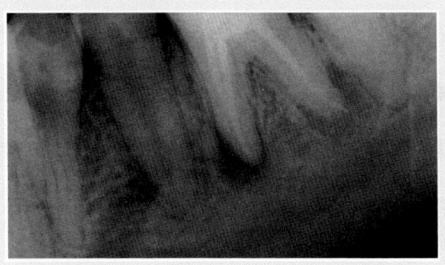

Other CBS Titles by the Same Author

- **Textbook of Operative Dentistry,** 2nd Edition
- **Pre-Clinical Conservative Dentistry**
- **Community Dentistry**

Fundamentals of
DENTAL RADIOLOGY
Fourth Edition

Vimal K Sikri

MDS, DOOP (PU), DEME (AIU), FICD

Principal
Punjab Government Dental College and Hospital
Amritsar

CBS Publishers & Distributors Pvt Ltd

New Delhi • Bengaluru • Chennai • Kochi • Mumbai • Pune
Hyderabad • Kolkata • Nagpur • Patna • Vijayawada

Disclaimer

Science and technology are constantly changing fields. New research and experience broaden the scope of information and knowledge. The author has tried his best in giving information available to him while preparing the material for this book. Although, all efforts have been made to ensure optimum accuracy of the material, yet it is quite possible some errors might have been left uncorrected. The publisher, printer and the author will not be held responsible for any inadvertent errors or inaccuracies.

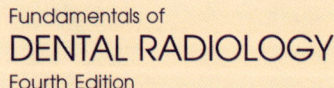

Fundamentals of
DENTAL RADIOLOGY
Fourth Edition

ISBN: 978-81-239-1791-7

Copyright © Author and Publishers

Fourth Edition: 2010

Reprinted: 2015
First Edition: 1992
Reprinted: 1996, 1997

Second Edition: 1999
Reprinted: 2001, 2003

Third Edition: 2006
Reprinted: 2008

All rights reserved. No part of this book may be reproduced or transmitted in any form or by any means, electronic or mechanical, including photocopying, recording, or any information storage and retrieval system without permission, in writing, from the author and the publisher.

Published by Satish Kumar Jain and produced by Varun Jain for
CBS Publishers & Distributors Pvt Ltd
4819/XI Prahlad Street, 24 Ansari Road, Daryaganj, New Delhi 110 002, India.
Ph: 23289259, 23266861, 23266867　　Website: www.cbspd.com
Fax: 011-23243014　　e-mail: delhi@cbspd.com; cbspubs@airtelmail.in.
Corporate Office: 204 FIE, Industrial Area, Patparganj, Delhi 110 092
Ph: 4934 4934　　Fax: 4934 4935　　e-mail: publishing@cbspd.com; publicity@cbspd.com

Branches

- **Bengaluru:** Seema House 2975, 17th Cross, K.R. Road, Banasankari 2nd Stage, Bengaluru 560 070, Karnataka
  Ph: +91-80-26771678/79　　Fax: +91-80-26771680　　e-mail: bangalore@cbspd.com
- **Chennai:** 7, Subbaraya Street, Shenoy Nagar, Chennai 600 030, Tamil Nadu
  Ph: +91-44-42032115　　Fax: +91-44-42032115　　e-mail: chennai@cbspd.com
- **Kochi:** 36/14 Kalluvilakam, Lissie Hospital Road, Kochi 682 018, Kerala
  Ph: +91-484-4059061-65　　Fax: +91-484-4059065　　e-mail: kochi@cbspd.com
- **Mumbai:** 83-C, Dr E Moses Road, Worli, Mumbai-400018, Maharashtra
  Ph: +91-22-24902340/41　　Fax: +91-22-24902342　　e-mail: mumbai@cbspd.com
- **Pune:** Bhuruk Prestige, Sr. No. 52/12/2+1+3/2 Narhe, Haveli (Near Katraj-Dehu Road Bypass), Pune 411 041, Maharashtra
  Ph: +91-20-64704058/59, 32392277　　Fax: +91-20-24300160　　e-mail: pune@cbspd.com

Representatives

Hyderabad	0-9885175004	**Kolkata**	0-9831437309, 0-9051152362
Nagpur	0-9021734563	**Patna**	0-9334159340
Vijayawada	0-9000660880		

Printed at: Paras Offset Pvt. Ltd., C-176, Naraina Industrial Area Phase-I, New Delhi

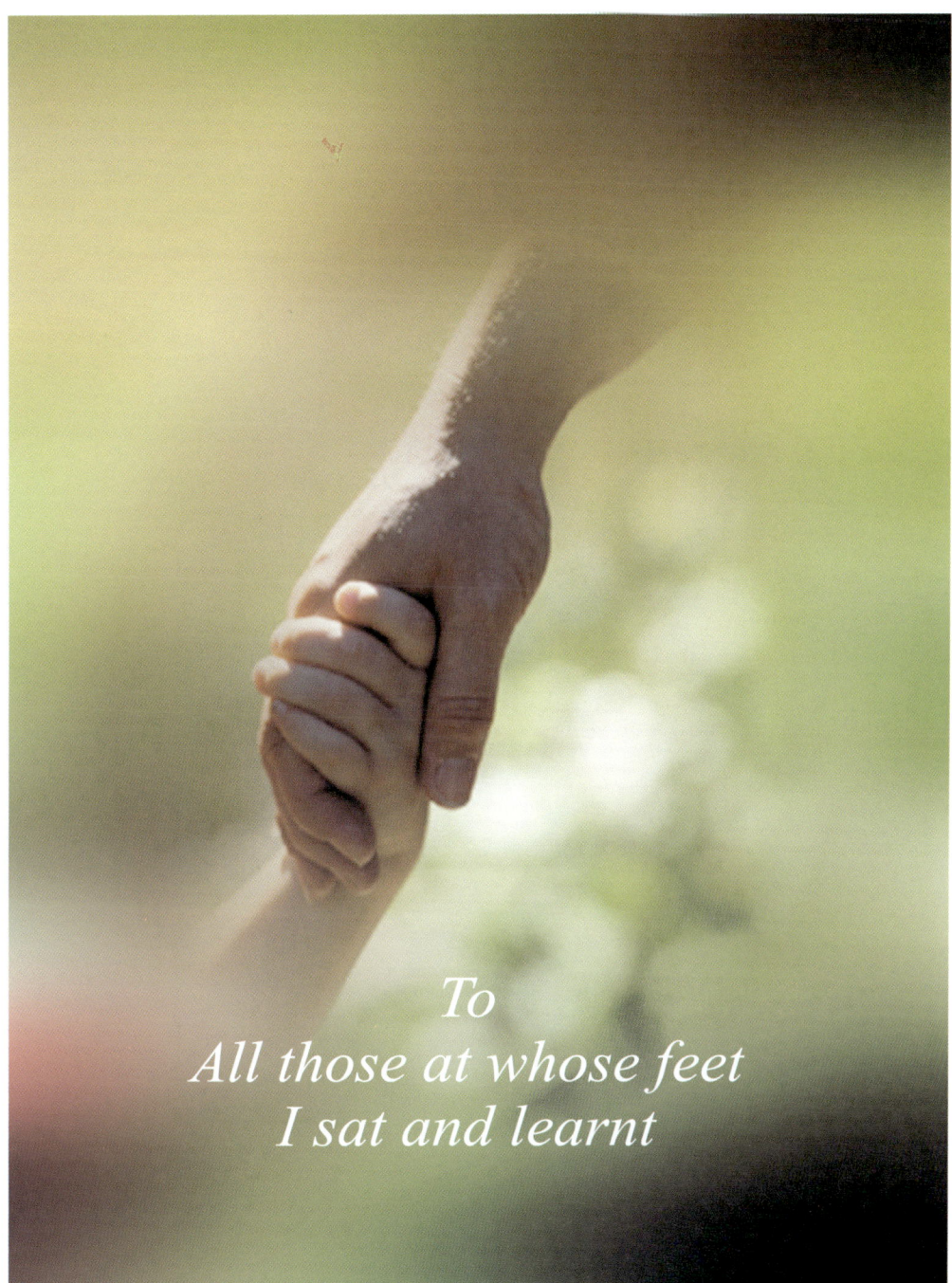

To
All those at whose feet
I sat and learnt

Foreword

Human ingenuity has led the X-rays to such heights that they are now considered as inseparable diagnostic aid in the field of dentistry.

Right from the time Dr. Kells took first dental X-ray, people in dental profession realised that the use of X-rays as a diagnostic medium has bright future.

Early workers, however, had not the slightest idea of their being so injurious to living tissues. They did not use any shield and in the process many lost their lives. Dr Rapar was perhaps the first person describing the ill-effects of X-rays and the means to protect both patients and the operators.

Dentists and the assistants are doing irreparable damage by not properly shielding themselves from the X-rays; some even hold X-ray films in patient's mouth. Such people should in all fairness, be warned of the consequences.

Dental radiographs have become inseparable modality in diagnosis of practically all dental ailments. And, with time, there is a marked improvement in the quality of X-ray techniques.

This textbook, prepared by Dr Sikri, I personally consider a commendable effort. He has given each phase of radiology in a very simple and lucid manner. Any person in dental profession will be benefited by this. He has given special attention to photographs for better understanding and he has also included a chapter on 'Multiple Choice Questions'.

I feel this book might be considered as a fundamental in radiological techniques and interpretations.

I wish the author and the book a success.

Dr. SS Dua
Principal
DAV Dental College
Yamuna Nagar 135 001

Preface to the Fourth Edition

The best moments in a father's life are to relish growth of his children. The child *Fundamentals of Dental Radiology*, born in early nineties, after undergoing a series of threats and opportunities, has grown to the level of the fourth edition. I am whole-heartedly indebted to God and also the blessings of my parents for the present edition in your hands. The readers' suggestions and criticism always help in improving the substance; credit goes to the readers for their valuable suggestions.

I hope the present edition will fulfill the requirements of all the teachers and the students alike. An attempt has been made to clarify every phase of the subject.

I am grateful to Dr Vandana Kumar, Assistant Professor, Oral Pathology, Radiology and Medicine, University of Missouri, for adding, "Cone Beam Computed Tomography (CBCT)" along with her cases in the field. The chapter "Advanced Imaging Modalities" has been expanded keeping in view the necessity of present-day radiology.

Dr Mohan Gundappa, Professor and Head, Saraswati Dental College, Lucknow, and Dr Soheyl Sheikh, Professor and Head, MM Dental College, Mullana, deserve special appreciation for their keen interests and contribution to this edition. I am thankful to Dr Vimal Kalia, Professor and Head, BRS Dental College, Panchkula, for rearranging chapter on "Imaging of Maxillary Sinuses".

I am thankful to Dr Jeevan Lata, Professor and Head; Dr SPS Sooch, Associate Professor; and Dr Nitin Verma, Demonstrator, Department of Oral and Maxillofacial Surgery, Government Dental College, Amritsar, for arranging radiographs for the present edition. I am also thankful to my students, Dr Gulvinder, Dr Amrit, Dr Payal, Dr Preeti, Dr Meenu, Dr Ibadat, Dr Pulkit, Dr Nalini, Dr Monica, Dr Kavita, and Dr Dheeraj for checking the typescript. Mr GB Singh did wonderful job on Corel diagrams, thanks dear.

With all humility, I hope the readers will find the book worth reading because of the lucid language and self-explanatory photographs. New illustrations have been added to simplify the text. My sweet wife, Dr Poonam, always encouraged and supported me during the upbringing of the book. My dear sons, Ankit and Arpit, need special thanks as they always helped me during checking of the typescript.

I request the readers to critically evaluate the text and send me their comments since their analytic suggestions would help me improve upon the book.

Vimal K Sikri

Preface to the First Edition

The idea of writing a book on radiology came to me when I was first given this subject to teach undergraduates. I had to consult many books and, so much so, many a time, I had to write to Dr. A.B. Surveyor, my unseen mentor, for clarification. All these difficulties coupled with my deep desire to be communicative inspired me to write a book on radiology in a very lucid and clear style and in as simple language as possible.

The scope of dental radiology has widened immensely in the recent past and a single book can no longer cover completely all the aspects of this constantly expanding subject. All care has been taken to present the subject with a view to helping the student community in particular and the practitioners in general. What prompted me to embark on this project is to help the people in dental profession meet their needs which remained unfulfilled hitherto. To attain clarity, I have pressed into service the following devices. First, the text is presented in a very simple language along with self-explanatory drawings and X-ray pictures. It is believed that this will help dental students grasp the subject easily. Secondly, the importance has been given to the chapter of 'Interpretation of Radiographs' because of the vastness of knowledge involved in it. An attempt has been made to present all the photographs depicting normal and abnormal structures. Thirdly, I have included the recent and the latest radiographic techniques though briefly. Finally, the chapter on 'Multiple Choice Questions' in radiology would be of special interest to students appearing in various competitive examinations.

An attempt has been made to clarify every phase of the subject. References, except those related to specific occasions, have been deleted. However, the reader will find a list of suggested readings at the end of the book. This textbook, though comprehensive, is concise and is expected to prove effective and useful for classroom teachings.

I am indebted to Dr. SS Dua, Principal, DAV Dental College, Yamuna Nagar, my revered teacher for creating in me the interest of writing and reading. I am also indebted to Dr. A. B. Surveyor, previously Professor and Head, Deptt. of Radiology, Nair Dental Hospital and College, Mumbai, for his encouraging letters.

I am thankful to Dr. Thukral, Assistant Professor of Radiology for his brotherly help. I am also thankful to Mr. Satjit Grewal and Mr. Girdhari Sharma for their help in taking radiographs, Mr. Kuldip Singh Neelon for drawings, Mr. Avinash for photographs and Mr. Ashwani for overall help. I acknowledge gratefully the assistance of my students Dr. Vimal Kalia, Ms. Moushmi, Ms Sangeet, Ms Sanjana and Ms Surinder to name a few. Appreciation is expressed to my colleagues Dr. Ravi, Dr. Bal and Dr. Bhupinder for their valuable criticism. I am indebted to Prof. O.N. Gupta of D.A.V. College, Amritsar and Prof. J.S. Walia of Khalsa College for Women, Amritsar for their analysis.

Finally, I am beholden to my wife, parents and brothers for their unstinted support, without which the book of this magnitude would not have been possible.

Vimal K Sikri

Contributors

Dr. Karthikeya Patil
Professor and Head
Department of Oral Medicine and Radiology
JSS Dental College, JSS Nagar
Mysore (Karnataka)

Dr. Soheyl Sheikh
Professor and Head,
Department of Oral Medicine and Radiology
MM Dental College and Hospital
Mullana, Ambala (Haryana)

Dr. Vimal Kalia
Professor and Head
Department of Oral and Maxillofacial Surgery
and Dean Academics
BRS Dental College
Panchkula (Haryana)

Dr. Sumeet Sandhu
Professor and Head
Department of Oral and Maxillofacial Surgery
SGRD Dental College
Amritsar (Punjab)

Dr. Vandana Kumar
Assistant Professor
Oral Pathology, Radiology and Medicine
School of Dentistry
University of Missouri
Kansas City, Missouri, USA

Dr. CS Saimbi
Professor
Department of Periodontology
KG Dental College
Lucknow (UP)

Dr. (Mrs) Poonam Sikri
Professor and Head
Department of Periodontology
Seema Dental College and Hospital
Rishikesh (Uttarakhand)

Dr. Mohan Gundappa
Professor and Head
Department of Conservative Dentistry and
Endodontics
Saraswati Dental College, Lucknow (UP)

Contents

C

1

Basis of Radiology

Perhaps the common saying '*I treat and He cures*' is true, but His curing and our treatment, undoubtedly, depend on one factor and that is proper diagnosis. For proper diagnosis of any case in dentistry or in medical profession at large, the radiographs play a very important role.

Radiographs have been regarded since long as an invaluable boon to mankind thus giving him a sixth sense. The radiographs are considered as an indispensable adjunct in oral diagnosis and play a role in detecting, evaluating and even treating various lesions of the teeth and the oral cavity.

Radiographs are always interpreted and never read. We do not read the radiograph; only interpret the various structures. For proper interpretation, basic factors of black and white must be understood which are the fundamentals in radiology.

If an unexposed film is developed, only the clear transparent base remains, i.e. no X-rays are fallen on the film. The film will be white or clear. And when the film is exposed to X-rays and is developed, it has a dark shadow depending upon the exposure time and the site where X-rays have fallen.

How much X-rays are absorbed by the film during exposure will depict as the relatively dark and white shadow. Clear film implies that no rays have fallen over it while black indicates that the film is exposed to X-rays.

If we expose any substance over the film, viz. a coin or a piece of bone, the resultant picture will be the white area in the centre and black all round. In case of bone, however, certain dark lines may be seen in the white area. Histologically, these are bony trabeculae. The relative whiteness of bone and coin will also differ. This is because the absorption of X-rays varies with different structures. Greater the physical density of the substance, the greater is the power to absorb X-rays, i.e. denser the substance more white appearance over the film (Figs 1.1 and 1.2A to C). The structure of the teeth and the periodontium is presented in Fig. 1.3.

Metals are whiter than enamel and enamel appears whiter than dentine and so on. Pulp is black in appearance. Air, fluids and soft tissues do not absorb X-rays and therefore appear black. Certain terms are commonly used in radiology

1

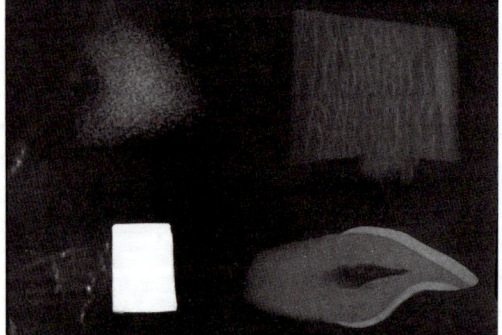

Fig. 1.1: Objects of different densities appear differently on radiograph. Clockwise from top left: tricalcium phosphate powder; a piece of bone; section of tooth and a metallic piece

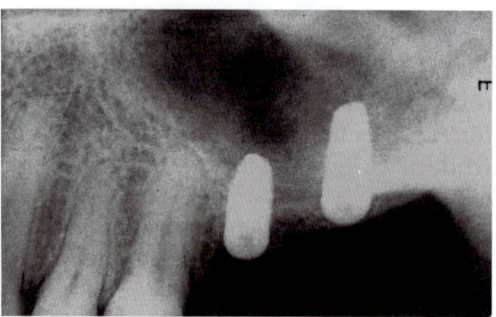

Fig. 1.2A: Implants appear as radiopaque. Radiolucent area over implants is maxillary sinus

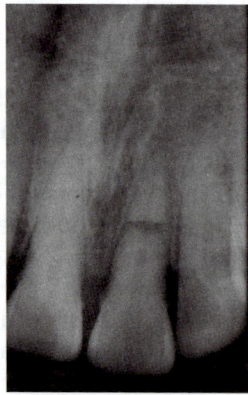

Fig. 1.2B: Horizontal fracture of root appears as radiolucent line

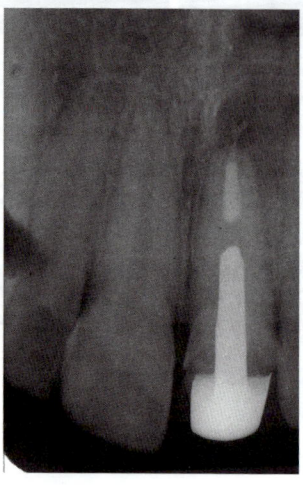

Fig. 1.2C: Metallic post and core appear radiopaque. Little less radiopaque over the post is gutta-percha

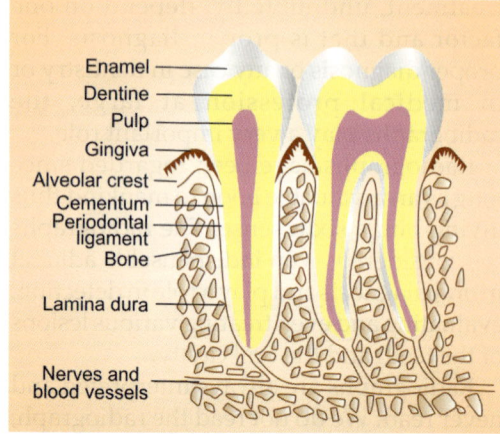

Enamel
Dentine
Pulp
Gingiva
Alveolar crest
Cementum
Periodontal ligament
Bone
Lamina dura
Nerves and blood vessels

Fig. 1.3: Structure of teeth and periodontium

concerning these black and white appearances. Substances or tissues which absorb more X-rays than others are called *opaque* or correctly *radiopaque*. The greater the thickness and density, the more radiopaque is the material and resultant white shadow over the film. Wherever there is complete absorption of X-rays such as caused by metallic fillings or coins, there occurs no action of X-rays over the film and the resultant shadow is white or *radiopaque*. Contrary to this, whenever there is no absorption of X-rays the resultant area appears black over the film and is called *radiolucent*, e.g. soft tissues, fluid, air, etc.

Certain other routinely used terms must also be made clear. A radiograph should have maximum detail with right amount of contrast and sharpness without distortion.

Detail is that quality which concerns with visualising fine structures under examination, e.g. in a radiograph of bone if the internal structures are portrayed normally, the radiograph is said to have good detail.

Contrast is the difference of density between black and white areas. The radiograph is said to be 'sharp' if the line of demarcation between objects of varying densities is clear.

Definition has also been used for details and sharpness. If all the structures are portrayed normally, the radiograph has good definition. The right amount of contrast is that which serves to bring out the detail in fullest possible manner.

In order to make a perfect radiograph, the position of the patient, film–object distance and object–tube distance should be kept properly (details in Chapter 6).

Distortion may be sidewise or lengthwise. It usually occurs due to improper placement of films, improper direction of X-rays or patient's instability during exposure. These factors affect collectively and even singly.

Radiographic studies or interpretations depend upon a thorough clinical knowledge of the underlying structures and the possible pathologies which may change these structures. Radiographic evidence, if taken at its face value may be misleading and many a time leads to serious errors. Limitations of radiographs of not being three-dimensional, and presence and superimposition of anatomical landmarks create difficulties in interpretation. As said earlier, these are adjunct to diagnosis and not the final diagnostic tools.

Study of anatomy with complete knowledge of underlying structures is mandatory for interpretation. A great degree of skill is required to distinguish normal from the abnormal. Experience no doubt helps but regardless of the experience of a person, new structures or artefacts appear which routinely fail to be explained.

Many a times it is impossible to determine by radiographic methods alone, whether a given appearance is abnormal or normal. Just by seeing the radiograph the operator decides and declares that the surgical intervention is necessary which is a wrong practice. However, clinical examination along with radiographic interpretation is a must for making final decision.

Radiographic evaluation or follow up examination is necessary before a final conclusion is drawn. Pre-operative, post-operative and follow up radiographs along with clinical examination is necessary before arriving at the final diagnosis.

Examination of radiograph in daylight is to be avoided. Light falling on eyes from the sides of the film reduces the accuracy of the vision. Examiner should use a viewing box which emits diffused light only over the area of radiograph. Magnifying lens should be used. Attention should be given to every part of the film from one corner to the other. Most of the times when one abnormality is seen, we stop examining the radiograph which is not a good practice. Other lesions should also be recognised or looked for which later on may prove to be of great significance.

Personal opinion should not be expressed if the examiner is unsatisfied with the quality of radiograph because of any reason such as faulty radiograph, defective light, shortage of time, etc.

Finally, the radiographic interpretation depends not only on clinical knowledge but also on mental state of the examiner, his physical well being and last but not the least, his mood.

DEFINITIONS

Radiology

It is the study and use of radiant energy including roentgen rays, radium and radioactive isotopes as applied to medicine and dentistry.

Radiology is a broad term, which embraces two main fields:

- Diagnostic radiology
- Therapeutic radiology

We are concerned mainly with the first aspect, i.e. diagnostic radiology. *Radiography* is the actual process of making radiographs. Trained technicians are required for these purposes.

Roentgenology

Roentgenology is the study and use of X-rays or roentgen rays as applied to medicine and dentistry. Sometimes the term *radiodontics* is used. This includes radiology of jaws and teeth, which is a misnomer because teeth and jaws cannot be separated from the human body. Modern dentistry, based on fundamental principles of human biology, has evolved as an independent and indispensable partner of medical field.

PHYSICAL MAKE-UP OF MATTER

A general understanding of physical make-up of matter is important to understand radiology and its principles.

Atom is considered to be the smallest component of matter, however, it can be further reduced to smaller particles, i.e. electrons, protons and neutrons (Fig. 1.4). An atom basically consists of two parts: centrally located nucleus and the electrons orbiting around it. Nucleus consists of *protons* (positively charged particles), neutrons (neutral particles) and many other smaller particles. All the particles in the nucleus are bound by strong nuclear forces. Number of protons is specific for each atom, which is its atomic number. Usually, the neutrons are equal to protons in lighter elements but in others the neutrons are more.

Electrons revolve around the nucleus in definite orbits (Fig. 1.4). Orbits can be one or more depending upon the atom. The inner circle or orbit is K and then L, M, N and so on. The number of electrons in dissimilar atoms varies. All forms of matter are merely different arrangements of these three, i.e. electrons, protons and neutrons. Electrons remain in constant motion because they are constantly repelling each other. They are held within the atom by the counter attractive force of protons. If this force is disturbed, the electrons are removed from their orbits, the atoms become positively charged. This is now known as +ve ion and is unstable. The free electron is called the –ve ion and the two known as *ion pair*. The production of ion pair or the dislodging of

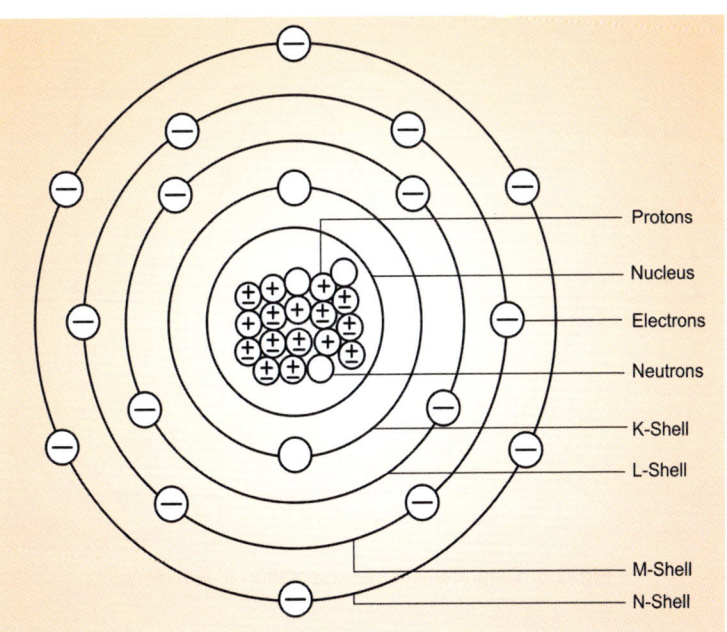

Protons

Nucleus

Electrons

Neutrons

K-Shell

L-Shell

M-Shell

N-Shell

Fig. 1.4: Fundamental concept of matter. Diagram of an atom

1

electrons from the orbit is known as ionisation.

Ionisation is the basis of good and harmful effects of X-radiations and other radiations.

TYPES OF RADIATION

From the technical view-point, radiations are of two types:

- **Particulate radiations:** These radiations have solid subatomic mass such as alpha (protons), beta (electrons) and gamma (neutrons) particles. Radium and radioisotope radiations are particulate in nature.

- **Electromagnetic radiations:** These radiations have no particle or mass but are pure energy waves. These are a combination of electric and magnetic energy. X-radiations belong to this group.

It is not fully known whether these electromagnetic radiations are actually waves of energy or individual units of energy called photons.

If radiation is considered as waves, it is measured by its length and if it is considered as bundles of photon energy, then it is measured in *ergs*. Preferably, we consider the concept of energy wave. Height of the wave is called the *crest* and the depth of wave is called *trough*. Distance between one crest to the other is called the wavelength and is abbreviated by the Greek letter lambda (λ) (Fig. 1.5).

X-radiations have a very short wavelength measured in Angstrom depicted as Å ($1\text{Å} = 10^{-8}$ cm).

1

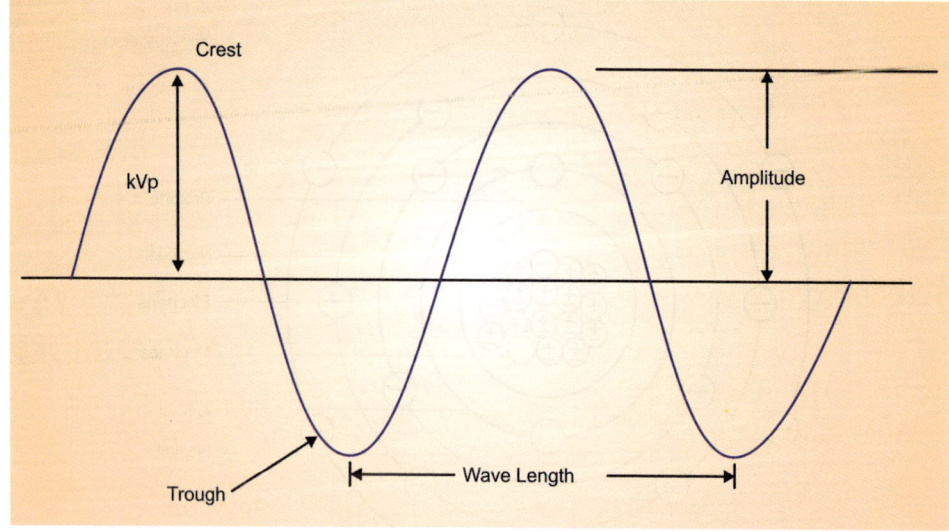

Fig. 1.5: Diagrammatic representation of wavelength

The difference in electromagnetic spectrum between visible light, X-radiations and other radiations is in their wavelengths.

The shorter the wavelength, the more the energy it bears. It is that energy which imparts power to penetrate matter. Other waves with different wavelengths are there in the universe, which also have the effect on the body depending upon their wavelengths and frequencies.

In contrast, if we take the 'quantum theory', it assumes that transfer of energy by electromagnetic radiations is not in the form of waves but as a flux of quanta or photon (bundle of energy). Each photon travels with the speed of light and contains a specific amount of energy. Unit of photon energy is electron volt (eV). Photon with shorter wavelength has higher energy.

CONCEPT OF ELECTRICITY

A simple review of the basic electrical terms is a prerequisite to study the X-ray machine

and its working. The electric circuit of the X-ray machine is depicted in Fig. 1.6.

Electric Current

Electric current is the flow of electrons through a circuit. Alternatively, motion of electric charge constitutes an electric current. A metallic conductor consists of a large number of free electrons (in the outermost shell) which move at random like the molecules of the gas enclosed in a container.

An electric current in a conductor is the movement of the free electrons from one part to the other. It may be considered similar to the flow of water in a tube. Since a difference of pressure is necessary between the two ends of a tube to make the water flow through it, similarly electrical pressure (potential difference) is necessary across the ends of the conductor for the electric current to flow through it. Metals are the most commonly used substances for electrical

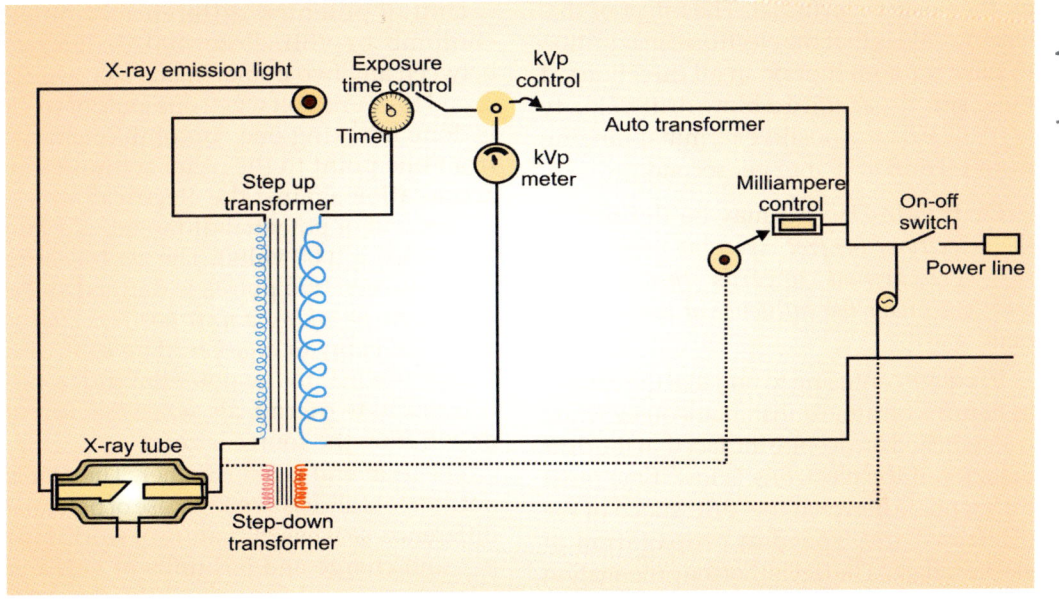

Fig. 1.6: Basic electric circuit of dental X-ray machine

conduction. However, the liquids and gases can also conduct electricity.

Current Strength

The strength of the electric current is defined as the rate of flow of electric charge across any section of the conductor. If q units of electric charge flow across any section of the conductor in t seconds, the strength of current is given by $I = q/t$.

The electric current is said to be steady if the rate of flow of charge does not change with time, otherwise it is said to vary. For flow of the current what is required besides a potential difference is the presence of charged particles or charge carrier such as electrons in metals. In order to maintain a flow of current between two points, a constant difference of potential has to be maintained between them. It can be done only by some external means such as battery, supply mains, etc.

In a metal there are free electrons. Since they possess thermal energy, they are in a state of continuous motion just like the molecules of a gas. They keep on colliding with the atoms, gaining and losing kinetic energy. The individual electrons drift slowly along the conductor with a speed of 1/100 cm/second, but the impulse due to its movement is nearly 1,86,000 miles/second.

When an electric field is applied, applying potential difference at the ends of the conductor, say copper wire, the electrons flow continuously from the negative terminal through the copper wire to the positive terminal and then through the battery to the negative terminal. They are repelled by negative terminal and attracted

1

by the positive terminal. The effect of this electric field is that the electrons, in addition to their random motion in all directions at huge speeds, acquire a blow drift velocity (v_d) towards the positive terminal ranging from 1.0 mm to 10 mm per second.

Drift velocity (v_d) may be defined as *the velocity of the free electrons with which they get drifted towards the positive terminal under the influence of the external field.*

It is quite confusing to find that the electric bulb turns on almost instantaneously when it is switched on despite the fact that the drift velocity of the electrons is low. One must differentiate between the 'drift speed of the electrons' and 'speed of propagation of electric effect'. The fact is that the propagation of an electric impulse takes place with a speed of the order of speed of light.

Ampere is the unit of current. *An ampere is the strength of current flowing in a wire when a charge of one coulomb flows across any section of it per second.* Ampere (1820) has said that the direction of the current is the direction in which the positive charge would move under the action of an electric field.

Current can be direct current or alternating current. An alternating current may be defined as *a current, which continuously changes its magnitude and periodically reverses its direction.* A current of constant magnitude and flowing in the same direction is called *direct current.*

Potential Difference or Voltage

Potential difference between two points in an electric field may be defined as *the amount of work done in moving a unit positive charge from one point to another without any acceleration against the electric force.*

Unit of potential difference is joule/coulomb or volt. Potential difference between any two points in an electric field is said to be one volt when one joule of work is done in taking one coulomb of charge from one point to the other without any acceleration against the electrical forces. Bigger unit of potential difference is 1 kilo volt (1 kV = 1000 volts). The *electromotive force* between two points is defined as *the work done in taking a unit positive charge from one point to another.* The emf of a source is equal to the potential difference between its two terminals, when the current drawn from the source is zero.

The term **emf** is a misnomer. The emf is not a force at all. It is a special case of potential difference, so it has the nature of work done per unit charge and has units of volt and kilovolt.

Galvanometer

It is a basic instrument for electrical measurements. It is a sensitive current detector. It produces a deflection proportional to the electric current flowing through it.

Ammeter

It is a low resistance galvanometer which is calibrated to measure the current directly in amperes. An ammeter is always connected in series in a circuit so that whole of the current to be measured should be able to pass through it.

Voltmeter

It is a high resistance moving coil galvanometer which is calibrated so as to measure the potential difference in volts. Voltmeter is always connected parallel with the circuit between the two points across which potential difference is to be measured.

Ohm's Law

The relation between potential difference and current strength through a conductor was described first by a German physicist, George Ohm, which is called Ohm's law. This law states that *provided the physical conditions (temperature, mechanical stress, etc.) of a conductor remain unchanged, the current flowing through it is always proportional to the potential difference between its two ends*. If V stands for potential difference between the ends of the conductor and C the current flowing through it, then:

$$V \alpha \, C \text{ or } \frac{V}{C} = R$$

where R is constant known as electric resistance. Its value depends upon the dimension, nature and temperature of the conductor.

Transformer

It is a device which can either increase or decrease the voltage. *Step-up* and *Step-down* transformers are available which increase and decrease the voltage respectively. A transformer is composed of two coils of electric wires insulated from each other. Magnetic field from one coil induces electric circuit in the second coil. Number of turns in one coil (conduction coil) and the number of turns in the second coil will determine what kind of transformer it is. The *autotransformer* makes one coil do the work of two coils (Fig. 1.7). This is used where minor change in voltage is required. The autotransformer selects the voltage from the kVp dial and applies it to the 'high voltage' transformer establishing potential difference between cathode and the anode.

Rheostat

It is a variable resistance used in a circuit in order to regulate the strength of current. It consists of a hollow porcelain tube on which is wound a length of wire of material like eureka, constantin and manganin, etc. The winding is done in such a manner that the various turns do not touch each other. Two

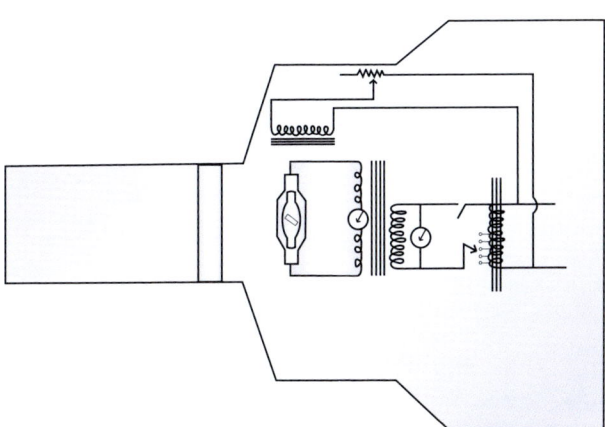

Fig. 1.7: Step-down transformer

1

terminals are connected at the two ends of the wire near the base of the tube. Over the porcelain tube is fixed a metallic bar parallel to the length of tube. A jockey can slide along this bar and makes contact with the different positions of the wire of the rheostat. There is a terminal at one end of the bar. The length and the diameter of the wire used in the rheostat depend upon the maximum resistance to be introduced in the circuit.

Resistance is directly proportional to the length of wire.

Bibliography

1. Aleox RW, Collett WK: A speciality of dental radiology is needed. *O Surg, O Med, O Path* 1972;33(1):130.

2. Dagering CI, Busenar RH: A roentgenographic film density study of dental restorative material. *O Surg, O Med, O Path* 1962;15:944.

2

Production of X-rays

The discovery of X-rays, like several other discoveries in the history of science, was 'accidental'. In November 1895, Wilhelm Conrad Roentgen, a Professor of Physics at Wurzberg University, Germany; was studying the effect of electric discharge through gases at very low pressure. Previous to this, Crooke, Hittorf and others were experimenting on fluorescence. On applying high potential difference between the electrodes, Roentgen found that the fluorescent screen covered with barium platinocyanide lying near the tube became luminous and a photographic plate lying in a closed box had become fogged. He realised that as current is passed, something comes out from the Crooke's tube, which causes the plate to glow. He covered the tube with thick black paper which was opaque to both visible and UV-light, but it made no difference in the glow of the fluorescent screen. As the nature of these radiations which caused fluorescence, etc. was not known at that time, they were named as X-rays ('X' being designated for unknown).

With more research and study of these rays, it was found that these radiations could penetrate several objects which were opaque to ordinary light. Roentgen was able to produce images of certain objects by placing them in the path of X-ray beam. He took the first radiograph of his wife's hand. Prof. Roentgen was awarded the Nobel Prize in 1901.

Within two weeks of the discovery of X-rays, Otto Walkhoff, a colleague of Roentgen, did the first dental radiograph. He exposed himself for 25 minutes and could get a crude form of the shadow. He had to suffer a lot because of radiation hazards. Kells was the one who popularised X-rays in dentistry. With all these, started the era of modifications and requirements, which led to the present radiology. Rollin Williams developed the first X-ray unit.

The discovery of X-rays is considered to be the most significant event in modern science, not only because it lead to important diagnostic applications but also it plays a vital role in therapeutics.

Soon after the discovery of X-rays their relation with other forms of radiation was the subject of keen interest. It was shown that these rays and light travel in straight line with the same speed, affect the photographic plate, cause fluorescence in certain materials and remain undeflected by electric or magnetic field. But they do differ in certain properties viz., extent of penetration, effect on photographic plate, etc. Haga Wind and other investigators performed several experiments in which they passed X-radiations through exceedingly narrow slits, a few thousandths of a millimeter wide. Such experiments were repeated by several investigators with modified techniques and the results indicated that their wavelength is of the order of 0.2–10Å. Ennis is of the view that X-rays with wavelength 0.8–1.0Å are used in dental radiography, which have higher penetrating powers.

From the study of optics, we know that suitable gratings can diffract light if the width of its elements is of same order as the wavelength of light. It was unthinkable to diffract X-rays because construction of such a small grating was not possible at that time.

However, it was known that the atoms in a crystal are arranged in a geometrical space lattice in which the grating between the atoms was of the order of 10^{-8} cm. These considerations inspired Voulance to suggest that a crystal should act as a three-dimensional diffraction grating for an X-ray beam.

Keeping this in mind an experiment was performed in which X-ray beam was directed upon the crystals of zinc sulphide. The apparatus is shown in Fig. 2.1.

The X-ray beam from the target of an X-ray tube is collimated in two lead screens

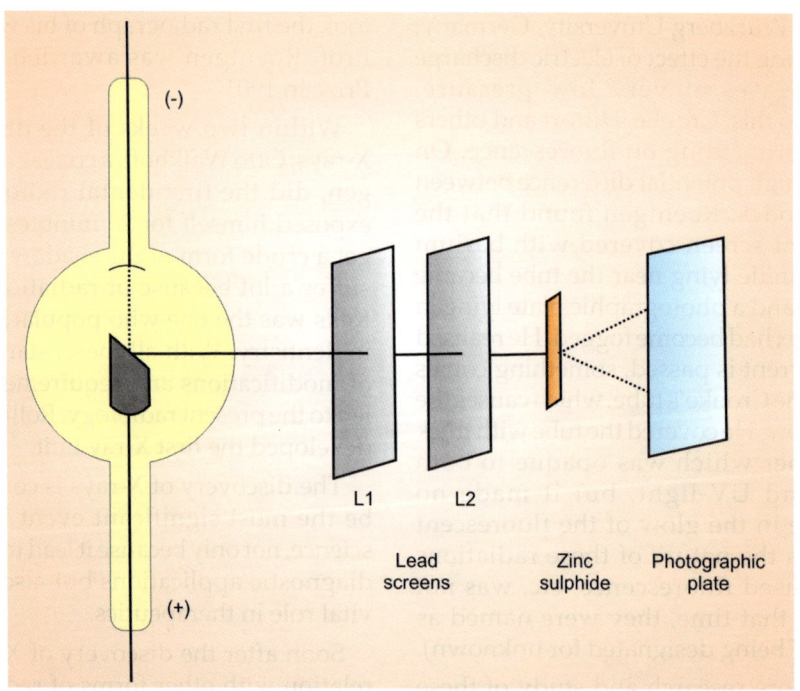

Fig. 2.1: Diffraction of X-ray beam using zinc sulphide crystals

L_1 and L_2 and then passed through zinc sulphide crystals. It was observed that the major part of the beam goes straight through the crystals to cause a spot at the centre. Besides this central beam, a number of relatively weak beams emerge in various directions to produce a group of other symmetrically arranged spots on the film around the central spot. This pattern is known as *Lane's pattern* (Max Von Lane) and this shows the diffraction of X-rays.

Regarding reflection of X-rays, *Bragg's law* is applied. He imagined three-dimensional crystal lattice to be divided into a number of different sets of parallel planes so that all the lattice points be on one of the planes and no point lies outside them. Each diffraction spot was produced by the interference between the rays reflected from a particular set of parallel planes within the crystal, which was rich in atoms.

Consider a set of parallel atomic places whose spacing is d and let a narrow X-ray beam fall upon these parallel planes at a glancing angle D. Each parallel layer in the given set gives rise to the reflected wave front (Fig. 2.2).

Two parallel rays X_1 and X_2 are reflected by two atoms A and B respectively. The distance between two lines is d. The additional path travelled by the ray reflected from the second layer is equal to CB + BD. The condition thus, is:

$$CB + BD = n\lambda$$
or $$2d \sin \phi = n\lambda$$

where n is an integer.

This is known as *Bragg's equation* and satisfies the reflection of X-rays from a set of atomic planes.

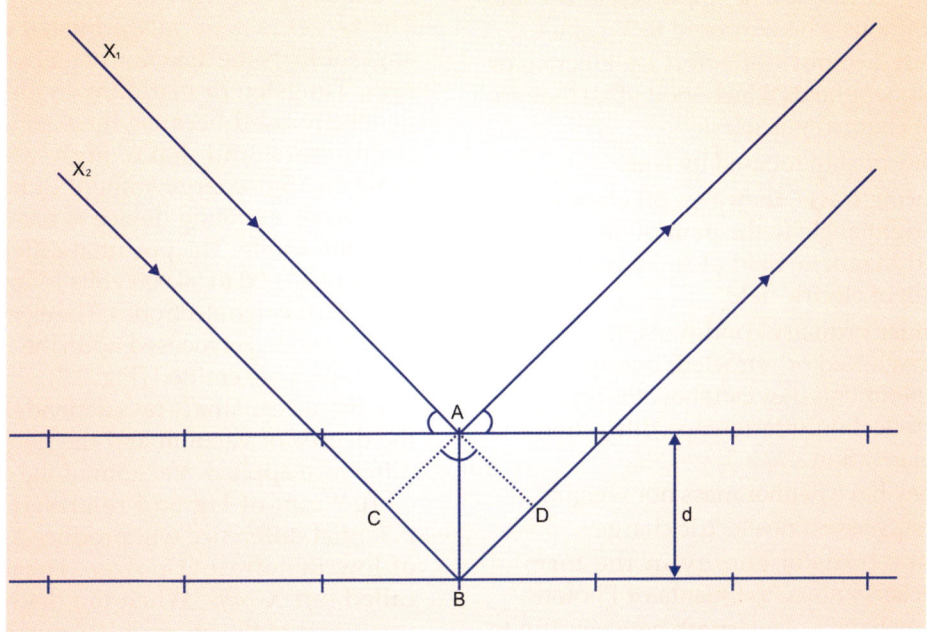

Fig. 2.2: Reflection of X-ray from lattice planes in a crystal

PROPERTIES OF X-RAYS

- X-rays travel in straight lines in wave motion with a speed that equals the speed of visible light, i.e. 1,86,000 miles/second or 3×10^8 m/sec.
- They are highly penetrating rays, which can pass through several materials which are opaque to ordinary light. It is this property of X-rays penetrating different materials to different depths which is being used in radiology to diagnose various lesions viz., fractures, presence of foreign bodies, etc.
- They ionise the gas through which they pass.
- They affect the photographic plate like visible light but the effect is much more intense.
- They cause fluorescence in several materials. Plates coated with barium platinocyanide zinc sulphide, etc. become luminous when exposed to X-rays.
- They are not deflected by electric or magnetic fields which shows that they are not charged particles.
- They are not focused by lens.
- During travel, they give off electric field at right angle to the path of propagation and magnetic field at right angle to the path of electric field.
- Under ordinary conditions, they cannot be reflected or refracted; but by suitable experiments they can show the properties of reflection, interference, diffraction and polarisation.
- They have neither mass nor weight.
- They possess no electric charge
- They transfer energy in the form of packets known as Quanta or Photons.
- They have a wavelength between 10Å to 0.01Å (Å= Angstrom)

- They cannot be detected by the human senses, namely sight, sound, smell, touch or taste.
- No medium is required for propagation.

PRODUCTION OF X-RAYS

Two types of tubes are employed:
   I. Gas tube
   II. Coolidge tube.

I. Gas Tube

Two types of gas tubes are available. These tubes are no longer used these days and are of historical interest only. Gas tubes are further of two types: (a) Crooke's tube; (b) Snooke's hydrogen tube.

a. **Crooke's tube:** It consists of glass tube fitted with three side tubes. One tube holds the soldered aluminium cathode C and the opposite tube anode or target T. The target is generally adjusted at an angle of 45° to the direction of the cathode rays. Tungsten or platinum anodes are generally used because they are good conductors and have high atomic numbers. Since large amount of heat is produced, a cooling device is provided with the anode. The potential difference of about 40,000 to 50,000 volts is applied between the two electrodes. The electrons from cathode get focused upon the target and X-rays are emitted (Fig. 2.3).
The character of the X-rays depends upon the degree of vacuum and the potential difference applied. Vacuum of the order of 10^{-3} mm of Hg and relatively low potential difference will produce X-rays of low penetrating power. These are called *soft X-rays*. When the degree of vacuum is of the order of 10^{-4} mm of Hg and high voltage is applied, X-rays

emitted are highly penetrating. Such X-rays are called *hard X-rays*, which have shorter wavelength than soft X-rays.

During operation of the tube the mixture of gases present in this tube gets ionized. This leads to gradual fall of pressure and more and more voltage is required to operate the tube. Ultimately the gas pressure in the tube becomes so low that it becomes impossible to maintain the discharge. To overcome this difficulty, a softening device is used. A side tube *R* with platinised asbestos is used in which the gases have been occluded. When due to extremely low pressure, the discharge does not pass across the main tube; it establishes itself across the tube *R*. The asbestos gets heated and the occluded gases are diffused into the tube, thereby increasing the pressure inside.

When the voltage across the tube is increased, there is increased ionisation of gases and the intensity of X-rays increases. At the same time, the energy of striking electrons also increases, so the X-rays emitted are of high penetrating power. It is seen that the voltage variation affects both the intensity and the quality of the X-rays.

b. **Snooke's hydrogen tube:** This is exactly the same as that of Crooke's tube; the only difference is that in place of a mixture of gases only hydrogen is used. With increased hydrogen content the tube is called *hard tube* and with decreased hydrogen content it is called *soft tube*.

Drawbacks

• It is not possible to have control on the quality and intensity of the X-rays separately.
• The softening device is not very efficient. There is limit to an increase in gas pressure by this method.

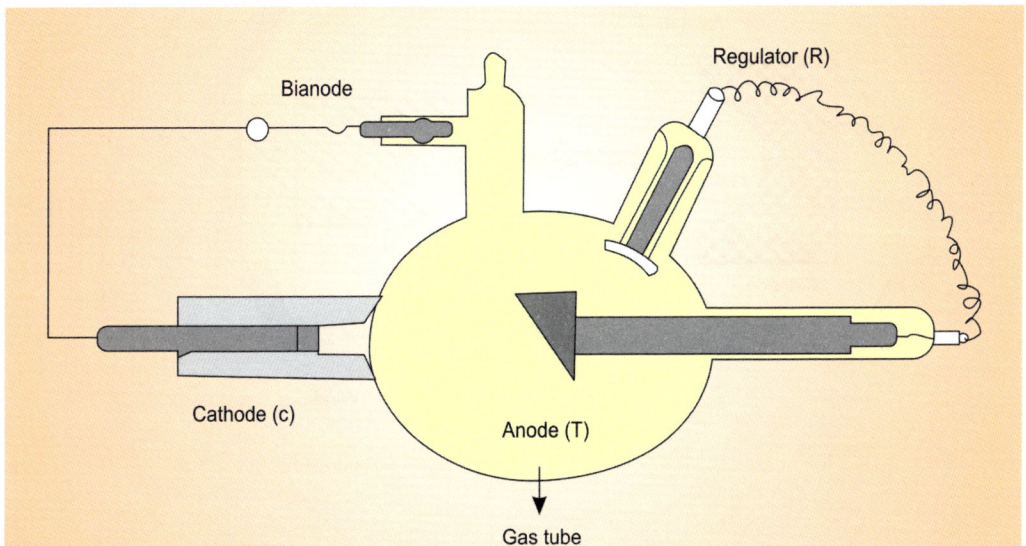

Fig. 2.3: Crooke's tube

- In Crooke's tube, gases cannot be controlled. So, uniformity in X-ray production is not maintained.

II. Coolidge Tube

It is also known as *Hot Cathode tube*. It was designed by William David Coolidge in 1913 and is still being used with a few modifications. It differs from the gas filled X-ray tube in respect that electrons are produced not by ionisation but by heating a filament in vacuum to about 2000°C (Fig. 2.4).

It consists of a double walled glass tube which is exhausted to nearly perfect vacuum. Glass tube is thinner or single walled at the site of X-ray emissions. The basic apparatus consists of:

- a cathode
- an anode
- a radiator

A Cathode

The cathode is composed of two parts:

- A molybdenum cup
- The filament

The filament is a coil of wire approximately 0.2 cm in diameter. When the current is applied, the filament is heated to incandescence. The hot filament emits electrons at a rate proportional to its temperature. The emission of electrons from the cathode is known as *Thermionic emission*. The current or the milliamperage controls

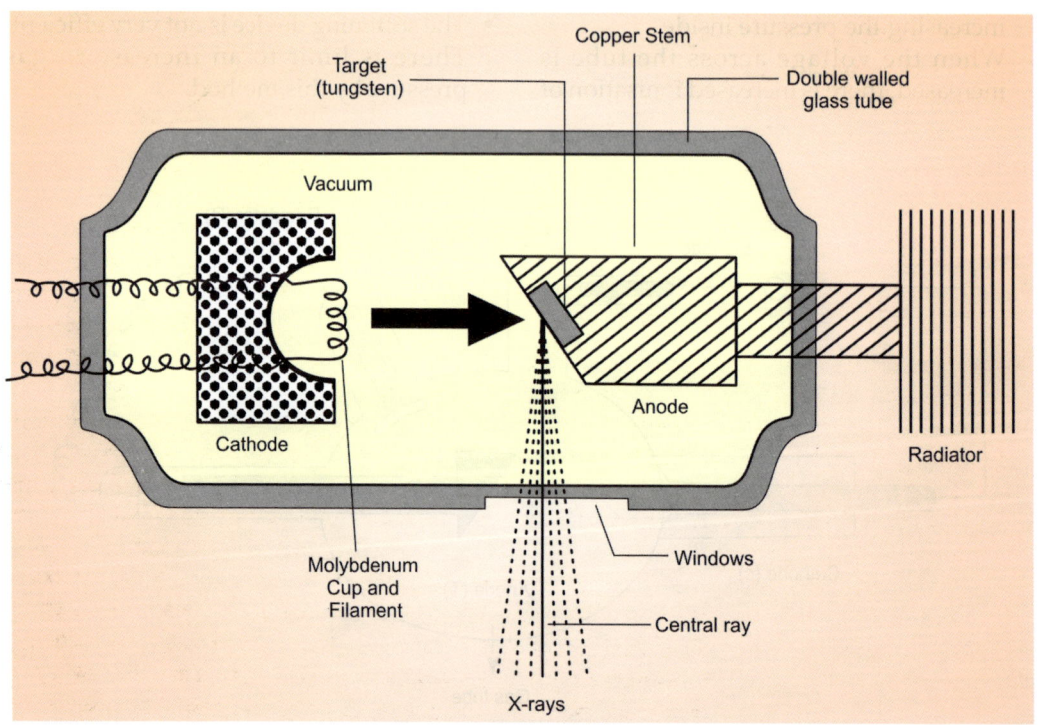

Fig. 2.4: Coolidge tube

the quantity of electrons which in fact controls the tube current, i.e. the future number of X-ray photons subsequently to be produced. The filament is fitted in a negatively charged concave reflector cup of molybdenum. The cup focuses the electrons emitted by the incandescent filament into a narrow beam. These days rectangular cups are being used in place of rounded cups. The high negative charge of the molybdenum cup repels the negatively charged electrons, which form an electron cloud around the filament. The positive charge of the anode attracts them. Complete vacuum in the tube facilitates the movement of the electrons otherwise they may strike the gas molecules.

An Anode

Anode is composed of a copper stem to which is attached the tungsten target. The area where electrons strike is known as the focus. So, in routine it is called *focal spot*. The copper stem in which the tungsten target is embedded, helps in conducting away the heat energy generated when the electrons from the cathode strike the target.

PROPERTIES OR REQUISITES OF TARGET METAL

- It should have high atomic number. Higher the atomic number, denser is the metal. We require sufficiently dense metal to stop the high-speed electrons. Although the atomic number of tungsten (74) is lower than platinum and lead but other properties of tungsten make this metal superior over the others.
- It should have low vapour pressure at high temperature. Since electron beam is directed to a very small area, some of the atoms may reach the vapour state, so blisters may be formed.

- It should have high melting point. Since most of the energy is converted into heat, the melting point of the target metal must be high. Tungsten fulfils this, as its M.P. is 3370°C, which is quite higher than others.

- It should have a high degree of thermal conductivity, since most of the heat generated is passed to the radiator or other cooling device. However, the thermal conductivity of tungsten is low, the tungsten target is fitted in a copper stem, which is a very good thermal conductor.

LINE FOCUS PRINCIPLE

The quality of X-rays is dependent in part on the geometry of the target. The sharpness of the image increases as the size of the focal spot decreases. But the disadvantage of a small focal spot is that a lot of heat is generated, which decreases the life of the focal spot. To take advantage of the smaller focal spot, the target is placed at an angle of 45° with respect to the central ray of X-ray beam. By this angulation the actual spot remains large (1.0–3.0 mm), allowing for dissipation of heat, while the effective focal spot is small (0.1–1.0 mm), which keeps the X-ray image sharp. In recent machines the angle is kept at 20° (as compared to 45°) with the central ray. However, the angulation of the focal spot is limited by what is known as the HEEL EFFECT, which states that, as the angulation of the focal spot is further increased (e.g. from more than 20°) then the number of X-rays from the cathode side of the focal spot increases. These kind of X-rays are weaker and detrimental to both patient and the image. Hence, the angulation of the focal spot is set at 20°.

2

A Radiator

Since 99.9% of the kinetic energy of the electrons is converted into heat energy, some cooling device is required which will dissipate heat. The radiator is connected with the copper stem, which is a good conductor of heat, dissipating it to the radiator.

Another method of dissipating heat from the focal spot is to use a rotating anode. As a result of the arrangement, the electrons strike successive areas of the target as it rotates. This effectively widens the focal spot and dissipates heat over the expanded area. Such rotating anodes are seldom used in dental X-ray machines. The few models of cephalostat machines have a rotating anode. The insulating oil in the X-ray tube head also helps in dissipating the immense heat generated.

X-ray machine also has some accessories which are included in the set up.

a. **Timer:** X-ray machines are provided with a time control device to control the X-ray exposure time. Usually the machines are provided with timers, which are calibrated in fractions of second. Some other machines provide timers according to the impulses per exposure. The number of impulses divided by 60 (the frequency of power source) gives the exposure time in fractions of a second. Thus, 30 impulses is equivalent to half a second exposure. Before the timer is set or high voltage is applied across the tube, the filament must be at the proper operating temperature to ensure the proper rate of electron emission. Filament should not be subjected to the prolonged heating as it may lead to filament burn out, which is a common cause of failure of the X-ray tubes. The timer should have a long cord which will take the operator away from the X-ray machine itself.

b. **Transformers:** Proper current to heat the filament and the potential difference between the anode and cathode are provided by *step-up* and *step-down* transformers. The transformers adjust the current flow through the filament, its heating and thus, the quality of electrons emitted by the filament. These electrons travel from cathode to anode and are called tube current. Ammeter measures the intensity of current which ultimately measures the tube current.

Autotransformers are also used. They control the voltage between anode and cathode of the X-ray tubes. They perform both step up and step down functions.

Points to Remember

1. The step-down transformer decreases the incoming 110–220 voltage to 3–4 volts, which is required to heat the filament, thus facilitating the phenomenon of thermionic emission.
2. The step-up transformer increases the incoming 110–220 voltage to 65–100 kVp required for X-ray production.
3. The autotransformer stabilizes minor fluctuations in the current.

WORKING OF THE TUBE

As the filament is heated by the supply of current and the high voltage from the transformer is applied between the two electrodes, the electron beam gets accelerated towards the anode. These attain large velocity depending upon the magnitude of the voltage applied. The rectangular or C-shaped molybdenum cup focuses the electrons to a small spot on the target. When these high velocity electrons strike the target focus, the X-rays are produced. Adjusting the current flowing through the filament by means of a rheostat can control the intensity of X-rays. If the filament is heated to a higher temperature, it emits a large number of electrons and hence the intensity of the X-rays is increased. If, however, the voltage across the tube is increased, the electrons attain a greater energy before striking against the target, so the high energy rays with better penetrating power are emitted. It becomes possible in this tube to have a separate control over the quality and intensity of X-rays. This will overcome the main drawback of the gas tube.

Points to Remember

1. The C-shaped cup around the filament is made of molybdenum. Molybdenum is so chosen because of its negative charge. Since the electrons emitted from the heated filament are also negatively charged, the molybdenum cup repels the electrons so that they form an electron cloud around the filament.
2. The current controls the quantity of X-rays. The more the current, the more is the heating of the filament. Hence there are more electrons, which eventually lead to more X-rays.
3. The voltage controls the quality of X-rays. The more the voltage, the more is the kinetic energy of the electrons. Hence the X-rays produced have greater energy.
4. X-rays are produced in the anode target when the electrons strike the target. This happens in the following ways:

   a. *Bremsstrahlung Radiation*
   This is also known as "Braking Radiation". Around 70–80% of the X-rays are produced in this fashion.

When the high speed electrons hit the target, some electrons hit the nucleus of the target atom directly and cease to exist. Their kinetic energy is converted to and released as an X-ray photon. The energy of this X-ray photon is equal to the kinetic energy of the electron that has hits the nucleus.

Alternatively, some high speed electrons, while missing the nucleus, may pass close to the nucleus of the target atom. When this happens, the path of the electron gets deviated. In this process of deviation, the electron loses some energy. This energy is released as an X-ray photon.

The radiation produced in these above two ways is known as Brehmstrahlung radiation (Fig. 2.5).

   b. *Characteristic Radiation*
   Now, when a high speed electron strikes an electron in a shell of the target atom, it displaces the electron and creates a vacancy in the shell of the target atom. To stabilize the atom, an electron from an outer shell comes and occupies the vacancy. In this process, some energy of the electron is lost. This energy is released as an X-ray photon. Radiation produced in this manner is known as 'Characteristic Radiation' (Fig. 2.6).

ROENTGENOLOGICAL ACCESSORIES

Fluoroscope

A fluoroscope is a device which enables one to see at once the shadow of the object exposed to the X-rays. These shadows are transitory and seen as long as the X-rays are passed. The object to be examined is placed

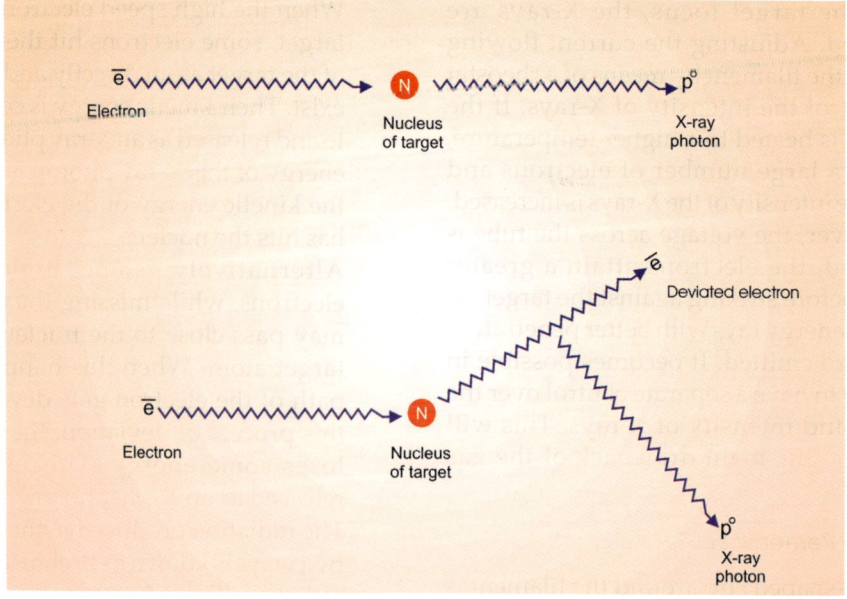

Fig. 2.5: Bremsstrahlung radiation

between the X-ray tube and the screen; X-rays penetrate according to the relative densities of the object and produce shadows on the screen. This is of little use in dentistry.

Diaphragm

It is a device, which absorbs approximately 90% of stray and secondary radiations emanating from the X-ray tube. This permits direct rays to pass through and act on the film. Without the use of a diaphragm, the picture may be foggy and poor in contrast; while the use of a diaphragm will produce better images superior in contrast and detail. Diaphragm is used along with long cone techniques; target film distance is 25 inches (described in Chapter 6). The exposure time is also increased accordingly. Diaphragm is preferably used where superior contrast is required.

Intensifying Screen

An intensifying screen is a device used to intensify the photographic effect of X-rays thereby shortening the time of exposure.

When X-rays strike the emulsion of film, the absorption of energy is only 1% and the rest 99% of the energy is wasted. It is the absorption that governs the formation of image later on. Thus, any method devised to utilise part of this 99% waste energy is advantageous to us. It is well known that certain chemicals have the property of absorbing roentgen rays and emitting their energy as ordinary light. This property is called *fluorescence*. These phosphors (substances having the property of fluorescence) are used in intensifying screens for use in combination with X-rays (Fig. 2.7A and B).

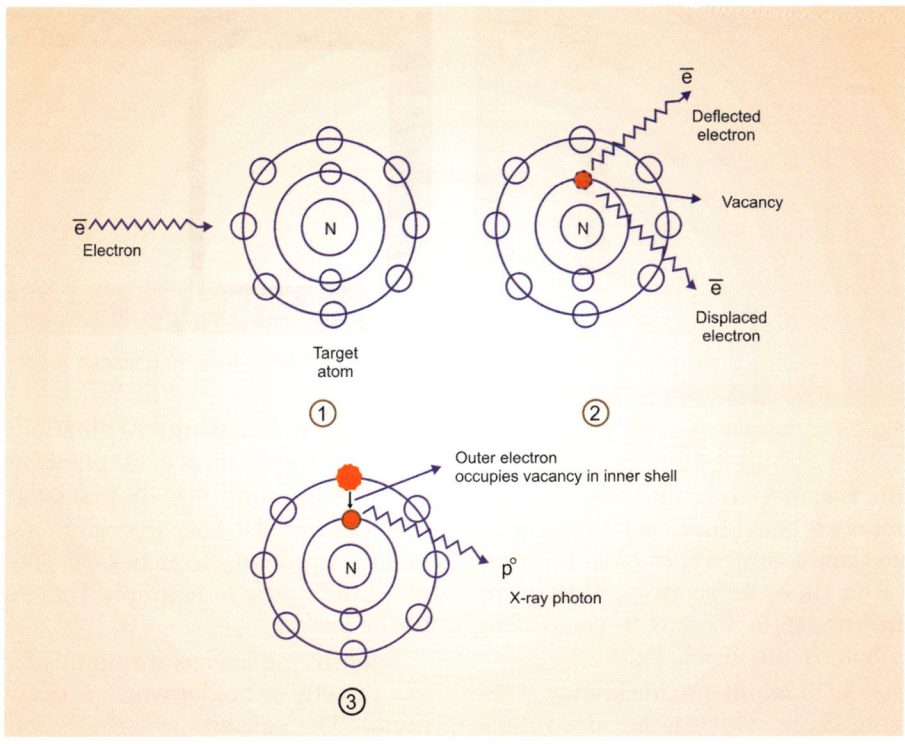

Fig. 2.6: Characteristic radiation

Intensifying screens are used in combination with films for all extraoral radiography including panoramic and cephalometric. Intensifying screen is available in three speeds, i.e. slow, intermediate and fast. Slow speed intensifying screens produce better results because of the coating of the crystals. They are usually not used with intraoral films because of loss of resolution. It definitely serves the diagnostic requirement, decreasing 85–90% of the patient's dose.

Composition

It consists of a base, a phosphor layer and also a protective coating.

Base: The base is made up of plastic polyester of 0.25 mm thickness. This provides mechanical support for the phosphor layer.

Phosphor layer: This layer consists of light sensitive phosphor crystals. An X-ray photon, which is absorbed in the intensifying screen will generate many light photons. Collectively they will affect the photographic plate.

Earlier phosphors being used were barium platinocyanide, cadmium tungstate and zinc sulphide, etc. Calcium tungstate is frequently used because it is quite stable and does not deteriorate under the X-ray bombardment.

2

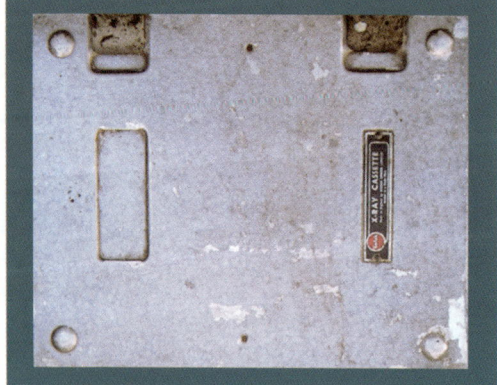

Fig. 2.7A: Intensifying screen (closed)

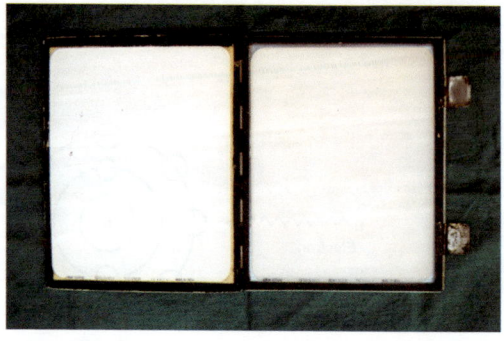

Fig. 2.7B: Intensifying screen (open)

In the recent years, a number of new phosphors are being used, notably terbium activated lanthanum oxybromide. These are about four times more efficient than the calcium tungstate screens in converting X-ray photons into visible light.

A layer of titanium dioxide known as the reflecting layer, which is not used these days, was used previously in between phosphor and the base.

Protective coating: A plastic coat of about 8 μm is placed over the phosphor layer to provide protection to the phosphor layer.

It is essential to keep intensifying screens clean of any debris, scratches, etc. These may affect the future radiograph. These should not be folded.

Intensifying screens are mounted in pairs in a cassette or holder which is made up of metal. The cassette is light proof when closed. Very rarely flexible cassettes are used but usually the cassettes are rigid.

3

Production of a Radiograph

Many factors are responsible for the production of a good radiograph. Some of the factors are in the hands of manufacturers while the others are related to the operator's skill and the technique.

These are divided into three basic groups:
- I. Factors relating to X-radiations
- II. Factors relating to object
- III. Factors relating to image recording

I. FACTORS RELATING TO X-RADIATIONS

a. Exposure time

It is one of the foremost factors controlled by the operator. Exposure time is the interval during which the X-rays are passed over the object and the film. Keeping all other factors constant, variation in exposure time can lead to a great variation in the results. Kilovolts peak (kVp) and the milliampere (mA) are the related factors. Exposure time is multiplied with milliamperage to produce a common factor, which denotes mAs (milliampere second).

An increase in the exposure time will lead to increased passage of electric current through the filament in the X-ray tube. This enhances the emission of electrons, thereby, increasing the production of X-rays. In simple terms increased exposure time will produce more X-radiations but of the same intensity.

Exposure time mainly affects the:
- Density
- Contrast

Density is the change in combination of lightness and darkness in a radiograph. As the exposure time is increased, the density will be increased and vice versa. If a light film is to be changed to a dark film, the exposure time is to be increased and vice versa.

Contrast is the distinction made by the eye between objects of varying densities. Contrast increases with increase of film exposure. Minor changes in the exposure time may lead to changes in the film which are practically insignificant.

b. Milliampere

It is the amount of current which is passed through the closed circuit in an X-ray tube

23

3

and is directly proportional to the rate of production of X-rays. Increased current will lead to increased number of electrons possessing greater energy, thereby, leading to the production of X-rays with greater penetration power.

c. Kilovoltage

It is the difference of potential between the anode and the cathode of X-ray tube. The higher the kVp (kilovolts peak), the greater the potential difference, more will be the attraction of electrons by the anode and greater will be the energy possessed by the photon. Thus the greater kilovoltage will produce X-radiations with more penetrating power.

kVp affects the exposure time. When kVp is increased, there occurs greater energy in the photons and the less such photons are required to expose the film. An increase of approximately 15 kVp necessitates halving of exposure time and a decrease of 15 kVp is compensated by doubling the exposure time to maintain the film density. kVp also affects the radiographic contrast. Lower the kVp, greater is the contrast. Increased kVp increases the amount of scattered radiations and thus further reduces the contrast.

The higher kVp produces more penetrating X-rays and when more penetrating X-rays are used, X-radiations reach the film with lesser absorption by the object. The higher the kVp, less is the skin dose and greater is the depth dose of X-rays.

d. Tube Film Distance

The distance from the target to the X-ray film or object greatly affects the intensity of radiation. This relationship is stated in the Inverse Square Law which states, *Intensity of radiation (Photons/unit area) is inversely proportional to the square of the distance, measured from the source of radiations to the point of radiation intensity measurement.*

$$I\alpha \frac{1}{(D)^2} \; ; \; I_a \, \alpha \, \frac{1}{(D_a)^2} \text{ and } I_b \, \alpha \, \frac{1}{(D_b)^2}$$

$$I_a = k \, \frac{1}{(D_a)^2} \qquad (i)$$

$$I_b = k \, \frac{1}{(D_b)^2} \qquad (ii)$$

Divide (i) by (ii)
$$\frac{I_a}{I_b} = \frac{(D_b)^2}{(D_a)^2}$$

I = Intensity
D = Distance

If intensity is decreased, exposure time is to be increased to compensate for the quality of the image. In other words exposure time is proportional to the square of distance measured from the tube to the film.

$$\frac{\text{Old exposure time}}{\text{New exposure time}} = \frac{(\text{Old distance})^2}{(\text{New distance})^2}$$

Other factors such as mA and kVp must be kept constant when this formula is applied to change in the tube-film distance or the exposure time.

Long tube film distances assist in reducing patient's exposure in extraoral radiography. In X-ray therapy (therapeutic radiography) long tube-skin distances are used for the treatment of deep lesions, while short tube skin distance is used for surface lesions.

The effect of mA upon TFD (Tube Film Distance) is the same as the effect of exposure time. It is noted that as TFD is increased, X-ray beam courses a larger area of the film (Fig. 3.1). This can be controlled by using a collimator—a device which limits the character of X-ray beam.

e. Collimation

Collimation refers to the control of the size and shape of the X-ray beam. When an X-ray beam is directed to a patient, most of the energy is wasted and the rest or very little is available to form the image. Scattered radiations generated by the wasted energy may reach the film but serve no useful purpose. These radiations only add fog to the film thus decreasing the overall quality of the film.

The detrimental effect of scattered radiations on the formation of images can be minimized by reducing the amount of scattered radiations and also by preventing them reaching the film.

Collimation refers to reducing the formation of scattered radiations by placing a radiopaque barrier containing an aperture in the path of the beam. Collimation thereby reduces the patient's exposure and increases quality of the image. Different types of collimators are available viz. (a) Rectangular collimator, (b) Tubular collimator, and (c) Diaphragm collimator, which are used in dentistry (Fig. 3.2).

Rectangular collimator limits the size of the X-ray beam to the size of the film. Rectangular collimator is the most suitable to be used, as it reduces the area of exposure on the patient's face, thus contributing to reduction of radiation exposure of the patient. This point is demonstrated in Fig. 3.3.

Tubular collimator is simply a tube lined by a radiopaque material or constructed of a radiopaque material.

Diaphragm collimator consists of a thin plate (1/6th of an inch) of radiopaque material (usually lead) with an aperture or hole in its centre. The shape of the X-ray beam is determined by shape of the hole. The diaphragm is placed over the opening of the tube.

When the X-ray beam size is restricted to the smallest possible area, the amount of tissue being irradiated can be minimized. By

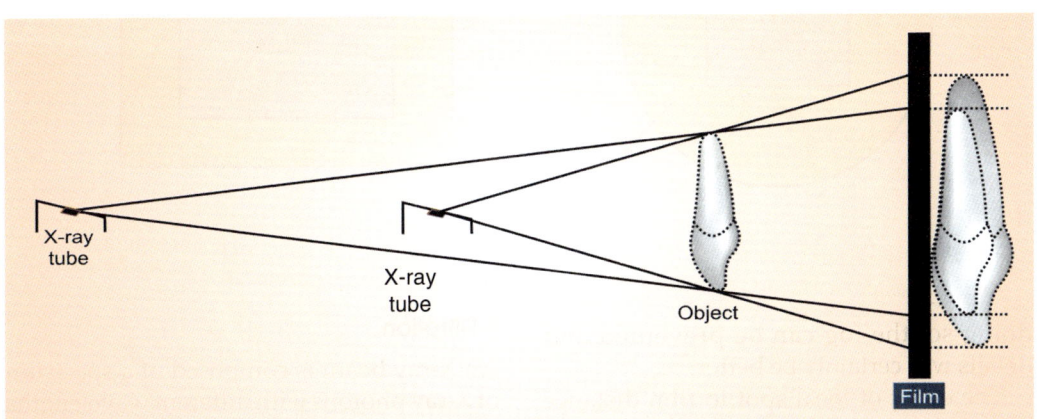

Fig. 3.1: Comparison of 8-inch and 16-inch tube film distance

3

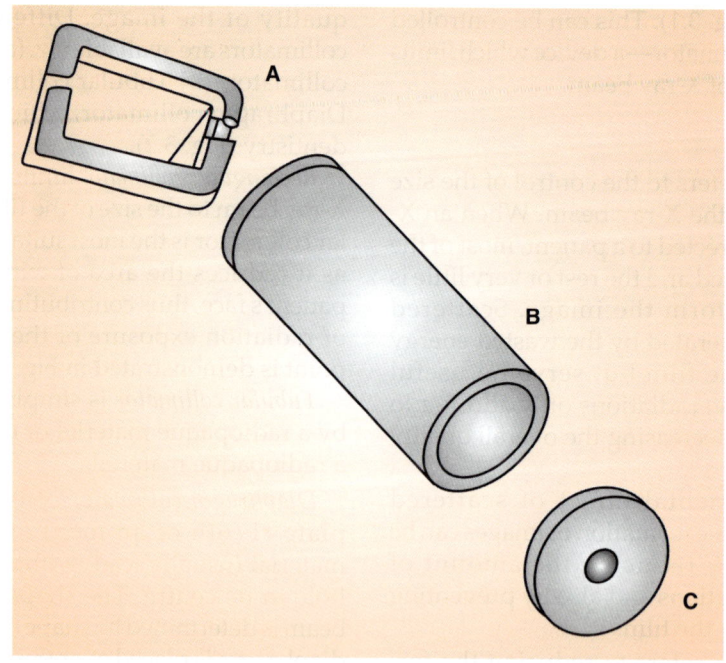

Fig. 3.2: Collimators. (A) Rectangular; (B) Tubular; (C) Diaphragm

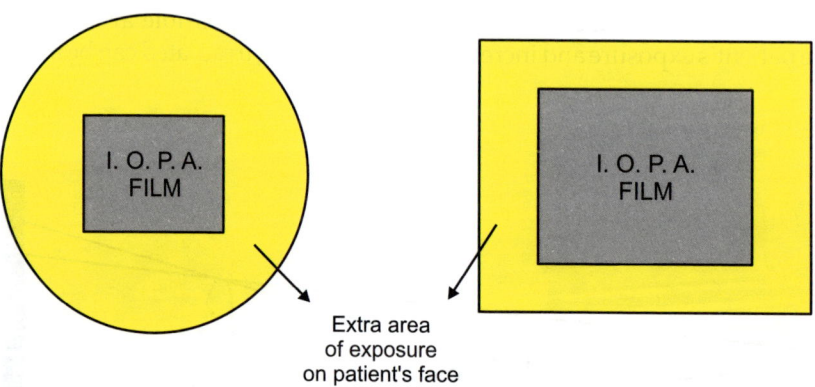

I. O. P. A.
FILM

I. O. P. A.
FILM

Extra area
of exposure
on patient's face

Fig. 3.3

doing so, the fog can be prevented and details will certainly be better.

The effect of focal spot to film distance with and without collimation on the volume of tissue irradiated is depicted in Fig. 3.4.

f. Filtration

An X-ray beam is composed of a spectrum of X-ray photons with different wavelengths and penetrating powers. X-ray beams with definite penetrating power are useful in

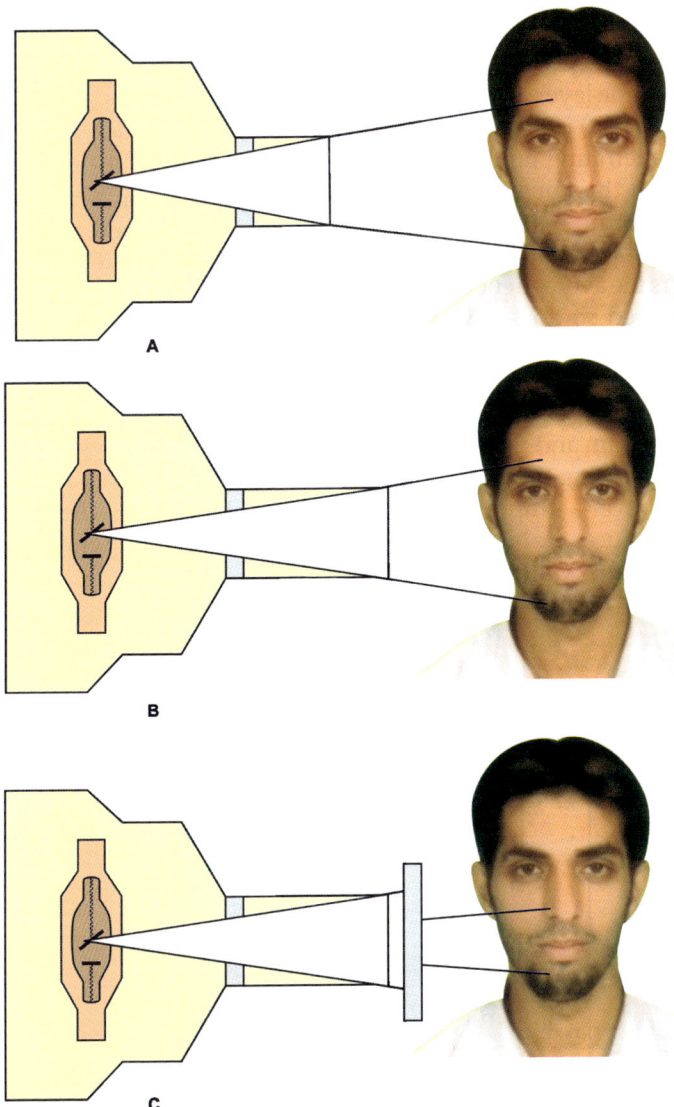

Fig. 3.4: Volume of tissue irradiated because of the effect of focal spot to film distance and collimation. (A) Short distance : large area; (B) Increased distance : lesser area; (C) Increased distance and collimation: further reduces area for irradiation

making an image while others (of low penetrating power) contribute to patient's exposure with no effect on the film.

For patient's safety and otherwise, the quality of X-radiations can be increased by removing the less penetrating photons. This is accomplished by placing aluminium filters in the path of X-ray beam (Fig. 3.5).

Quality of X-ray beam can be determined by determining its half-value layer. In other words, *Half Value Layer* (HVL) is the useful way to designate the penetrating power of X-ray beam. HVL is the thickness of an absorber, usually aluminium, required to reduce the number of X-ray photons passing through it by one half. As the average energy of X-ray beam is increased so does HVL. 'Quality' is often used to refer to the mean energy of an X-ray beam.

Successive layers of filtering material are placed in the path of the beam and then the amount of X-ray energy passing through it is measured and plotted over a graph. The thickness of filter which reduces the incident beam to one half of its original value, is the HVL. Usually 2.0 mm filter is required in dentistry.

Contrast and the quality of film is increased with the use of filters while density is affected because increased filtration may result in absorption of some of the useful penetrating X-rays. Therefore, when filtration is increased, a slight increase in exposure time is required.

Filters are generally placed at the inner end of the cylindrical collimator or adjacent to the diaphragm.

II. FACTORS RELATING TO OBJECT

Two factors play an important role in radiography of the object. The quality of the X-ray film image depends upon the following:

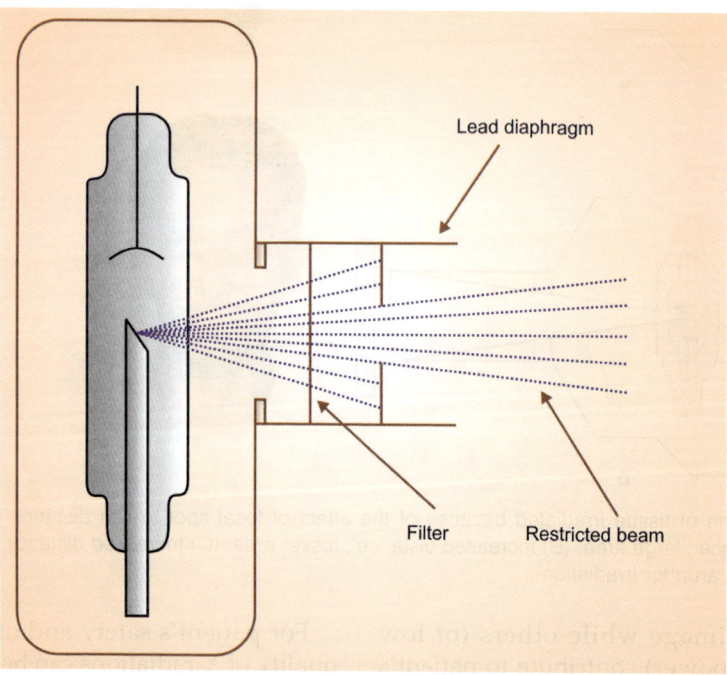

Fig. 3.5: Collimation and filtration of X-ray beam

a. **Thickness of the object:** The X-radiations are passed on to the film after some of the energy is absorbed by the object. For thicker objects more radiations are required to get through the object to the film.

The latent image is formed only when certain amount of radiations have fallen on the film. Whenever the object thickness is increased, it is advisable to use higher kVp. Higher mA or increased exposure time can also help but by increasing kVp, patient's exposure time is decreased and the blurring due to movement is minimized. Increased object thickness usually produces increased secondary radiations. Absorbing screens are used with the X-ray film to minimize the effect of secondary radiations.

b. **Density of the object:** Density may be defined as the mass per unit volume of an object. X-rays are absorbed proportionately to the total mass (density × thickness). In intraoral radiography, secondary radiations can be minimized by the use of small X-ray beam. Proper collimation of the X-ray beam is essential to minimize the production of secondary radiations since they can change the image to a great extent (Fig. 3.6).

Most of the film packets contain a lead sheet or other radiation absorbing material,

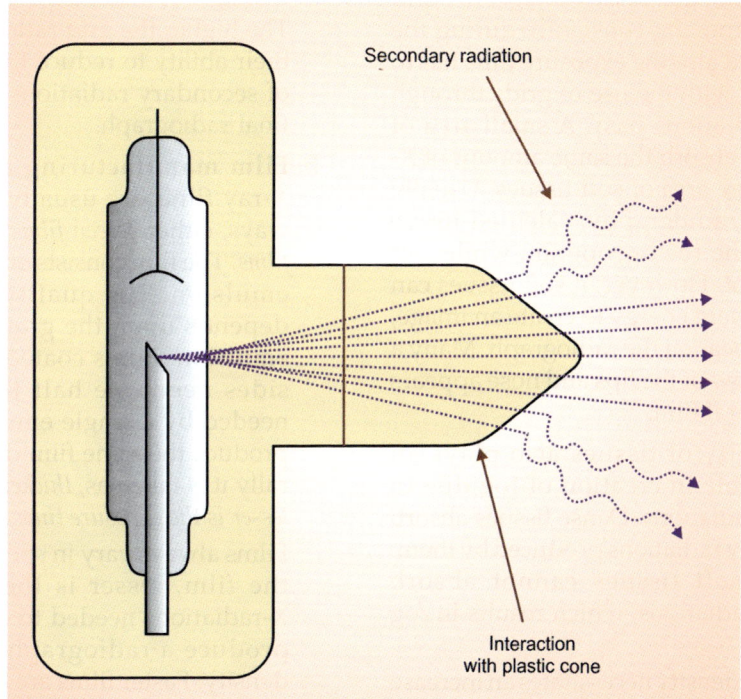

Secondary radiation

Interaction with plastic cone

Fig. 3.6: Production of secondary radiation resulting from interaction of the primary beam with the cone

3

which partially or totally absorbs the secondary radiations. The living tissues and also the X-ray film is protected by the use of protective sheets behind the films.

In extraoral radiography, the same principles and techniques are utilized but in addition to these, certain other methods are employed. One of the methods is the use of grid. The grids are designed to separate at a particular tube-grid distance. The grid is placed between the object and the film. The grid consists of a base to which strips of lead are embedded.

Most of the secondary radiations originating in the object are absorbed by the lead strips. One disadvantage of using a grid is the production of dull white lines, which represent lead strips on the final radiograph.

To overcome this disadvantage, the grid can be kept moving constantly during the exposure; and also the exposure time has to be increased with the use of grids through which X-radiations pass. A small area of enamel may absorb the same amount of X-rays as a large area of soft tissues. Usually in intraoral radiography, calcified tissue appears in the roentgenogram while soft tissues do not. However, if soft tissues can absorb sufficient energy to create an image, they will appear on the radiograph. Many a time, a shadow of the lips and nose appears on the intraoral film.

The density of tissues also plays an important role in creation of fog due to secondary radiations. Dense tissues absorb the secondary radiations produced by them. However, soft tissues cannot absorb secondary radiations, which results in fog formation.

Increased density necessitates an increase in mA, kVp or exposure time.

III. FACTORS RELATING TO IMAGE RECORDING

As X-radiations are passed through an object towards a film, a latent image is formed which is processed to form a radiograph. Many factors control the production of this image and the final radiograph. These are:

a. **Secondary radiations:** The secondary radiations reach all parts of the film and produce a film fog in the radiograph. Consequently the final image shows poor contrast.

Since the secondary radiations usually originate from the object itself, some devices are used to reduce their production.

The effectiveness of a grid depends upon the grid ratio, which is the distance of lead strips over the base. The higher the grid ratio, the better is their ability to reduce the production of secondary radiations affecting the final radiograph.

b. **Film manufacturing and storage:** X-ray films are usually used in two ways, either *screen films* or *non-screen films*. The film consists of a base and an emulsion. The quality of the film depends upon the grain size of the emulsion. Films coated on both the sides need one half the exposure needed by a single emulsion film to produce the same film density. Generally it is taken as, *thicker the emulsion, lesser is the exposure time required.*

Films always vary in speed. The faster the film, lesser is the amount of X-radiations needed to expose it and produce a radiograph of required density. Faster films are designated as D, E and F and as they utilize less exposure time, the patient and operator have less chance of radiation hazards. Faster films, however, produce less sharp images due to the increased size of silver grains.

Whenever fast films are used, precaution in the developing procedures must be followed, as these films are very sensitive in the dark room.

Storage of films is also very important. Stored films, when exposed to humidity, excessive temperature and stray radiations produce foggy results. These should always be stored in a cool place, preferably in a dark room, and placed inside a lead box or any other device, which can protect the film from stray radiations. Expiry dates of films should be noted and the films should be used before their expiry date.

c. **Use of intensifying screens:** Intensifying screens are used to intensify the image and reduce the exposure time. These are used usually with extra oral films. The screen and the film is kept tight in a box. They consist of fluorescent material, which when exposed to radiations emit blue or violet light. The collective effect of these two on the X-ray films reduces the exposure time.

Screen films are usually used when X-ray films alone will require long exposure time and the patient will be irradiated for a longer period as during examination of the skull or thicker body parts.

The speed of the screen also varies depending upon the crystal size. Larger the crystal size and thicker the layer, the greater is the speed of the film. Larger crystals are more efficient than smaller ones; however, large crystals expose larger areas leading to dull images. Compromise between the image sharpness and the exposure time is to be made while selecting the screens.

Contrast is also affected with the use of screens. Contrast is greater when screens are used.

d. **Processing of films:** All the factors and the precautions taken during exposure etc. are of little value if the films are not processed properly. Good quality radiograph cannot be produced without a good darkroom equipment and a good technique. Time and temperature range should be tackled carefully with optimum temperature being 65–70°F and the time 4–5 minutes.

Films developed at higher temperatures show greater contrast and vice versa.

Excessive developing leads to increased fog. When a film is not properly processed, i.e. lesser time taken at any stage during developing, fixing and washing, discolouration results. Films, which are left in fixer solution for longer time, lose density.

Many other types of errors and artefacts are produced without the proper use of developing procedures. These are discussed in detail in Chapter 7.

Bibliography

1. Geleskey DE, Baker CG: Energy selective filtration of dental X-ray beams. *O Surg, O Med, O Path:* 1981;52:565.
2. Okano T, Grondahl HG, Grondahl K: Effect of quantum noise in the detection of incipient

proximal caries. *O Surg, O Med, O Path:* 1982; 53:212.

3. Richards AG: Technical factors that control radiographic density. Symposium on oral roentgenology. *Dent Clin North Am:* 1961;5:371.

4. Stenstrom B, Henrikson CO, Holm B, Richter S: Absorbed doses from intraoral radiography with special emphasis on collimator dimensions. *Swed Dent J:* 1986;10:59.

5. Stephen RG, Koyon SL, Reid JA: An investigation of potential application of intensifying screens in intraoral radiography. *O Surg, O Med, O Path:* 1982;54:591.

6. Weissman DD, Longhurst GE: Clinical evaluation of a rectangular field collimating device for periapical radiography. *JADA:* 1971;82:580.

3

4

Radiobiology

The branch of science which studies the effect of radiations on the human body or living tissues is known as radiobiology. These effects can be physical, chemical or both.

The basic unit of life is the cell. It is estimated that the adult human body consists of about 10^{14} cells. In human body the smallest cell is the platelet having diameter 3–4µ. Nerve cell is the largest having length of 75 cms while the width is 100µ.

Cell consists of the nucleus and the cytoplasm. Certain cells do not contain nucleus, for example red blood cells (RBCs). Nucleus is the centre of control of cellular activities while the cytoplasm containing organelles, controls the synthesis of energy transfer and conversion.

In the human body certain cells are always in the process of division to replace worn out cells while others (e.g. red blood cells) are differentiated, perform special functions and are not dividing.

There are two types of cell division:
- **Mitosis:** In mitosis each daughter cell has the same number of chromosome pairs as the parent cell. Such types of cells are called zygotes.
- **Meiosis:** In meiosis each daughter cell has half the number of chromosomes of the parent cell and also they occur singly and not in pairs. Such types of daughter cells are known as gametes.

The nucleus consists of chromosomes, which contain the genes, characterising the genetic or hereditary traits. DNA carries the genetic material and constitutes the genetic component of cell.

INTERACTION OF RADIATION WITH THE CELLS

Radiations affect the cells either directly or indirectly.

a. **Direct action:** The sensitive volume in the cells (e.g. molecule, atom) is changed by direct absorption of energy from the radiations. Direct action is explained in terms of *Target theory*, where the sensitive volume is assumed as the target and production of the ionization in it as the 'hit'. In case where a single hit is sufficient to produce an inactivation, the number of the surviving cells will decrease exponentially with dose.

b. **Indirect action:** The sensitive volume is inactivated by transfer of energy from another volume which in turn has absorbed energy from the radiations. In other words, while in the direct action the volume which absorbs energy is the volume which is inactivated, in indirect action, the volume which is inactivated is not the volume which absorbs the energy.

In simple words, direct means radiations have direct effect and indirect means radiations cause destruction through chemical decomposition of various enzymes, etc. Usually the cell dies at the time of mitotic division due to radiations.

The degree of cell alteration depends upon the irradiation. In any case where there are number of similar cells, the destruction of some of them do not have any deleterious effect on the body. Subjective symptoms occur only when large number of the cells are destroyed which are either irreparable or the adjoining cells cannot take up their function.

RADIOLYSIS OF WATER

Human tissues consist of 85% of water. Consequently on irradiation, most of the energy will initially be deposited in H_2O, only a small proportion will be taken up by the materials such as skin, bone, etc. When water molecules are irradiated, ionization takes place as follows (Fig. 4.1):

H_2O loses an electron and becomes H_2O^+

$$H_2O \xrightarrow[\text{Radiation}]{\text{Ionizing}} H_2O^+ + e^-$$

The electron can be captured by another H_2O molecule to give a negative molecule.

$$H_2O + e^- \longrightarrow H_2O^-$$

This completes the formation of an ion pair. Until this, the stability of molecule is maintained and comes under physical changes. After that the chemical changes occur.

$$H_2O^+ \longrightarrow H^+ + OH^+$$
$$H_2O^- \longrightarrow H^- + OH^-$$

Free radicals have an odd electron (surplus or deficient), which are highly reactive entities. They have a life-time of about one microsecond and attack most of the organic substances. The free radicals can react with proteins, carbohydrates, hormones and enzymes resulting in their breakdown.

The presence of oxygen at the time of irradiation acts as a sensitizing agent. The effect of radiation becomes low as the amount of the oxygen contained in the surrounding tissues is decreased. This is known as the *oxygen effect.*

VARIABILITY IN TISSUE SENSITIVITY

Certain tissues are more susceptible to radiations as compared to the others. Degree of susceptibility, however, depends upon cellular differentiation and cellular reproduction. Following are the tissues in order of their susceptibility to the radiations:
- Blood forming cells
- Reproductive organs
- Bone and glandular tissues
- Epithelium of alimentary canal
- Skin and muscles
- Nervous tissues.

The radiosensitivity of various tissues of interest to the dental surgeon is depicted in Table 4.1.

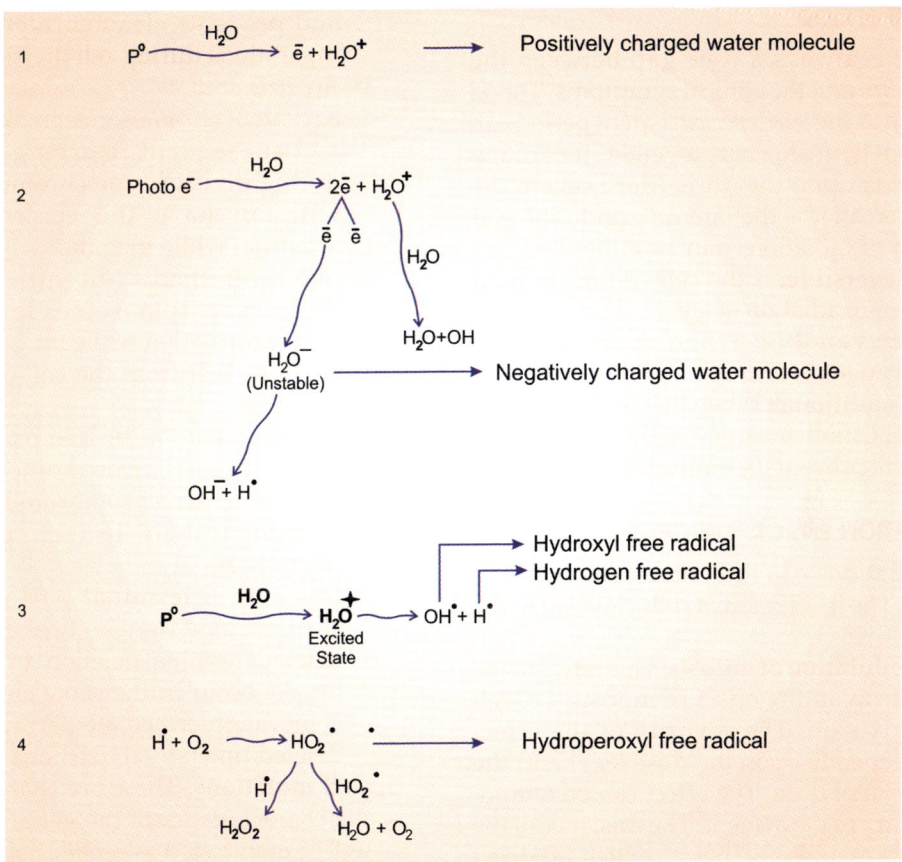

Fig. 4.1: Radiolysis of water

Intensity	Effect
• High radiosensitivity	• Bone marrow
	• Basal cell of oral mucous membrane
	• Inner enamel epithelium of developing tooth
• Intermediate radiosensitivity	• Fine vasculature
	• Growing cartilage
	• Growing bone
	• Salivary glands' parenchymal cells
	• Fibroblasts
• Low radiosensitivity	• Cranial nerves
	• Muscles
	• Surface cells of oral mucous membrane

Table 4.1: Radiosensitivity of various tissues

4

LATENT PERIOD

There is always a time gap between the exposure and the clinical symptoms. This is known as the *latent period*. Latent period can be from hours to years together. It partially depends upon the dose. More severe the dose, smaller is the latent period. The end results of radiations may be either:

i. **Reversible:** If the cells return to their pre-irradiation stage.

ii. **Irreversible:** When the permanent change occurs.

iii. **Conditional:** When they are so affected that another similar and/or small dose will prevent their return to the normal.

RADIATION EFFECTS ON CELLS

X-radiations can affect the cells in many ways. The irradiation of cells can lead to the following:

1. **Inhibition of mitosis:** This refers to the delay in the onset of mitosis, i.e. cell division. The severity of the effect depends upon the dose level and the rate of dose. The effect can be temporary or permanent. The existence of the threshold dose below which no delay occurs suggests the interference with some metabolic process.

2. **Chromosome aberrations:** Radiation can cause breakage in chromosomes. Usually the breaks may restitute and the damage may not be manifested. It may result in some part of the genetic material not being transferred to the daughter cells. Sometimes breakage occurs and union takes place at levels other than the normal resulting in mutation.

Types of aberrations

a. *Stickiness*: This leads to formation of temporary or permanent bridges and prevents clean chromosome separations during cell division.

b. *Acentric or dicentric chromosome*: As a result of chromosome breakdown and subsequent re-arrangement during division, one chromosome will not have the centromere (acentric) while the other will have two centromeres (dicentric). The dicentric chromosomes leads to bridge formation while the acentric one gets lost from the cell during division.

c. *Translocation:* The broken part may join another chromosome (unilateral) or two chromosomes may exchange their broken pieces (reciprocal).

d. *Deletion:* A terminal part of the chromosome may be broken and deleted (terminal deletion) or if two breaks occur in the same chromosome, an intermediate part may be deleted (interstitial deletion).

3. **Cell mutations:** These are changes in the characteristics of the gene, which will be manifested as genetic defects (it refers to cell and not hereditary).

4. **Cell death:** Irradiation can result in the death of the cell and this may be due to changes in the physical properties of vital cell structure.

Lymphocytes, oocytes and spermatocytes are killed by a few hundred rads while the organs where the rate of cell division is low, require several thousands of rads to cause death.

BIOLOGICAL EFFECTS OF RADIATIONS

These can be considered in two aspects:

A. **Somatic:** Somatic effect is that which occurs in exposed individuals.

B. **Genetic:** Genetic effect is that which is manifested in the future generation of the exposed individuals.

Biological effects can also be categorized into:

a. **Stochastic effects:** For which the probability of an effect occurring rather than its severity is regarded as a function of the dose without threshold.

b. **Non-stochastic effects:** For which the severity of the effect varies with the dose for which a threshold may matter.

Examples of stochastic effects are:

• Carcinoma
• Leukaemia
• Hereditary effects

Examples of non-stochastic effects are:

• Cataract
• Shortening of life span
• Infertility.

Lethal dose: Let us study the unit of X-radiations.

• *Roentgen*, a unit of exposure is the amount of radiation absorbed in air at a given point.

• *Rad* is the unit of absorbed dose. It is the amount of radioactive energy absorbed per gram of tissue or any material.

• *Rem* is the product of absorbed dose and the modifying factor. Rem indicates the potential degree of danger to health.

The radiation sensitivity or response varies considerably from one species to another. To compare the radiation response the term lethal dose is used. This is designated as LD 50/30. This is the whole body acute dose required to kill 50% of the exposed organisms within 30 days after irradiation. LD 50/30 for humans is 400–600 rem. It is much higher in fish (700 rem) snail (10,000 rem), and amoeba (1,00,000 rem).

A. SOMATIC EFFECTS

Somatic effects can be classified into acute and chronic effects:

• *Acute effect* will be manifested within a few hours to a few days of acute irradiation and the severity of the effect will depend on the dose and the dose rate.

• *Chronic effects* are mainly due to low levels of irradiation for longer periods, or chronic irradiation.

Dose levels have been established, below which no effect is expected to be observed in persons irradiated. No harmful effect can be seen if patients and operators maintain these doses.

For convenience, effects of radiation, both somatic and genetic, can be studied under two heads:

I. Acute
   i. Large area of the body
   ii. Small area of the body
II. Chronic
   i. Large area of the body
   ii. Small area of the body.

Acute radiation affecting large area of the body: Such type of effects are never seen in dentistry. These are only possible in nuclear accidents and atomic bombardments. With a large amount of the radiations, the following effects are seen.

0–25 rem = no possible effects

25–50 rem = minor blood changes

50–200 rem = vomiting, etc. severity rises with dose. No deaths

200–300 rem = 20% of deaths can occur after six weeks.

400–700 rem = Hematological changes: No survivals.

Above 700 rem = CNS changes—death within few hours

Acute radiation affecting small area of the body: Such type of effects are seen in cases of treatment of malignant tumours. Large doses upto 6000 R are administered in short span of 3–10 days. This results in the death of the irradiated cells. Acute reactions do occur over skin and other parts resulting in skin erythema and even bone marrow depression. In dentistry, many radiographs are required only in case of root canal therapy. However, skin reactions vary from individual to individual depending upon the threshold. Usually 250 Roentgen is considered as the *Threshold Erythema Dose* (TED). In dentistry exposures are kept ½ of the TED.

4

OSTEORADIONECROSIS

The term implies an infection in bone rendered necrotic by ionizing radiation. This is frequent complication in the treatment of cancer of the oral cavity by irradiation. Because of its high mortality rate, it is the duty of the dentist to prevent its occurrence.

Osteoradionecrosis results from either of the following or in combination:

a. Radiation in massive doses
b. Partial necrosis of bone
c. Trauma which causes infection.

Radiation is delivered as a therapeutic measure for cure of malignant tumor of oral cavity in areas such as:

- Tongue
- Floor of the oral cavity
- Salivary glands
- Sinuses and neoplasms, etc.

Sometimes even small, superficial lesions of the face may cause osteoradionecrosis of mandibular and maxillary bones. Necrosis and ulceration of soft tissues occur two to three months after the irradiation.

Bone, because of its histological architecture, is highly susceptible to radiation. Radiation further leads to its vascular damage and interference with its nourishment. Radiation primarily leads to thickening of the periosteum and strangulation of blood vessels, which combine and ultimately lead to the depletion of blood supply to the bone. The chances of necrosis are enhanced by the fact that most of the patients are well past middle age, a stage where a certain degree of osteoporosis and arteriosclerosis are almost always there. The dentist must realize that the patients can function well with undernourished and partly necrotic mandible and maxilla. So infection and trauma should be avoided. Extractions and other procedures are not indicated for such patients.

Poor oral hygiene, periodontal diseases, residual roots, caries, etc. are local factors which must be eliminated prior to irradiation in order to prevent *osteoradio necrosis*. Systemic diseases, which also affect the state of health of the oral cavity, such as diabetes, anaemia etc. are also some of the predisposing factors. Questionable teeth, which can cause infection later on, must be removed prior to irradiation. Usually any bone receiving 5000–6000 rads radiations may not be able to recover from trauma and in case of the mandible, it must not exceed 2500 rads. The patient should be put on thorough oral hygiene measures, viz., mechanical and chemical plaque control. Preventive measures should be followed until and unless the extraction becomes necessary. If at all extraction is to be executed, it should be carried out under antibiotic cover and thorough sterilization.

It may also be understood that a tooth in reasonably good condition may deteriorate after irradiation. Saliva is diminished and enzymes are altered. Teeth may become brittle and prone to caries. Dentist must question the patients before extractions regarding their irradiation dose and time.

Radiographic Appearance

The X-ray picture in the case of osteoradio-necrosis is very deceptive before infection. Trabecular pattern, size and configuration of medullary spaces show normal appearance. Once the infection gets established, ragged radiolucent areas can be seen. Clinically, the patient experiences excruciating pain and there can be a suppurative discharge from the sequestrated sites (Fig. 4.2).

Chronic Radiation Affecting Large Area of the Body

This type of hazard is seen usually in workers (occupational hazard) or exposure received by a group of population.

In dentistry, occupational hazard is associated with X-ray machine operators. A

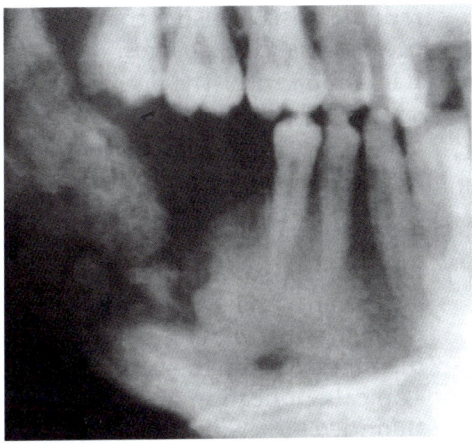

Fig. 4.2: Osteoradionecrosis (irregular, ill-defined, 'moth-eaten' appearance in body of right mandible)

committee on radiation protection had set a *maximum permissible dose* (MPD) as 1.2 R/week and 0.6 R/week previously; but now 0.3 R/week is the MPD.

However, the total accumulated dose should not be more than 5 R/year. What matters is the total accumulated dose which is given to the tissues one over the other. Patients feel nervous, apprehensive and tired. Nausea, vomiting and other GIT disturbances follow.

Accumulated MPD over the years is:
$$MPD = (N - 18) \times 5 \text{ rems}$$
where N is the age in years.
This is always greater than 18.

Chronic Radiation Affecting Small Area of the Body

Small doses of X-radiations when given to the smaller areas can lead to various types of hazards such as:

- **Radiation burns:** This effect is seen especially in cases where the operator holds the film in the patient's mouth. The small amount of the radiation received today plus the amount received yesterday and so on, until the tissues have received an amount that produces an erythema. Appearance is something like sunburns.
  - Skin becomes dry, slightly discolored and patient feels burning sensations.
  - Nails become friable with ends broken.
  - Cuticle around the nails is also affected.
  - Slight change is evident in blood supply of the sebaceous and sweat glands.
  - In later stages cracks appear, which may lead to malignant changes.

- **Loss of hair (alopecia):** Loss of hair (alopecia) can result because of too frequent or too long exposure to the roentgen rays. Although the loss of hair is not permanent, however, one must be vigilant.

- **Cataract:** Cataract can result from chronic exposure of X-radiations in and around the eyes.

- **Effect on oral mucous membrane:** The mucous membrane shows areas of redness and inflammation. With repeated exposures pseudo-membranes are formed because of breakdown of the mucous membrane. Secondary infection by *Candida albicans* is a common complication. Usually the mucous membrane heals rapidly once the irradiation is over. Otherwise after a few months, the mucous membrane will tend to become atrophic and relatively avascular.

- **Effect on the taste-buds:** Taste-buds are very sensitive to radiation and soon degenerative changes begin. Loss of taste is very common. Alteration in saliva may account for overall reduction of the taste sensitivity.

- **Effect on the salivary glands:** Salivary glands come under exposure during treatment of cancer in the oral cavity and oropharyngeal region. There occurs acute inflammation involving serous acini. A marked increase in the serum amylase has been reported. As the exposure progresses, the glands demonstrate degeneration. The salivary changes have a marked influence on oral microflora and even on the dentition. Increase in *Streptococcus mutans, Lactobacillus* and *Candida* has been reported. Xerostomia has also been reported.

- **Effect on the teeth:** The growth is retarded when teeth are irradiated during their development. If the radiation precedes calcification, the tooth may be destroyed. After calcification, if irradiation continues, malformation can result. The root development is retarded. In some instances the tooth erupts prematurely. Fully developed teeth are usually very resistant to the X-radiations.

- **Effect on the bones:** In dentistry, mandible is most susceptible among bony tissues to be irradiated frequently during the treatment for the cancers. The predominant change occurs in the marrow, where a progressive loss of vascular and haemopoietic elements may occur. There occurs lack of osteoblastic activities. The lacunae of the compact bone are empty indicating early necrosis. A marked decrease in the vascularity of bone because of irradiation decreases the capacity of bone to resist infection. Osteo-radionecrosis is also a complication because of such exposures.

- **Radiation caries:** The decrease in the salivary flow, its pH and buffering capacity coupled with increased viscosity are the complications of radiation exposure which lead to rampant type of carious lesions. The histological features of these carious lesions are similar to those of typical carious lesions; however, they can be distinguished by their rapid attack. Topical application of 1.0% sodium fluoride (1.0% NaF) and proper oral hygiene measures can reduce the radiation caries.

B. GENETIC EFFECTS

Most of the studies, regarding effect of radiations on the reproductive system have been conducted mainly on animals and rarely on human beings. Gene mutations do occur depending upon the severity of dose. Radiations cause fragmentation of chromosomes and mutation of genes of sex cells, and these mutant genes with altered characteristics pass on to next generation.

From conception to age 30, genetic cells can be given 50R radiations and from 30–40, another 50R can be given. Most of the children are borne when the parent's age is below 30 years.

In case of dentistry, when the patient's teeth are exposed, it is said that 1/10000th of secondary/stray radiations are directed from face to reproductive organs in the males; and 1/7th of this in females. In children, the exposure is much more because of their short stature.

The human embryo is said to be the most sensitive especially during 15–42 days of its life. Therefore, X-radiations in pregnant women must be avoided.

With heavy doses, sterility in human beings has been reported.

RADIATION DETECTION AND MEASUREMENT

Detection and measurement of nuclear radiation must be accomplished by suitable instruments, since these radiations are invisible and their presence cannot be generally sensed by human perception.

All methods of detection of radiations are based on the ability of radiation to cause ionisation, i.e. to produce charged particles from originally neutral atoms and molecules.

A detection system consists of two parts:
- A device which responds to nuclear radiation
- A measuring part which indicates this response

Various radiation measurement units are available which differ in the ionisation media and the method by which the ionisation is directed. Various type of detectors are: (a) Gas filled detectors; (b) Ionization chambers; (c) Photographic emulsions; (d) Solid state dosimeters.

a. **Gas filled detectors:** It is generally of a cylindrical shape with a central rod electrode (Fig. 4.3). The central electrode and the outer sheath are separated by an insulator.

A variable positive voltage is applied to the central electrode with respect to the outer sheath. On exposure to radiations ion pairs are formed (ionisation). The numbers of ion pairs collected at different voltages are measured and five distinguishable regions of response can be noticed. They are:

i. *Region of recombination:* The applied voltage being low, some of the ion-pairs recombine to form neutral atom. Recombination usually decreases as the voltage is increased.

ii. *Ionisation chamber region:* All the ion pairs are collected as there would be no recombination. The number of ion pairs produced and collected depends upon the energy spent by the radiation inside the detection volume.

iii. *Region of proportionality:* The negative ions towards the central electrode are accelerated because of higher electrical fluid in the vicinity of central electrode. The electrons gain

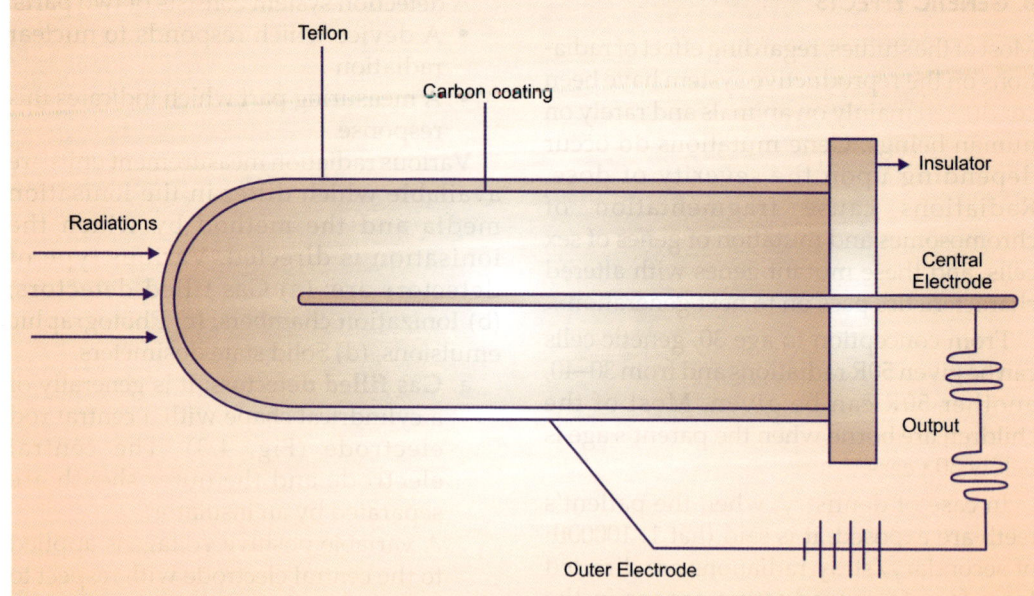

Fig. 4.3: Gas filled detector

sufficient energy to produce secondary ionisation when they interact with gas molecules. This results in an increase in the number of ion pairs collected, which is proportional to the energy dissipated by the incident particles inside the detector.

iv. *Region of limited proportionality:* The amplification is not constant and depends upon the energy dissipated by the incident particles.

v. *Geiger-Mueller region:* The sensitive region spread over the entire length of the chamber and there will be no difference in pulse heights for particles of different ionising abilities.

vi. *Region of continuous discharge:* Ionisation chamber region, proportional region and Geiger-Mueller

region are regions commonly used for radiation detection.

b. **Ionisation chamber:** In the measurement of radiation exposure, the ionisation chambers are filled with air generally at atmospheric pressure. The effective atomic number of the wall material should be close to that of the air. Materials such as graphite, bakelite, etc. satisfy this requirement. Ionisation chambers are also used for personal monitoring. They are called pocket dosimeters. It has built in capacitance which can be charged by the external potential. The reduction in voltage across the capacitance is a measure of the amount of ionisation and hence the quantity of radiation exposure. In the self-reading type of pocket dosimeter, a fibre electrometer with an eyepiece graticules are incorporated in the ionisation chamber capacitance unit. Total dose accumulated at a given date is mR, which can be measured. It indicates the total exposures as well as exposure in between. A pocket dosimeter can be recharged.

c. **Photographic emulsions:** Photographic film consists of the sensitive emulsion layer which on exposure to radiations forms a latent image. The radiations cause ionisation of silver bromide crystals. The films when processed show blackening and the amount of blackening is related to the quantity of radiations recorded. The amount of the blackening is in terms of the measured optical density and is defined as $\log_{10} (I_o/I_t)$ where:

I_o = Intensity of incident light
I_t = Intensity of transmitted light
The optical density is measured using an instrument known as dosimeter.

d. **Solid state thermoluminescent dosimeters:** Many thermolucent materials like LiF, Al_2O_3, $CaSO_4$, etc. are available. $CaSO_4$ is useful for dosimetry. These materials have the property of emitting light when exposed to radiations. The emitted light is proportional to the exposure to the radiations. These are used as personal monitoring services. Thermoluminescent dosimeters can measure gamma dose as low as 1R and as high as 10^5R.

PERSONAL MONITORING

Monitoring is the physical measurement of X-radiations. Personal monitoring is the evaluation of radiation doses received by the persons working in the department concerning radiation. A commonly used device is the film badges, which can be of different types. Films badges and thermoluminescent badges are commonly employed. With a film badge, a wide range of doses from 10 mR to 1000R of different types of radiations can be measured. This is worn on the chest and measures the whole body radiations under normal conditions. X-rays, β-rays, γ-rays, etc. are all measured with the film badges.

Cadmium can be used to detect the radiations of higher penetrating wavelengths (Figs 4.4A and 4.4B).

Advantages

- Permanent record can be kept
- All types of radiations can be differentiated

Disadvantages

- It cannot be read immediately
- It is not very accurate
- It cannot record accidental exposures

The second type of badge is the thermoluminescent dosimeter (Fig. 4.5). This consists of three $CaSO_4$ discs embedded in a metallic frame work and enclosed in a multifilter cassette. This can be used to monitor β, γ and X-radiations. This can cover wide range of doses from 10 m rem to 1000 rem.

Film badges can also be formed with the gradation of only copper over the film. Stepwise increased thickness of copper is placed over the film (Fig. 4.6).

AREA MONITORING

Area monitoring is the assessment of radiation levels at different locations in the vicinity of radiation sources. On the basis of this measurement, protection measures are taken. The most commonly used area monitoring device is the survey-meter based

4

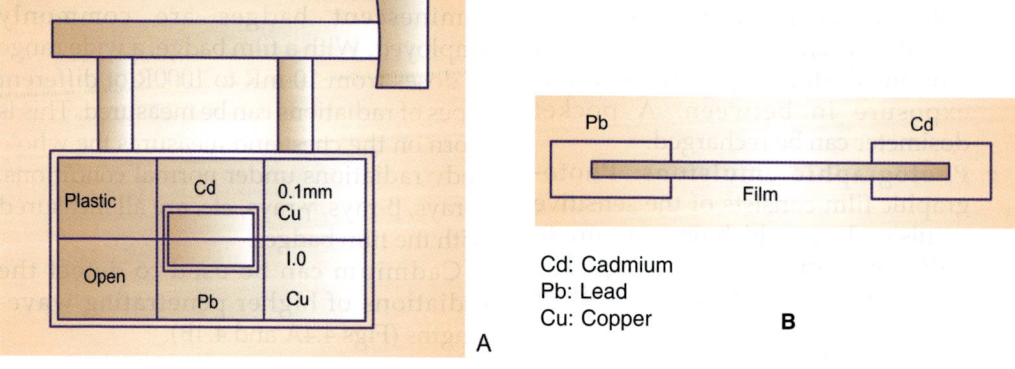

Figs 4.4A and B: Types of film badges

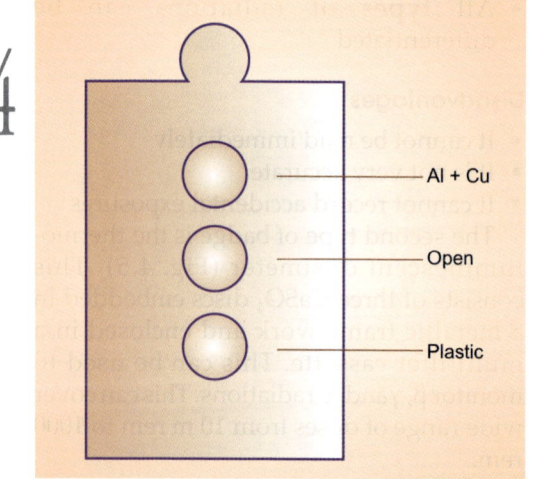

Fig. 4.5: Thermoluminescent dosimeter

on the ionisation chambers. The chamber is provided with a window and by opening the window β-radiations can be measured. This meter usually does not function at the high radiation levels.

RADIATION PROTECTION

The philosophy of radiation protection follows the principle of ALARA (*as low as reasonably achievable*). Even with a single periapical film, the exposure to the patient is 217 mR. According to the ALARA principle, the exposure to X-radiation is to be reduced as far as possible. The three basic parameters which affect radiation doses are described as follows:

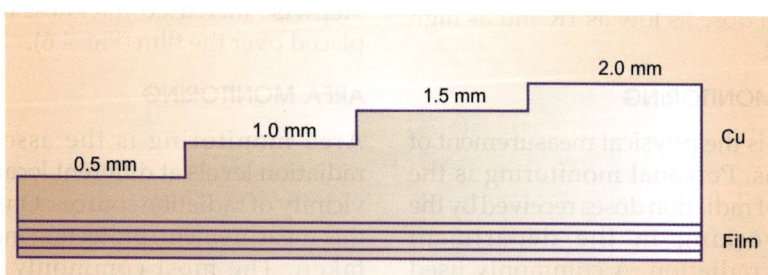

Fig. 4.6: Stepwise increase of copper thickness

i. **Shielding:** Various shielding materials are used such as iron, lead, concrete wall and hard plastic, etc. As the thickness of the shielding interposed between X-ray beams and the *point of interest* (e.g. location of the operator) is increased, the exposure rate decreases exponentially. The thickness of the shielding material, which reduces the intensity of the radiations to half its original value (50%) is defined as the *half value thickness* (HVT) of the material. Exponential attenuation is seen in the case of X-rays and γ-rays and not for electrons as such. This implies that even a very large thickness of the shielding material will not completely attenuate the radiations to have zero intensity. It is pointed out that the X-radiations have a spectrum of energies and that the low energy or soft X-rays are preferentially attenuated than the hard ones. The basic rule is, larger the shielding thickness, lower the exposure rate.

ii. **Distance:** The exposure rate from a point source of radiations at a specified location varies inversely as the square of the distance. The exposure rates E_1 and E_2 at distances D_1 and D_2 are related as:

$$\frac{E_1}{E_2} = \frac{D_2^2}{D_1^2}$$

The practice of being as far away from the machine as possible should be encouraged. Basic formula is larger the distance from the source, lesser is the radiation dose.

iii. **Time:** For a uniform distance and shield, the exposure from a source at a point will be directly proportional to the time during which the exposure was on. Other things remaining constant, the exposure time must be kept to the minimum possible. Lower the exposure time; lower the radiation dose to patients and personnel.

PROTECTION OF THE PATIENT AND THE OPERATOR

Unless and until the lead apron (Fig. 4.7) or proper shielding is provided to the operator, the *installation* should be so arranged that the operator should stand as far away from the source as possible. Minimum of six feet distance is recommended.

The recommendation is that the walls of the operatory room should be sufficiently thick or covered with black paper so that someone occupying the adjacent room should not receive radiations greater than 10R/week.

- The rule of six feet distance and the proper angle of the operator with respect to X-ray tube must be followed. An angle of 135° to the central ray is recommended as a safer zone.

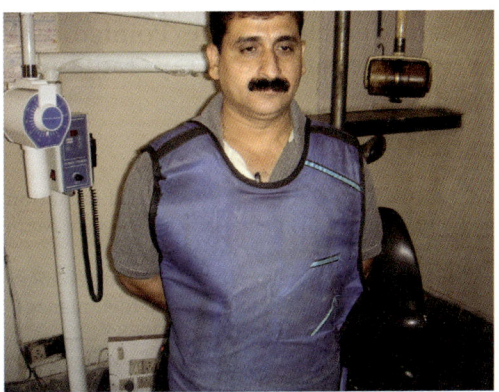

Fig. 4.7: Operator wearing lead apron

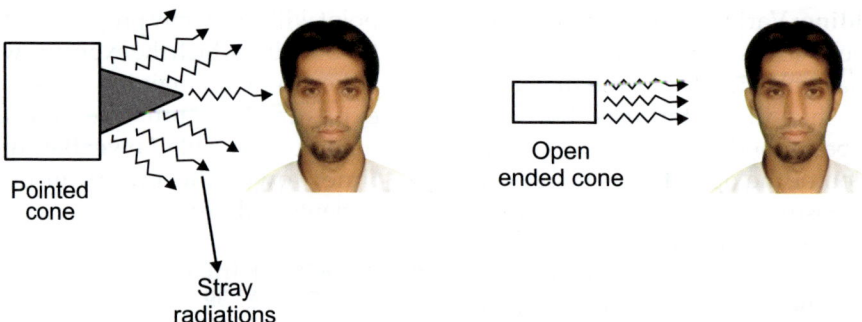

Pointed cone

Open ended cone

Stray radiations

Fig. 4.8: Stray radiations using pointed cone and open ended cone

4

- The operator should never hold the film in the patient's mouth.
- The tube should never be held by the operator during exposure.
- Personal monitoring devices should be used and checked every week.
- Protective guards especially around gonads should be used both by operator and the patient.
- Personnel working in X-ray department should be kept informed of various newer materials and equipment and also the various protective devices.
- Avoid the use of a pointed cone and use an open-ended cone. Pointed cone produces more stray radiations (Fig. 4.8).

Bibliography

1. Alcox RW: Biological effects and radiation protection in the dental office. *Dent Clin North Am* 1978;22:517.
2. Blozis GG, Robinson JE: Oral tissue changes caused by radiation therapy and their management. *Dent Clin North America* 1968;843.
3. Brown L, Dreizen S, Handler S, Johnston D: Effect of radiation induced xerostomia on human oral microflora. *J Dent Res*, 1973;54: 740.
4. Cole LJ, Nowell PC: Radiation carcinogenesis: The sequence of events. *Science*, 1965;150, 1782.
5. Colquitt, W.N. and Richards, A.G.: An old/new idea for reducing exposure to X-rays. *O Surg, O Med, O Path*: 1982;54;597.
6. Coucke ME, Dermant LR: Radiation dose in temporomandibular joint zonography. *O Surg, O Med, O Path*: 1991;71(B);756.
7. Farman AG, Farmann TT: A comparison of 18 different X-ray detectors currently used in dentistry. *O Surg, O Med, O Path*: 2005;99:485.
8. Frank RM, Herdly J, Phillipe E: Acquired dental defects and salivary gland lesions after irradiations for carcinoma. *JADA* 1965;70:868.
9. Manson-Hing LR: The fundamental biological effects of X-rays in dentistry. *O Surg, O Med, O Path*: 1959;12:562.
10. Marciani RD, Plezia R: Management of teeth in the irradiated patient. *JADA* 1974;88:1021.
11. Marx RE: A new concept in the treatment of osteoradionecrosis. *J Oral Max Surg* 1983;41: 351.
12. Marx RE, Johnson RP: Studies in the radiobiology of radionecrosis and their clinical significance. *O Surg, O Med, O Path*: 1987;64:379.
13. Nowak AJ, Creedon RL, Musselman RJ and Troutman, KC: Summary of the Conference on Radiation exposure in pediatric dentistry. *JADA*: 1981;103:426.
14. Payton HG: The effects of radiation on teeth. *O Surg, O Med, O Path*: 1968;26:639.
15. Richards AG: Roentgen ray doses in dental radiograph. *JADA*: 1958;56:351.

16. Richards AG : Secondary radiations and the dentist. *JADA*: 1958;57:31.

17. Richards AG: X-ray protection in the dental office. *JADA* : 1958;56:514.

18. Richards AG, Colquitt WN: Reduction is dental X-ray exposure during the past 60 years. *JADA* 1981; 103:713.

19. Stenstrom B, Hebrikson CO, Holm B, Richter S: Absorbed doses from intraoral radiography with special emphasis on collimator dimensions. Swed. *Dent J* 1986;10:59.

20. Underhill T, Chilvarquer I, Kimura K, Langlais PR: Radiobiologic risk estimation from dental radiology I. Absorbed doses from critical organs. *O Surg, O Med, O Path* 1988;111:66.

21. Underhill T, Kimura K, Chilvarquer I, McDavid DW: Risk estimation from dental radiology II. Cancer incidence and fatality. *O Surg, O Med, O Path* 1988:261:66.

22. Weyman J. The effect of irradiation on developing teeth. *O Surg, O Med, O Path* 1968; 623:25.

4

5

X-ray Films

Various types of X-ray films are available in the market having different shapes and sizes. The different shapes and sizes of X-ray films are required depending upon their use in particular conditions. The chemistry of the X-ray films also varies with subsequent variation in their properties.

X-ray films like photographic films, are composed of two major components, the base and the emulsion. The basic difference of an X-ray film and the photographic film is that in the former the emulsion layer is thicker and contains more silver. The basic constituents of base and emulsion are described below:

1. **Base:** The base of the X-ray film is approximately 0.2 mm thick and is made up of cellulose acetate or cellulose nitrate. Cellulose acetate is preferred because it is less inflammable. Recently, polyesters (polyethylene tera phalate) is being used as a base. The base is to support the silver halide grain and other parts of the emulsion, so a thin layer of adhesive is applied over the base. The base should be flexible, which will enable easy manipulation and it should be translucent, producing clear images.

2. **Emulsion:** The emulsion is a layer of silver halide particles supported by gelatin matrix. Silver bromide is the main constituent and silver iodide is added to a lesser extent. The approximate thickness of the silver halide particles is 0.7 mm. Silver iodide adds to the sensitivity of the film emulsion. It has also been established that sulphide contamination increases the photosensitivity. The emulsion layer can be on one side or both the sides of the X-ray films. Practically all the dental X-ray films contain emulsion on both the sides.

A protective coating of gelatin is placed over the emulsion coating. The gelatin helps to protect the film from damage by scratching and contamination. The X-ray films are manufactured with emulsions with different speeds. The speed or the sensitivity (higher the speed, the more sensitive the film is) depends on the temperature and the duration of heating to which the emulsion is subjected. Gelatin is first immersed in cold water. It absorbs water and swells. On heating, it gets dissolved forming gelatin solution. To this gelatin solution, silver salts are added. This is stirred vigorously and continuously, thereby not allowing the silver salts to settle down. The solution thus prepared is painted on the base.

The speed of the film depends upon:
  i. Duration of heating and temperature.
  ii. Larger the grain size, more sensitive the film, consequently the speed.

American National Standard Institute (ANSI) designates the speed of films from A to F, from slowest to highest speed respectively.

- **A or slow speed:** These are rarely used. These are coated on one side only. After developing, the film is read from the shiny surface.

- **B or medium speed:** Emulsion is coated on both the sides. Half the exposure time is required as compared to slow speed films. It has an embossed dot on one side of the film.

- **C or high speed:** This requires half the exposure time as compared to medium speed films. Sensitivity or speed depends mainly upon the size of silver halide particles. Larger the grain size, more sensitive is the film and a more sensitive film requires less exposure time.

However, as the grain size increases, image sharpness decreases. **Image sharpness** is defined as *the extent to which a radiograph will define a boundary between areas of different densities.*

Depending upon the grain size of silver halide particles, size D, E and F are also available which requires lesser and lesser exposure time respectively.

X-ray films can be intraoral and extraoral.

INTRAORAL FILMS

Intraoral films are used inside the oral cavity. These films are comparatively of smaller size. Intraoral films are usually coated on both the sides, which allows less radiations to form an image. Slow speed films are however, available with emulsion on one side only. Therefore they require more exposure time but also provide increased sharpness and are usually used where there is no concern for exposure time such as industrial applications. The corner of the film has a raised dot. The convex part of the dot is placed towards the tube and the concave part towards the patient's tongue. After the film is developed, the dot is used to identify the right or left of the patient. The concave part or the depression is kept towards the operator and the operators right and left is the patient's right and left.

Single film packets or sometimes double film packets are used. If two films are used, second film is used for keeping the duplicate records. The film (Fig. 5.1D) is enveloped in a paper on both sides (Fig. 5.1B) and an outer protective coating of moisture resistant paper (Fig. 5.1A).

Also, included in the film packet between the wrappers is a thin lead foil backing. The lead sheet is on the back of the film, which protects the film from secondary radiations (Fig. 5.1C).

Intraoral films are generally divided into three categories. The categorization is only on the basis of their clinical use; however, their make is identical. For convenience, the

5

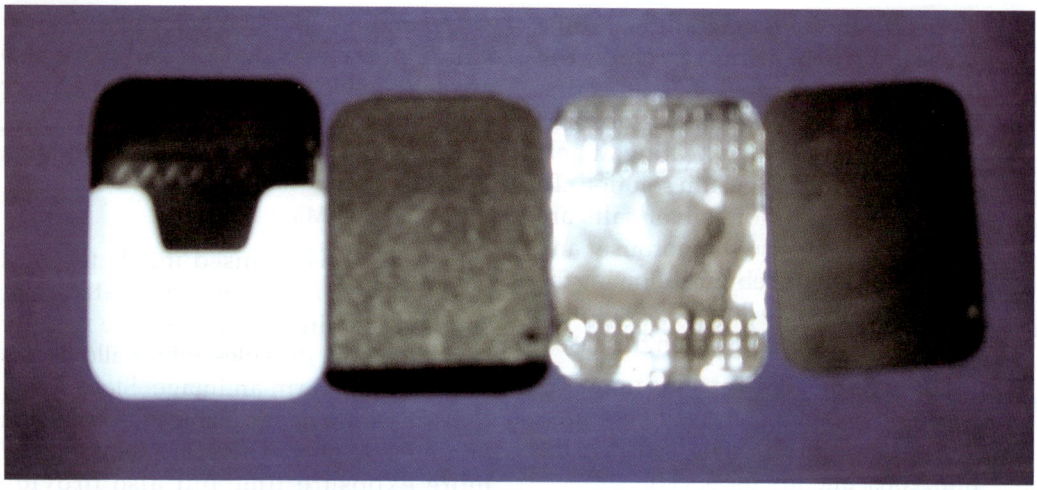

Fig. 5.1: From left (A) waterproof covering; (B) paper cover; (C) lead coating; and (D) X-ray film

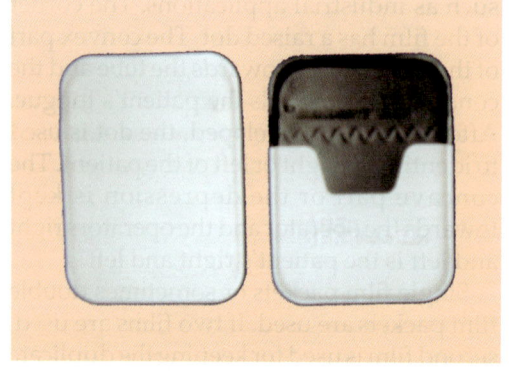

Fig. 5.2: Periapical film

intraoral films are designated by numbers as: periapical films (No. 1), bite wing films (No. 2) and occlusal films (No. 3).

a. Periapical Films

The periapical films are designated as No. 1. These films are utilized where radiographs of crowns, roots and periapical areas are required. One such film is sufficient for three teeth (Fig. 5.2). Periapical films are given number 1.0, 1.1 and so on. 1.0 is the periapical film for children (20 × 35 mm). It is also used in adults who have the problem of gagging. 1.1 is the periapical film for routine use whereas 1.2 is of slightly larger size. With these films, contrast and details are quite good. The film may be single or double in one packet.

b. Bite Wing Films

The bite wing films are designated as No. 2. These are further designated as 2.0, 2.1 and so on depending upon the size. 2.3 is used in anterior teeth because the vertical dimensions is greater than horizontal dimension. These are available in three sizes.

- For anteriors
- For premolars
- For molars

These films record the coronal portion of maxillary and mandibular teeth in one image. These are generally taken for periodic checkup to detect early caries and changes in periodontal tissues.

The film has a flap opposite its centre upon which the patient can bite occluding the upper and lower teeth. Flap is held in position and the patient is asked to bite the flap, which is kept in position using soft wax. Flap is first kept in mandibular teeth and the patient bites slowly. This is not disturbed until the X-ray is taken.

Bite wing films are used:
- To detect early caries and periodontal lesions.
- To see the penetration of caries on the proximal side.
- To see extent of pulp chamber.
- To see the permanent tooth bud in relation to the deciduous tooth.
  Mainly bite wing films are used for periodic checkup.

c. Occlusal films

The occlusal films are designated as No. 3. Right (R) and left (L) is marked on the films. The size of the film is four times the routine periapical films (60 × 75 mm) (Fig. 5.3). As the name suggests, the occlusal film is held in position by letting the patient bite lightly on the film to support it between the occlusal surface of each jaw.

These are used:
- To have a broad view of deciduous teeth for serial extractions.
- To view large areas with pathological involvement.
- To detect extent of fractures.
- To detect impacted or supernumerary teeth.
- Gross examination of maxilla and mandible.
- Localization of foreign bodies in glands.
- For determining the buccolingual relationship of the pathological lesions.

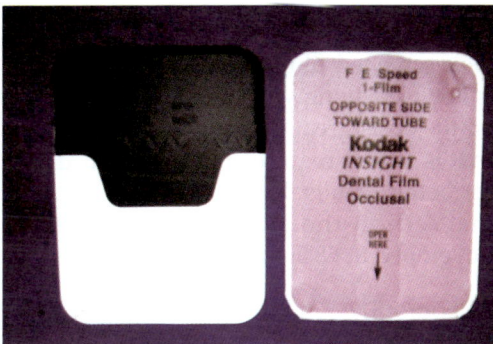

Fig. 5.3: Occlusal film

EXTRAORAL FILMS

As the name implies, these films are used outside the oral cavity. These films are comparatively bigger in size. These are used where:
- Patient cannot open the mouth.
- Temporomandibular joint radiographs are required.
- To detect pathologies of sinuses.
- Broad view of teeth and surroundings.
- To detect fractures of jaw.
- Gross view of impacted teeth.

Extraoral films are of following two types:

a. Screened

In these films intensifying screens are used on both the sides of the film. Intensifying screens are used along with the X-ray films. Intensifying screens along with the films are packed in plastic cassettes. The film should be in direct contact with the screens. There should be no space in between, otherwise image will not be proper. Depending upon the size of crystals these can be slow, fast or medium. With the use of screens, exposure time is decreased. These films are developed at 68°F for 5 minutes.

b. Non-screened

Non-screened films are used where screen is not used alongwith the film. Thickness of emulsion is greater in non-screened films, that is why it requires more exposure time for better results. Right (R) and left (L) are marked on the sides. These films are developed at 68°F for 8 minutes.

Bibliography

1. Horner K, Rushton, VE and Shearer AC: A laboratory evaluation of Ektaspeed plus dental X-ray film. *J Dent*. 1995;23:359.
2. Kaffe I, Littmer MM, Kuspet ME: Densitometric evaluation of intra-oral X-ray films : Ektaspeed v/s ultraspeed. *O Surg, O Med, O Path*: 1984;57: 338.
3. Mourshed F: Clinical evaluation of two bitewing instruments. *O Surg, O Med, O Path* 1971;34:972.
4. Price C: An evaluation of lead foil in dental X-ray film packets. 1st and 2nd. *British Dental Journal* 1972;133;300–343.
5. Svenson B, Lindvall M and Grondahl HG: A comparison of new dental X-ray film, Agfa AGevaert Dentus M4, with Kodak Ektaspeed dental X-ray films. *Dentomaxillofacial Radiology* 1993;22:7.
6. Watts DC, Mc Cabe JF: Aluminium radio-opacity standards for dentistry: An international survey. *J Dent* 1999;27:73.
7. Wenzel A: Bitewing and digital bitewing radiography for detection of caries lesions. *JDR* 2004; 83:C72.
8. Wong A, Monsour PA, Benford KE: A comparison of Kodak ultraspeed and Ektaspeed plus dental x-ray films for the detection of dental caries. *Aust Dent J.* 2002;47:27.
9. Wooten JW and Tarsitano JJ: Hard and soft tissue profile radiograph with one exposure. *O Surg, O Med, O Path* 1970;30:374.

5

6

Radiographic Techniques

Errors, however small they may be, are always grave, especially in radiology. Interpretation of radiographs being a science in itself, is not an easy job. A radiograph which is less than perfect in any sense cannot guide or assist in diagnosis; however, radiographs are important aids in diagnosis. Keeping in view the necessity and importance of a perfect radiograph, the techniques to be followed in exposing the films should be understood well before taking the radiographs. Prevention of distortion is the first step. This is achieved by proper placement of the X-ray tube in relation to the area under examination and to the film. The tube can be moved in two planes—vertical and horizontal depending upon the technique to the followed. The horizontal plane of movement of the tube is parallel to the plane of the floor. Before any rule governing the angulation of the tube is followed, it is necessary that the plane of occlusion (head of the subject) should be aligned parallel to the plane of the floor. In the *vertical plane*, the tube so moves that all its motions are in a plane perpendicular to the plane of the floor. In

this plane, tube moves with an angle which may be +ve or –ve with respect to the plane of occlusion.

X-ray beam is limited to two movements — a *vertical movement* which controls the longitudinal dimension of the resulting image (to prevent elongation and shortening), and a *horizontal movement* which controls the anteroposterior dimension (to prevent overlapping of one tooth shadow over the other).

Based upon these planes and the movement of the tube, two techniques are commonly used, which have their relative advantages and disadvantages.

BISECTING TECHNIQUE

Principle

The bisecting technique is based upon the principle of isometry given by Ceiszynski in 1907, which states that two triangles are always equal when they have two equal angles and a common side. The angle formed by the mean plane of the tooth and the mean plane of the film is bisected and the central beam is directed through the

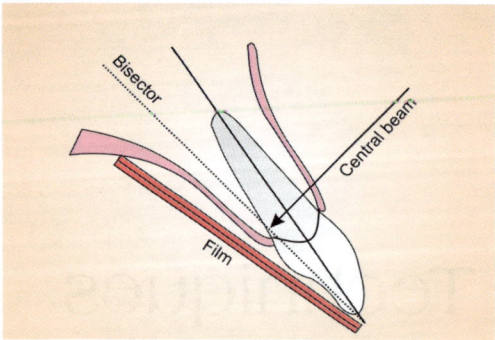

Fig. 6.1A: Bisecting technique

centre of the tooth perpendicular to that imaginary bisector (Fig. 6.1A).

The triangles formed by the tooth on one side of the bisector and by the film on the other side are equal. So the image formed will be of the same size as that of tooth.

In the following geometric diagram (Fig. 6.1B) the logic of the bisecting angle technique may be recognized.

AB = Length of image

AC = Actual length of tooth

AD = Line bisecting the angle between long axis of tooth and long axis of the film, i.e. ∠CAB.

CB = X-ray beam at 90° to the bisector line.

The above diagram has two triangles:

ΔACD and ΔABD. It has to be proved that AC = AB (in other words, the length of the tooth is equal to the length of its X-ray image).

Now, in triangles ACD and ABD, AD is common side. ∠CAD = ∠DAB, because AD is bisecting ∠CAB. ∠CDA = ∠BDA, because they are both right angles. Hence according to the ASA geometrical theorem (Angle-Side-Angle), the triangles ACD and ABD are congruent (equal). Hence AC = AB.

If the central beam is passed perpendicular to the long axis of the tooth, elongation of the image (Fig. 6.2A, B) will occur, and if the central beam is passed perpendicular to the long axis of the film, shortening will occur (Fig. 6.2C, D).

By following this basic rule, if the rays are directed perpendicular to the bisector plane, the image produced will be as near to perfect as possible.

Placement of the Film

The film should be placed in close contact with the tooth structure and alveolar mucosa and then the rays should be directed perpendicular to the imaginary plane bisecting the angle between the film and the tooth.

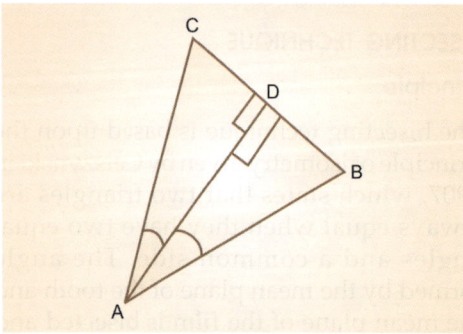

Fig. 6.1B

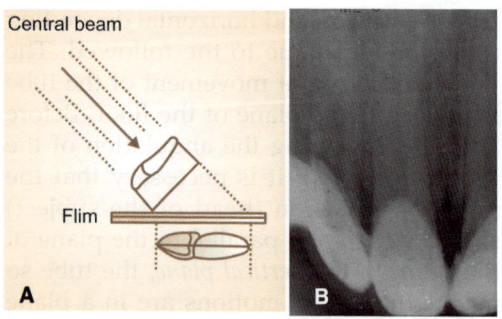

Figs 6.2A and B: Elongated image

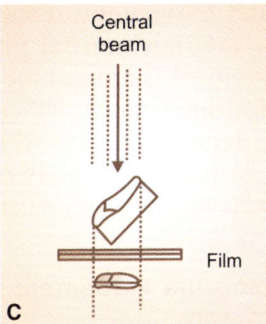

C

Central beam

Film

ii. *In mandibular teeth*, when the patient opens the mouth, the occlusal plane of lower teeth changes its position and therefore, does not remain parallel to the floor. So to place the occlusal plane of mandibular teeth in proper relationship to the floor, it becomes necessary to tilt the head backward. In mandibular teeth, the plane of occlusion vis-a-vis the floor is judged by the operator (Fig. 6.3B).

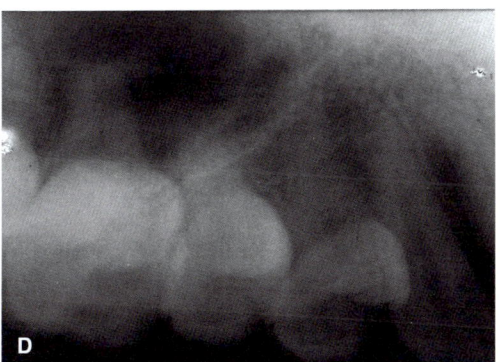

D

Figs 6.2C and D: Shortened image

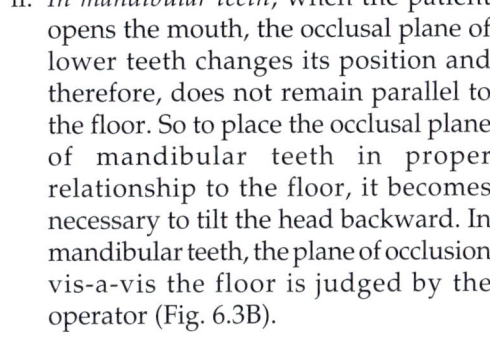

Fig. 6.3A: Patient's position for maxillary teeth

Position of the patient depends upon the following two planes.

a. Occlusal Plane

The occlusal plane is formed by the tangent passing through the occlusal surface of the maxillary and mandibular teeth when the teeth are in centric occlusion.

The occlusal plane should be aligned parallel to the plane of floor.

i. *In maxillary teeth*, an imaginary line drawn from the ala of nose to tragus of ear is almost parallel to maxillary occlusal plane (Fig. 6.3A).

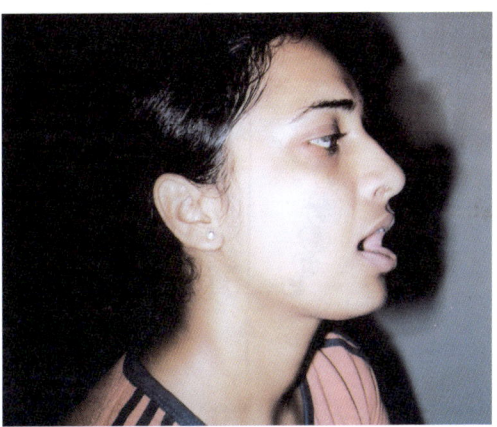

Fig. 6.3B: Patient's position for mandibular teeth

6

b. Median Sagittal Plane

The plane which is vertically passing through the centre of head is known as mid-sagittal plane. This plane should be perpendicular to the floor, no matter whether the head is tilted or not.

Adjusting these two planes is the first step in the production of the radiograph and any deviation from this adjustment will adversely affect the angulation.

Once these two planes are adjusted, horizontal and vertical positions of the tube are considered. Horizontal position of the tube should be such that the central ray is directed perpendicular to the mean antero-posterior tangent of the teeth under examination (Figs 6.4A and B).

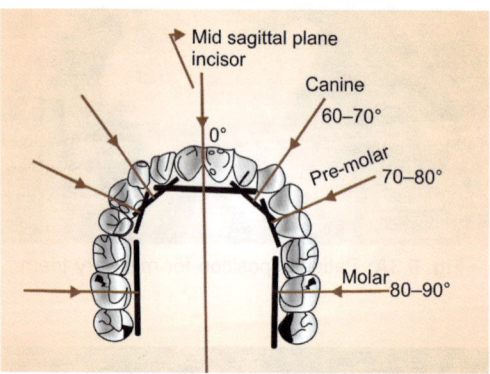

Fig. 6.4A: Horizontal angulations for maxillary teeth

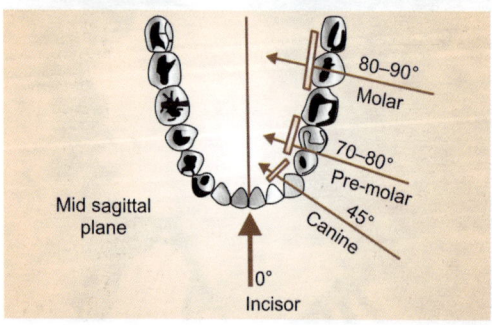

Fig. 6.4B: Horizontal angulations for mandibular teeth

Horizontal movement of the tube is around the median sagittal plane and vertical movement is around the occlusal plane. Vertical angulation is either positive or negative depending upon whether the tube head is facing towards the floor (positive) or facing upwards (negative) (Fig. 6.5).

Rules Guiding the Placement of Film in Oral Cavity

The operator is advised to follow certain rules while placing the film in the oral cavity. These rules are:

- Avoid mis-shaping the film. Films can be bent if necessary, but without crease.
- Carry the film into mouth by thumb and forefingers.
- Teeth under examination should be in the centre of the film.
- Position the lower margin of the film in such a way that 1/8th inch of periapical area is included.
- The index-finger of the patient will rest against the side of the face, other fingers extending in such a way that these should not come in between the path of X-radiations.

PLACEMENT OF THE FILM, ANGULATION OF THE TUBE AND DIRECTION OF RAYS FOR VARIOUS TEETH

Maxillary Central Incisors

The periapical film is grasped by the patient by his thumb and fingers. The film is in close contact with the teeth and alveolar mucosa. After adjusting the film, the operator will observe the imaginary line bisecting the plane of the film and the plane of the tooth. The rays will be passed perpendicular to this plane. The incisor teeth have a 15 to 20° inclination away from a true vertical. Care

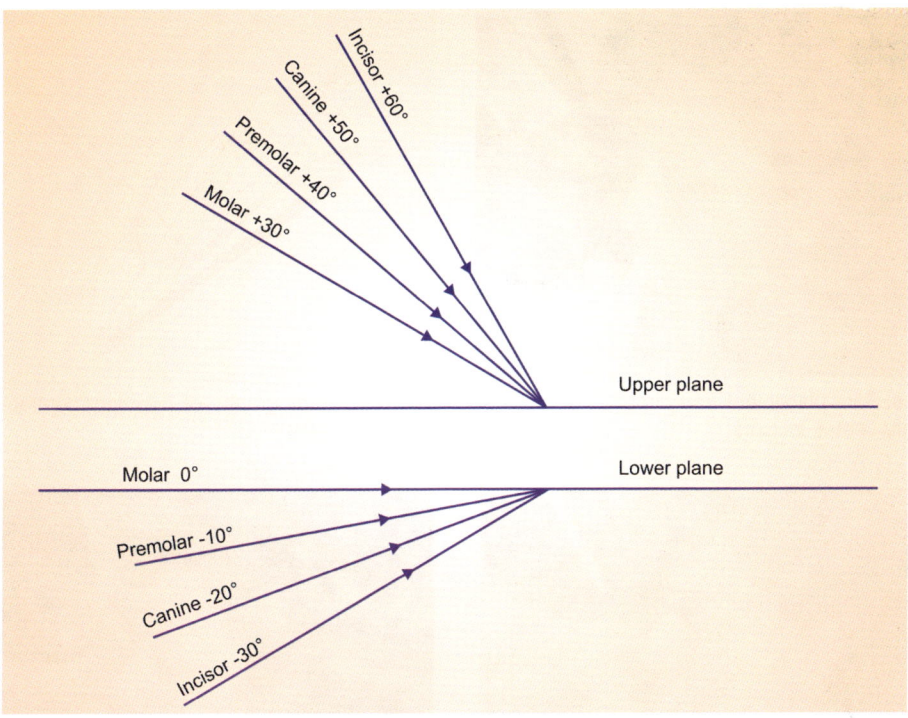

Fig. 6.5: Vertical angulations for different teeth

should be taken to visualise the imaginary lines accurately if optimum results are required. The predetermined angulation can be modified in accordance with the need. Horizontal angulation is 0°. Vertical angulation is 55–60° (Figs 6.6 and 6.7).

Maxillary Lateral Incisors

The film is so positioned that the inter-proximal surface between the central and lateral incisor is centered on the film.

Maxillary Canines

The technique is similar to the one used for maxillary central incisors. The film, however, is placed more apically keeping in view the long roots of canines. Bending of

the films may become necessary, however, crease is to be avoided. The central ray is passed at the tip of canine (Fig. 6.8).

Maxillary Premolars

The film placement for premolars requires certain modifications, because the operator stands on the right side of the patient. The anterior position of the film should be in the midline of canine. The film is held by the patient's thumb, the palm of the thumb should contact the film and palate at the upper border of the film, while fingers are rotated out of the visual field. Horizontal angulation and the vertical angulation are adjusted accordingly. The entry of X-rays should be through the inter-proximal spaces

6

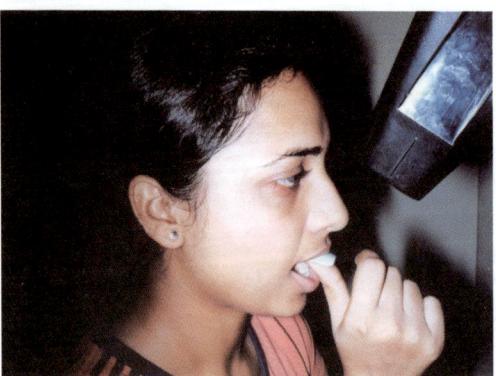

Fig. 6.6: Film placement and direction of tube for maxillary central incisors

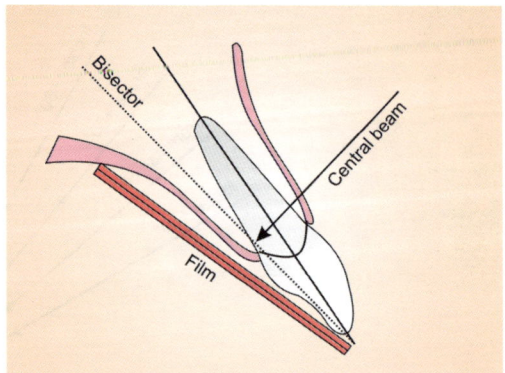

Fig. 6.7: Radiography of maxillary central incisor (diagrammatic)

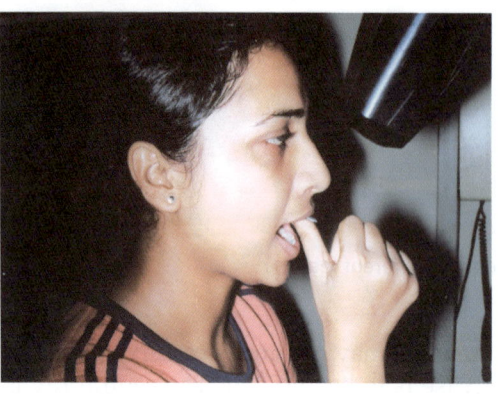

Fig. 6.8: Film placement and direction of tube for maxillary canines

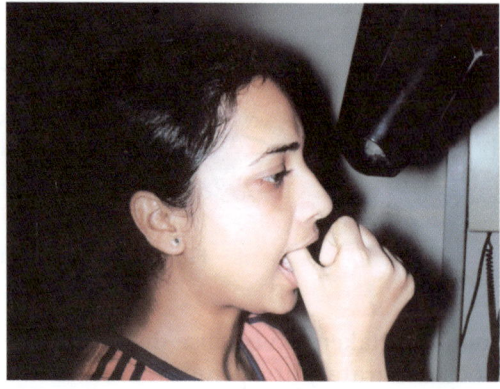

Fig. 6.9: Film placement and direction of tube for maxillary premolars

6

between canine and first premolar and between first and second premolars (Fig. 6.9).

Maxillary Molar Area

Film placement is the same as for premolars, except that the film is to be kept more distally. Rays are passed along the interproximal surfaces of first and second molars. Angulations are adjusted accordingly (Figs 6.10 and 6.11).

Mandibular Central and Lateral Incisors

The mandibular anterior films, especially the narrow films, are easily inserted. The lower border of the film is placed on the floor of the mouth, under the tongue. The palm of the finger tip should rest on the edges of the teeth and not on the film. The film should not be pressed along the lingual surfaces of the teeth. The remaining fingers are elevated in such a way so that they may not come in the operator's line of vision.

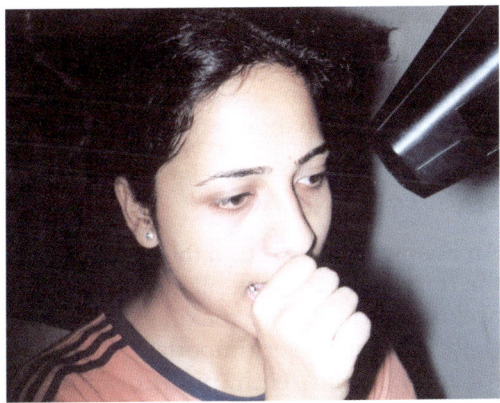

Fig. 6.10: Film placement and direction of tube for maxillary molars

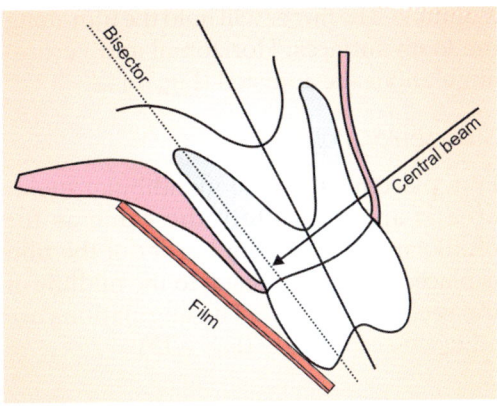

Fig. 6.11: Radiography of maxillary molar (diagrammatic)-Bisecting technique

Angulations are adjusted and the rays are passed along the symphysis menti (Fig. 6.12).

Mandibular Canines

The film is shifted towards the canine area. Care should be taken so that the long axis of the film should be along the long axis of the tooth. The rays should be directed along the

tip of the root after adjusting the angulations (Fig. 6.13).

Mandibular Premolars

The operators should stand in front of the patient. The film is grasped by the upper anterior corner with the left hand when the film is placed on left side and right hand when the film is placed on right side of the

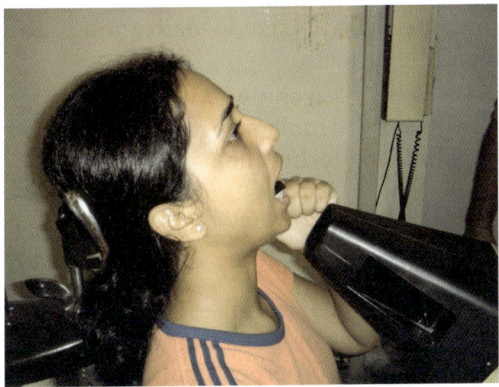

Fig. 6.12: Film placement and direction of tube for mandibular incisors

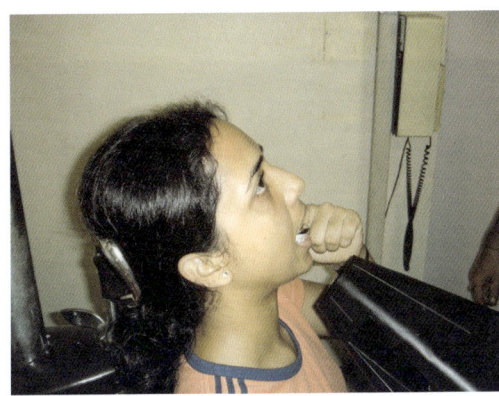

Fig. 6.13: Film placement and direction of tube for mandibular canines

mandible. The finger will hold the film along the tooth surfaces. Horizontal and vertical angulations are adjusted (Fig. 6.14).

Mandibular Molar Area

Film placement for the mandibular molar area is approximately the same as for premolars. The anterior border of the film is placed somewhat distal to the midline of the second bicuspid. The angulations are adjusted accordingly (Fig. 6.15).

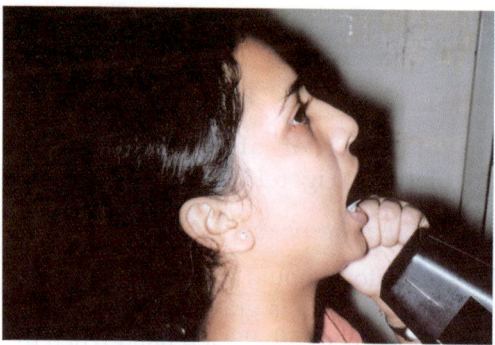

Fig. 6.14: Film placement and direction of tube for mandibular premolars

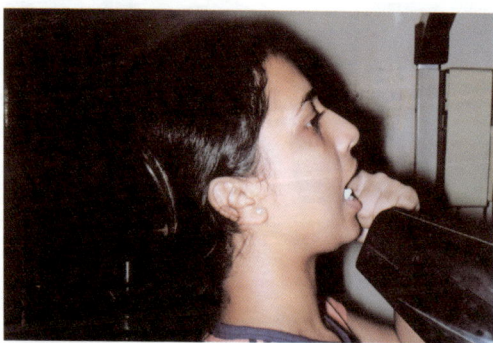

Fig. 6.15: Film placement and direction of tube for mandibular molars

Point of Entry of X-radiations

Once the head is placed in proper position and the angulations are adjusted, the point of entry of X-radiations and their duration are to be decided.

ALA-TRAGUS LINE

An imaginary plane from the ala of nose to the tragus of ear is the plane of maxillary occlusal surfaces. For maxillary posterior teeth, this plane is very important. However, for mandibular teeth, point of entry of X-rays is 0.5 cm above the lower border of the mandible.

For individual maxillary teeth, a plane is dropped from the outer canthus of eye, so that it crosses the ala-tragus plane at a certain point. This point of intersection is the point of entry of X-rays for the maxillary first molar. For second molar, 0.5 cm distal to it and for second premolar, 0.5 cm mesial to it is the point of entry. If a plane is dropped from the centre of the eye, the point where it intersects the ala-tragus plane is the point of entry for premolars. For canines, it is from the canine fossa and for incisors, it is from the tip of nose.

For mandibular teeth, it is less complicated because of easy visualization of the mandibular teeth.

Le Master's technique is employed for maxillary third molars (Fig. 6.16) (explained in paralleling technique).

PARALLELING TECHNIQUE

Principle

When the long axis of the film lies parallel to the long axis of the object/tooth and the rays are directed perpendicular to either of the two, the image produced is of the same size as the object (Figs 6.17 and 6.18).

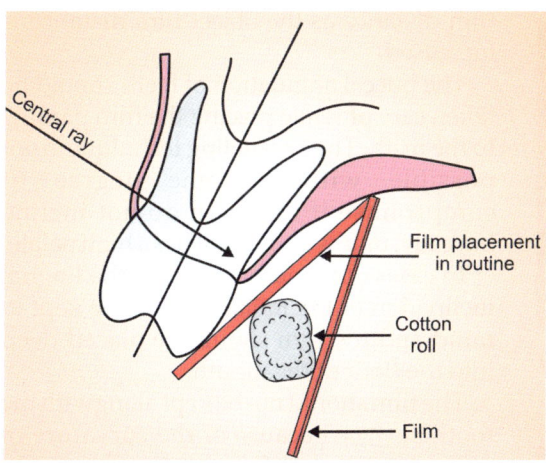

Fig. 6.16: Le Master's technique

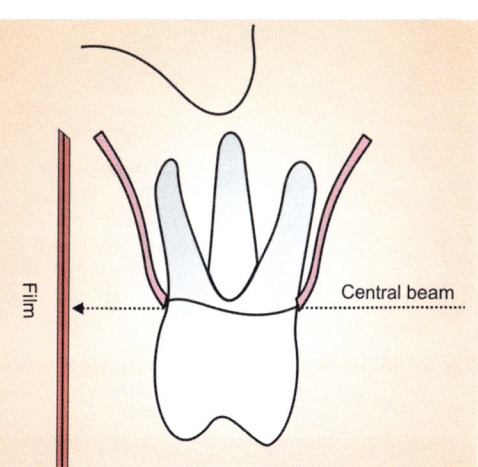

Fig. 6.18: Radiography of maxillary molar (diagrammatic)-Paralleling technique

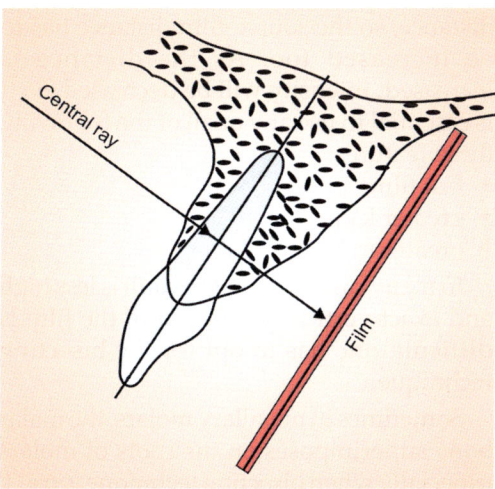

Fig. 6.17: Paralleling technique

Explanation

In dental radiology or otherwise only the central beam of rays can be made perpendicular to the long axis of the film, whereas other peripheral rays are divergent

as they emerge out of the target. As the rays have to move a longer distance, lesser will be the divergence of peripheral rays and lesser will be the elongation. The increased source-film distance becomes necessary because of the following reasons:

- To prevent magnification of the image during short tube-film distance; divergent rays tend to magnify the image.
- To prevent blurring of the image border.
  Distances of 16", 20", 24" and 30" are employed when long cone is used. The other name of paralleling technique is *long cone technique*. Long cone is useful in reducing the divergence of peripheral rays. The radiographic difference between bisecting and paralleling technique is depicted in Figs 6.19A and B.

Placement of the Film

The film should not be bent at any point. The film can be carried to the mouth with the help of thumb and fingers or throat sticks or hemostat. The planes and the tube movements are the same as those described

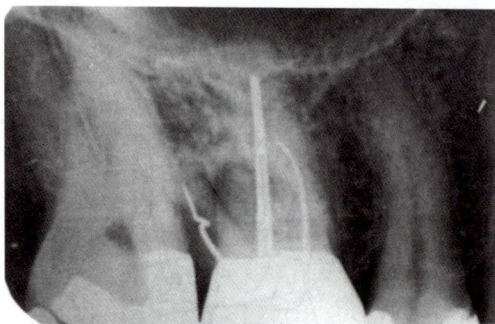

Fig. 6.19A: Radiograph following bisecting technique

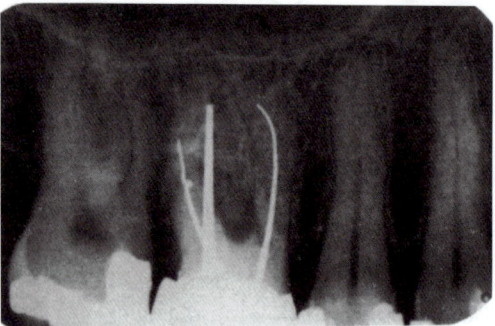

Fig. 6.19B: Radiograph following paralleling technique

for bisecting technique. The only difference, as the name indicates is the placement of the film which is kept parallel to the long-axis of the tooth.

The point of entry of X-radiations and the horizontal angulation are adjusted. Throat sticks and hemostat with rubber tubings are used to keep and hold the film in patient's mouth.

The film is placed as far palatally as possible in maxillary teeth till it can cover the periapical areas. This is especially true for maxillary canines and for maxillary molars where vault is low. The only factor to be kept in mind is to increase the source-film distance as the object-film distance is increased.

The buccal angulation of teeth should be taken care of while placing the film parallel to the teeth. The paralleling technique is not possible without some degree of compromise if the teeth do not incline buccally, unless the patient has a high palate.

In cases of mandibular teeth, the lingual inclination of the molars should be kept in mind and the film should be placed deep into the floor of the mouth.

The film should not be kept alongwith the tooth surface because of the curvature of palatal vault and floor of the mouth. In maxillary teeth, especially molars where the vault is low the film has to be placed towards the median palatine suture. Such a placement of the film increases the film object distance, so the source-film distance has to be increased too. As the distance is increased, intensity will be decreased, so it is essential to use any or all of the following three features:

• fast film
• greater kVp
• greater mA

In many cases, where the vault is less high and exact vertical placement of the film is difficult, one has to opt for the bisecting technique.

Sometimes in maxillary molars, the malar bone superimposes on the roots of molars especially when bisecting technique is used. In these cases paralleling technique is preferred.

In such cases, a compromise is made between the two techniques for better results.

It is called *Le-Master's technique* (Fig. 6.16). A cotton roll is kept between the film and the tooth to make the angle between them less-sharp. Two main disadvantages of the bisecting technique, which are overcome in the paralleling technique are:

i. Superimposition of zygomatic bone over the roots of maxillary molars.
ii. Distortion of the cervical area of the teeth and the alveolar crest area.

A significant improvement was accomplished by Richards, who developed a new X-ray tube head in which long cone is fitted inside the machine. The source-film distance kept inside the tube is 16". It produces better results.

Procedure of Film Placement and Angulation using Bite Wing Films

Bite wing films are useful especially to visualize inter proximal carious lesions and the underlying periodontal condition. Bite wing films with tags can be purchased from the market, though prefabricated tags are also available which can be fixed with routine periapical films. When the bite wing film is placed, the tag is folded upward against the film surface. The film is placed in mouth like any routine film except that deep placement in the floor is not required. As the tag is placed on occlusal surfaces, the patient is asked to slowly close the mouth. The upper surface of the film is kept away from the palatal surface by using tongue blade (Figs 6.20 and 6.21A to C).

A vertical angulation of 0–5° is used and the horizontal angulation is so adjusted that the rays pass through the inter-proximal spaces between the teeth under examination.

Procedure of Film Placement and Angulation using Occlusal Films

The occlusal film is inserted in the oral cavity with the film to be retained by patient's

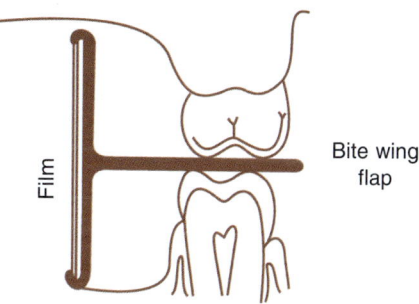

Fig. 6.20: Bite wing film placement

closing of the mouth (the technique is also known as *sandwich technique*). In the edentulous arch, the film is held against the maxillary ridge by the patient's thumb and on the mandibular ridge by the forefingers. The exposure side of the film is placed towards the teeth to be examined.

When the entire dental arch is to be observed, the rays are directed perpendicular to the centre of the film (Figs 6.22A and B, Figs 6.23A and B). Occlusal films can be used for a variety of purposes and for different purposes, different exposure sites and timings are recommended.

The projections used for occlusal films are:

i. **Anterior mandibular (mandibular symphysis):** The central ray is passed through the point of chin keeping an angulation of –55° to the occlusal plane (Fig. 6.24).

ii. **Cross-sectional mandibular (mandibular symphysis occlusal):** The central ray is passed through a point below the chin, and 3.0 cm posterior to the point of chin, keeping an angulation of 90° to the occlusal plane (Fig. 6.25).

iii. **Lateral mandibular:** The central ray is passed through a point 3.0 cm below the

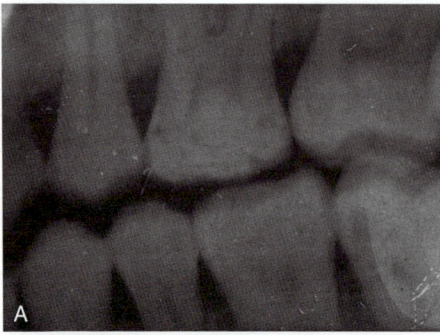

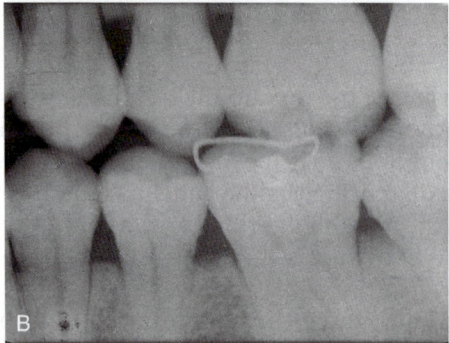

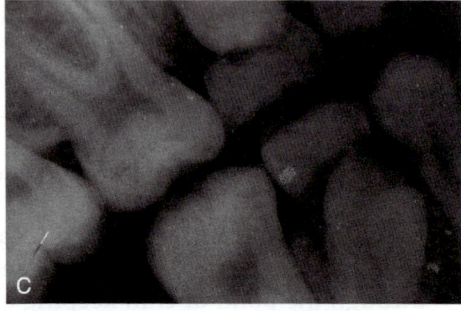

Figs 6.21A to C: Bite wing radiographs

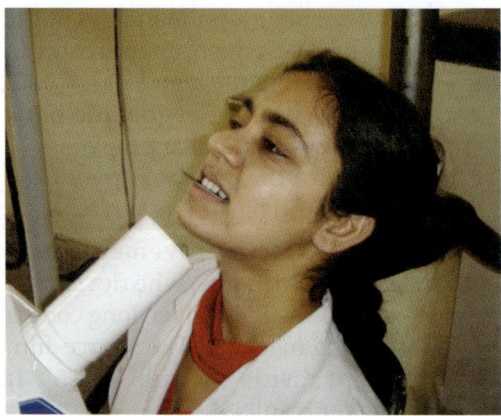

Fig. 6.22A: Film placement and direction of tube for mandibular occlusal

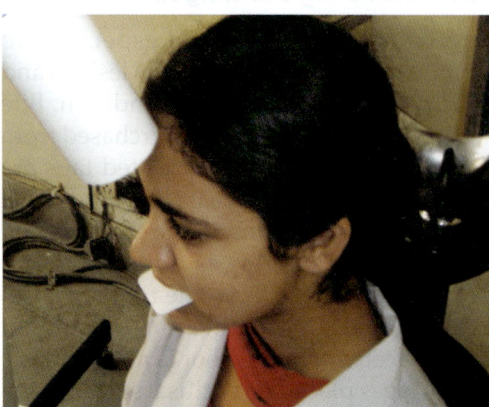

Fig. 6.22B: Film placement and direction of tube for maxillary occlusal

6

point of chin and 3.0 cm lateral to the midline, keeping angulation of –90° to the occlusal plane (Fig. 6.26).

iv. **Anterior maxillary:** The central ray is passed through the tip of nose, keeping an angulation of +45° to the occlusal plane (Fig. 6.27).

v. **Cross-sectional maxillary (topographic maxillary):** The central ray is passed through the bridge of nose, keeping an angulation of +65° to the occlusal plane (Fig. 6.28).

vi. **Lateral maxillary:** The central ray is passed through a point 2.0 cm below the lateral canthus of eye, towards the centre of the film, keeping an angulation of +60° to the occlusal plane (Fig. 6.29).

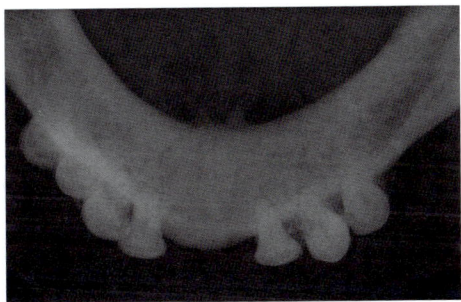

Fig. 6.23A: Occlusal radiograph of mandibular teeth

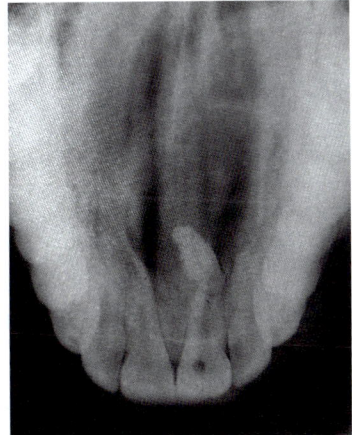

Fig. 6.23B: Occlusal radiograph of maxillary teeth

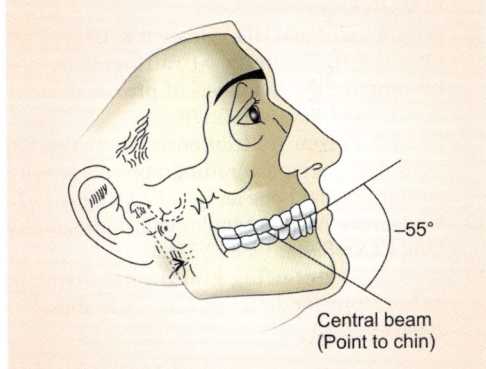

Fig. 6.24: Anterior mandibular projection (mandibular symphysis)

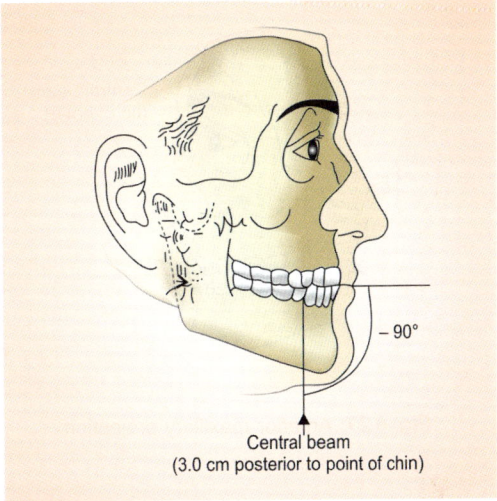

Fig. 6.25: Cross-sectional mandibular projection (mandibular symphysis occlusal)

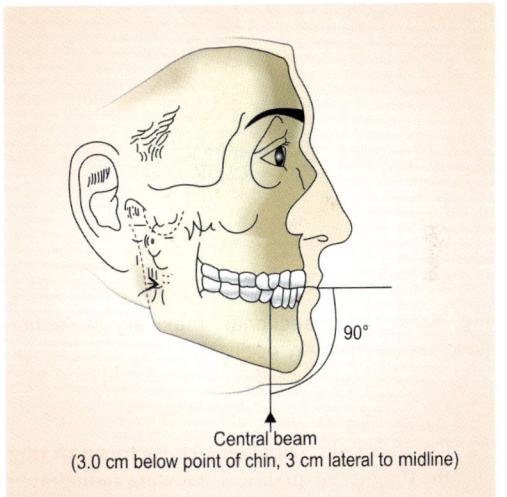

Fig. 6.26: Lateral mandibular projection

Bibliography

1. Bohay RN, Kogon SL, Stephens RG: A survey of radiographic techniques and equipments used by a sample of general dental practitioners. *O Surg, O Med, O Path* 1994;78:806.

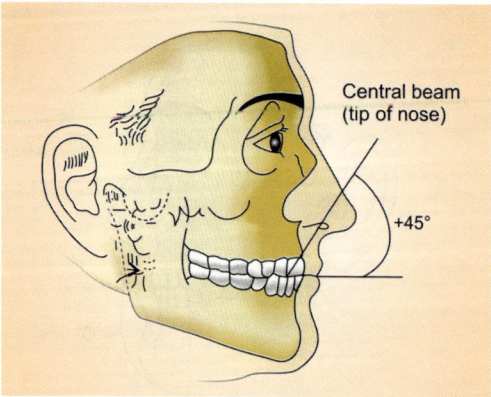

Fig. 6.27: Anterior maxillary projection

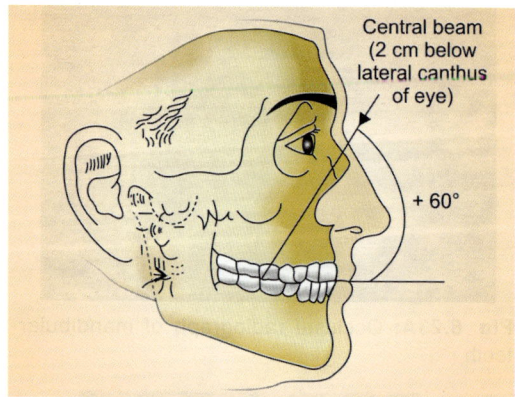

Fig. 6.29: Lateral maxillary projection

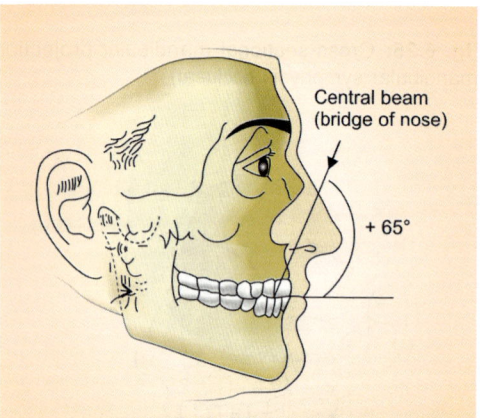

Fig. 6.28: Cross-sectional maxillary projection (topographic maxillary occlusal)

endodontic working length. *Int Endo J* 1992;25:279.

5. Grondel HG, Hollender L, Osvald O: Quality and quantity of dental X-ray examinations. *Dentomaxillofac Radiol* 1980;9:70.

6. Jones PE, Warner B: A teaching method for paralleling technique. *O Surg, O Med, O Path* 1976;42:126.

7. Kells CE: Thirty years experience in the field of radiology. *JADA* 1926;13:693.

8. Manson-Hing LR: On the evaluation of radiographic technique. *O Surg, O Med, O Path* 1969;27:631.

9. McDavid WD, Welander V, Pillai BK, Morris CR: The interrex: A constant potential X-ray unit for periapical dental radiography. *O Surg, O Med, O Path* 1982;53:433.

10. Mejare J, Grondal HG, Carlstedt K, Grever AC, Ottoson E: Accuracy at radiography and probing for the diagnosis of proximal caries. *Scand J Dent Res* 1985;93:178.

11. Read B, Polson A: Relationship between bite wing and periapical radiograph in assessing crestal alveolar bone levels. *J Period* 1984;55:22.

12. Updegreve WJ: Right angle dental radiography. *Dent Cl North Am* 1968;12:571.

13. Wenzel A: Bitewing and digital bitewing radiography for detection of caries lesions. *JDR* 2004; 83:C72.

2. Chadwick BL, Dummer PH: Factors affecting the diagnostic quality of bitewing radiograph: A review. *BDJ* 1998;184:80.

3. Council on Dental Materials : Instruments and Equipments. Recommendations in Radio-graphic Practice. *JADA* 1984;109: 764.

4. Griffiths BM, Brown JE, Hyatt AT: Comparison of three imaging techniques for assessing

7

Processing of X-ray Films

After an X-ray film is exposed to X-radiations, it is processed to have a visible image of the object which was exposed. The complete processing cycle comprises of development, rinsing, fixing, washing and drying. In automatic and computerized processing units, the rinsing is omitted and the films are squeezed after developing and fixing. In both the processes, the end result is a dry film with an image which can be viewed properly and can be stored.

FORMATION OF LATENT IMAGE

As the X-ray film is exposed to X-radiations, the photosensitive silver halide particles get chemically changed. Such inherent changes in the X-ray film collectively form the latent image. The silver bromide of the photographic emulsion consists of positive silver and negative bromide ions arranged in a geometrical pattern. This is known as *crystal lattice*. As the radiations fall on silver bromide, the electrons are emitted. These electrons travel with great speed within the confines of the crystal and collect at one

region, known as *electron traps*. These regions are also known as *sensitivity specks*, which can be produced at various stages of manufacturing. The electrons confer a negative charge at the sensitivity speck areas and this grouping of electrons is the first stage in latent image formation (Fig. 7.1).

The silver ions in the crystal have positive charge. Not all the silver ions are held in the lattice, some are free moving. These free moving silver ions are attracted to the negatively charged sensitivity speck areas and are neutralized. The silver atoms in the areas increase in number. This sequence repeats itself and the sensitivity speck has a number of atoms of silver and forms a part of the latent image. The cycle of events takes place very quickly, which clearly reveals the difference between the exposed crystals, which contain metallic silver atoms and the unexposed crystals, which do not contain metallic silver atoms.

ACTION OF THE DEVELOPER

The developer basically reduces the metallic silver of the exposed silver halide crystals.

67

7

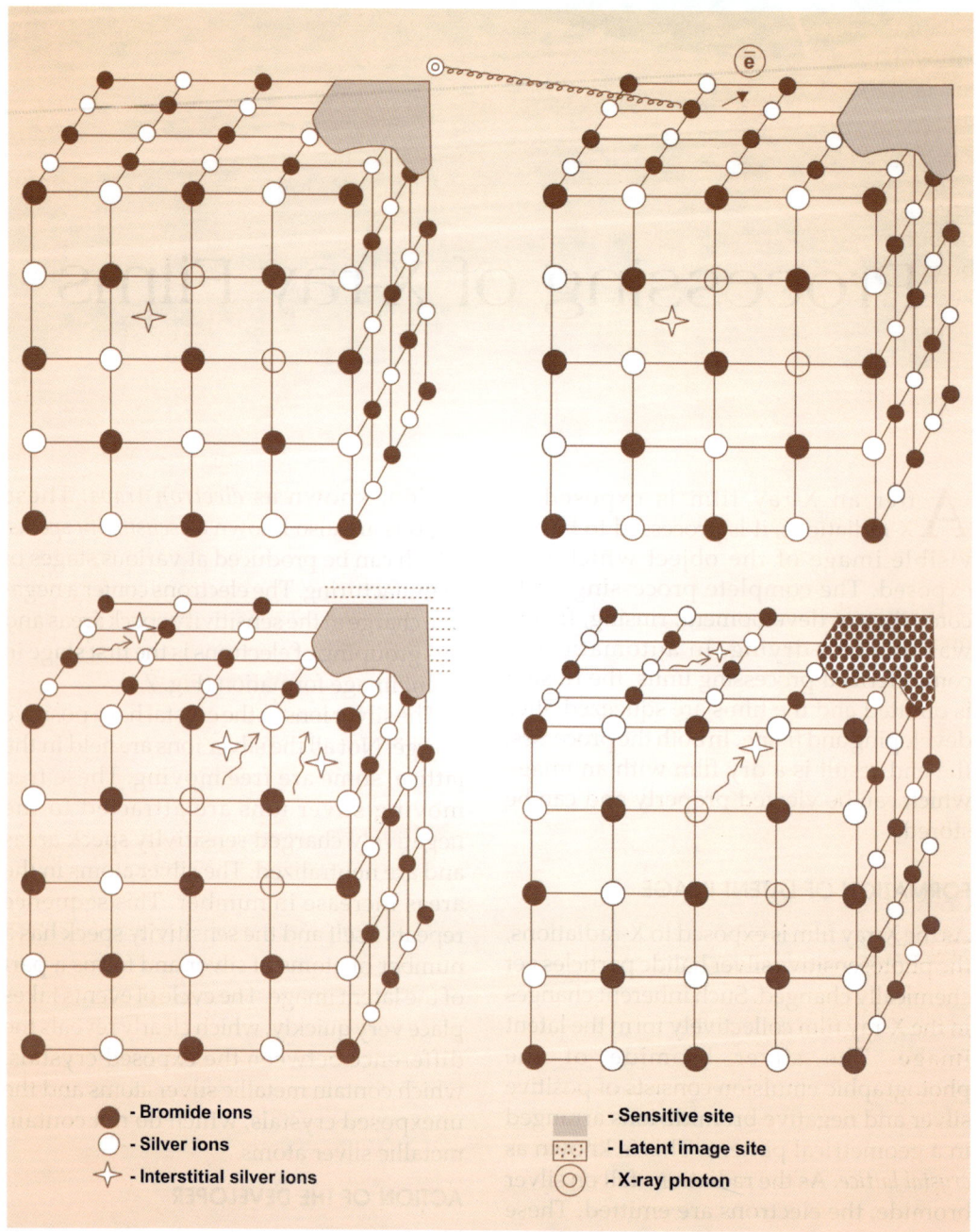

- **Bromide ions**
- **Silver ions**
- **Interstitial silver ions**
- **Sensitive site**
- **Latent image site**
- **X-ray photon**

Fig. 7.1: Formation of latent image

When the developer comes in contact with silver, it donates electrons to neutralize the silver ions. With this more silver ions are attracted into the sensitivity speck area and are neutralized by the developer. The negative bromide ions, which formed the crystal lattice with the positive silver ions disperse into the developer solution as free bromide ions, for they have no silver ions to keep them in place.

Usually, a negatively charged barrier of bromide ions surrounds each silver bromide crystal. This repels the developer. Only the exposed grains have sensitivity areas and constitute a weakness in the bromide ions barrier. Electrons from the developer gain easy access and reduce the exposed crystals to metallic silver.

In brief, the total action can be summed up as:

Silver bromide (AgBr) $\rightarrow$ Br$^-$ + Ag$^+$

Br$^-$ + light $\rightarrow$ Electrons emitted (e$^-$)

(e$^-$) Electrons + Ag$^+$ $\rightarrow$ Silver atom

Developer $\rightarrow$ gives Electron to Silver ions

(e$^-$) Electrons + Ag$^+$ $\rightarrow$ Silver atom

Constituents of the Developing Solution

The developing solution contains mainly five components:

a. Developer
b. Activator
c. Restrainer
d. Preservative
e. Solvent

Other additions such as water softeners, wetting agents and bactericidal agents are in traces. Aldehydes are used as hardeners in the developer. A pair of buffering agents is also added such as boric acid and sodium hydroxide.

a. Developer

A developing agent is a substance which is able to change silver halide into metallic silver. Chemically this is known as reduction. When reduction occurs, atoms or molecules gain electrons and when oxidation occurs, atoms or molecules loose electrons. Unexposed crystals without latent images are unaffected during developing.

Two types of combinations are usually used as developing agents:

i. Elon—Hydroquinone combination
ii. Phenidine—Hydroquinone combination.

The latter type (ii) of developer is 10–15 times more effective than the former. This combination does not exhaust as quickly as type (i) combination. Additionally they are less susceptible to the restraining effect of bromide concentration, which comes into play when the developer acts.

b. Activator

The developer is alkaline in nature. Maintaining its alkalinity is important. Too little alkalinity results in developer being sluggish in action and too much alkalinity makes it overactive.

The required pH range of X-ray developer is 10–11.5.

The alkalies used as activators are sodium hydroxide, sodium carbonate, potassium hydroxide and potassium carbonate. The potassium salts have an advantage over the sodium salts because of their higher solubility. Activator also serves to soften the gelatin so that the developing agents diffuse more rapidly into the emulsion.

7

c. Restrainer

Potassium bromide is added as a restrainer. One of the qualities of good developing agent is its ability to act on the exposed silver bromide grains more rapidly than on the unexposed. The restrainer prevents or check action on the unexposed grains and thereby prevents fog.

Without any restrainer, the developer will be too active and reduce the unexposed crystals too rapidly. Restrainer improves radiographic contrast by reducing fog. In type (ii) combinations, one more restrainer with potassium bromide can be added. This is benzotriazole. Organic restrainer can act efficiently at a much lower concentration than potassium bromide. These agents are also known as *anti-fog agents*.

d. Preservative

Developing agents are easily oxidised and readily absorb oxygen from air. A chemical, therefore, is necessary which checks their oxidation. Sodium sulphite and potassium sulphite are used for this purpose and are called *preservatives*. As the developing solution is oxidised, the developing agents produce certain oxidation products. Some of these can accelerate the process of further oxidation. Sodium sulphite or sulphonate are inert and the final oxidation products are not formed.

e. Solvent

The solvent used is always water, which has the advantage of being cheap and universally available. Distilled water is comparatively better. With the use of hard water, the salts can react with photographic chemicals and produce precipitates.

Water softeners are added in the developing solutions to eliminate the problem of precipitation. Only in extreme cases, water softener Calgon (sodium hexameta-phosphate) is added.

Added water should be clear and free from copper impurities, otherwise it will result in fog on the films.

DEVELOPING TIME

The developing time is that period, which the film spends in the developing solution to produce optimum results. In automatic machines, this time varies with the full cycle period of the processor. If the cycle time is 3.5 minutes, the developing time is 65 seconds, and if the cycle time is 110 seconds, developing time is 30 seconds. As the time shortens, the total time of the cycle decreases.

Developing time can also be defined as the period required for the image to develop optimum density and contrast.

Certain factors, which influence the developing time are:

a. Constitution of the Solution

The constitution of the developing solution significantly affects the resultant image, especially with regard to its density and contrast. So care must be taken regarding the following:

  i. Relative proportion of the developing constituents
 ii. Degree of alkalinity
iii. Combined fractions of all the chemical ingredients. An ideal developing solution should give high contrast, high speed and minimum fog. Presently, such problems are rare because almost all processing is done in automatic processor and even if carried out manually, the developing agents are compounded to meet all the needs.

b. Temperature of the Solution

The temperature of the solution has marked effects on the activity of the agents used. A developer is always more active if it is warm. It is established that lower temperature requires longer developing time and higher temperature needs shorter developing time.

Different developing agents are affected to different extents by changes in temperature, e.g. hydroquinone loses activity to a greater extent than others as the temperature of the solution falls. A developer temperature of around 31°C is the most widely used temperature in automatic processors. Raising the temperature in automatic processors is one of the methods by which the development time is greatly shortened.

c. Degree of Exhaustion of the Solution

The activity of the developer decreases with use as the composition of the solution alters with time. The reactions involved are given as under:

i. Developer which is in use: Developing agents + Silver Bromide → Silver ions + bromide ions + hydrogen ions + oxidised developing agents

ii. Developer which is not in use: Developing agents + Oxygen → Oxidised developing agents + hydroxyl ions.

The activity of the developing solution in the working tank of the machine must be kept constant by what is known as *replenishing*. The replenisher is added at a rate, which is proportionate to the rate of exhaustion.

Aerial oxidation and oxidation through normal development action have opposing effects on pH. Oxidation due to the use of developer causes decrease in pH while aerial oxidation of the developer causes increase in pH.

Used solutions are always less energetic than fresh ones. In practice, usually, as the solution exhausts, the development time at a given temperature must be increased to obtain optimum contrast and density.

REPLENISHER

Since the developing agents are used up, a replenisher containing the same ingredients in relatively higher concentration than the original solution is added every morning to make up for the depleted constituents of the developing solution. Also with use, there is increased concentration of bromide, which restrains the developer. Bromide, therefore, is not included in the replenisher.

The replenisher contains a high concentration of an alkali (usually sodium hydroxide) to offset or compensate for the fall in pH that occurs with the use of the developer.

Extra sulphate is also added to prevent the aerial oxidation of the replenisher and hence the developer.

A replenisher is designed to be used with a particular developer.

In order to effectively use a developing solution, it is necessary to simultaneously restore both the physical volume and the chemical quality (pH) of the depleted solution. The amount of replenisher added to restore the working level of the solution must bring sufficient regeneration to restore the activity of the solution.

d. Agitation of the Solution and the Film

Agitation of both the film and the solution has two prominent effects:

i. Shorter developing time

ii. Uniformity of development

This problem is minimised in roller type automatic processors as the film remains in continuous movement. In manual type of processors, continuous agitation is required, otherwise light and dark streaks are formed.

Light streaks are formed as follows: In heavily exposed areas, there is considerable reduction of silver bromide to silver, accompanied by the release of Br^- ions. Local Br^- concentration has a restraining effect on development. Agitation would sweep this Br^- concentration, whereas a static state would allow it to sink down and restrain the developer in areas vertically below the regions of high exposure. These areas, therefore, show light streaks.

Dark streaks occur in the following way: In the static state, the developer from areas which are lightly exposed is allowed to sink downward (developer being largely unused). Thus, in regions vertically below these areas, the developer is more active and dark streaks result.

Solutions which are not stirred properly result in uneven development. Chemical mixers with a mechanical action are useful for obtaining proper development.

FIXING

Fixing process is required to fix or make the image permanent by removing silver halide, leaving the metallic silver image unaltered against a translucent background. The main function of fixing is:

- To remove the unexposed, undeveloped silver-halide.
- To stop further action of the developer absorbed in the swollen gelatin of the film.
- To harden the films.

Hardening is important both to protect the film from damage and to control the extent to which it swells after absorbing moisture.

In manual processors, an intermediate step is required, which is known as rinsing. The main objective of rinsing is to prevent films from carrying active developer into the fixer.

The intermediate step is carried out:

i. To slow down the action of the developer by removing it from the surface. This is plain rinsing.

ii. To stop the action of the developer by neutralizing the emulsion layer. This is achieved by putting the film in an acid bath. Usually, plain bath is sufficient because the next step of fixing is acidic. The rinsing should be carried out in running water although just dipping in water will do. Spray rinses are advantageous, since the water is fresh, being provided by jet system.

The developing solution, if carried to the fixer, can result in:

- Dichroic fog
- Brown staining of the film (because of oxidation products)
- Increased alkalinity of the fixing solution as the developer is alkaline. In automatic developer, however, this is omitted. The developer is squeezed from the film after the development is over.

CONSTITUENTS OF THE FIXING SOLUTION

The fixing solution contains the following constituents:

a. Fixing Agent

The fixing agent is the constituent which converts silver halide into soluble complexes thereby removing it and leaving the metallic silver image. The most common fixing agent used is sodium thio-sulphate commonly known as hypo. The action can be simply put as:

Silver bromide + sodium thiosulphate → Sodium Bromide + sodium salt of mono argento-di-thiosulphuric acid

Ammonium thiosulphate is also used as fixing agent. The action can be expressed as:

Silver bromide + Ammonium thiosulphate → Ammonium bromide + Ammonium salt of mono argento-di-thiosulphuric acid.

The ammonium silver complex is highly soluble in water and can be washed out very quickly. Ammonium complex is less stable than sodium complex.

If films are not washed thoroughly, subsequent staining and deterioration of the image will be quicker with the use of ammonium salts.

b. Acid stabilizer and the Buffer

Rinsing is a must before fixing, otherwise slight degree of development may remain continuous even in the fixer. A developer carried to the fixer results in:

- Dichroic fog
- Brown staining because of the oxidation products of developer
- Formation of streaks

In order to save the film from these effects, the fixing solution contains acid which halts the action of developer. A weak acid (acetic acid) is usually used because strong acids can cause deterioration of the developer. There is a tendency on the part of thiosulphate solution to decompose and precipitate sulphur even with weak acids. To prevent this, a stabilizer like sulphite or bisulphite can be used.

Alternatively, sodium meta-bisulphite or potassium meta-bisulphite is used, which provide both acids and stabilizers.

Another ingredient used is buffer. The pH of the bath should be 4.0–5.0. To maintain this, sodium acetate and acetic acid or sodium sulphite and sodium bisulphite are used.

c. The Hardener

The emulsion layer of the film absorbs moisture and swells during processing. The swelling is marked during the water rinse and washing stages. Hardening of the emulsion during fixing has certain beneficial effects:

i. Gelatin absorbs less water and can be dried more quickly.

ii. The film becomes less susceptible to physical damage such as streaks, scratches, etc.

iii. Driers with higher temperature can be used.

Hardening agents are incorporated in the emulsion but it is necessary to obtain further hardening. Hardening agents are incorporated as constituents in fixing-bath. The hardening agents used are:

- Chrome alum
- Potassium alum
- Aluminium chloride

The pH of these hardeners is important. If the pH of hardening agent is too low, yellow sulphur is deposited in the solution and if the pH is high, hardening efficiency is lost.

- **Chrome alum:** Chrome alum as a hardener works effectively at pH 3.5 to 4.7. Above 4.7 there is little hardening effect. It is suitable for fixing solutions, which are to be used soon after preparation and are not to be used for long. Chrome alum as a hardener has one disadvantage—it does not keep its efficiency for more than few days.

- **Potassium alum:** Potassium alum works at pH 4.5 to 4.9. At pH above 5.5, white bloom (a precipitate of aluminium hydroxide with potassium hardener) may appear on the film.
- **Aluminium chloride:** Aluminium chloride works at pH 4.1–4.4. It is normally used with the rapid ammonium thiosulphate fixers.

d. Solvent

The solvent diluent for fixing solution is water. The type and quality of water which is preferred has been discussed in the text pertaining to the developer.

e. Other Additives

Boric acid is added as another additive, which acts as an anti-sludging agent, especially when the pH rises too high, particularly with potassium alum hardener. If not used, a sludge is formed in the fixing bath.

FACTORS AFFECTING THE USE OF FIXER

Several factors affect the rate of clearing and fixing the film in the fixer. These are:

a. Type of Fixing Agents Used

The commonly used fixing agents are ammonium thiosulphate and sodium thiosulphate. Among these two fixing agents, ammonium thiosulphate is more rapid in action than sodium thiosulphate when compared in equivalent concentrations.

b. Concentration of Fixing Agents

It is established that a higher concentration results in a shorter clearing time especially for wet films.

c. Temperature of the Solution

Usually at a high temperature, the diffusion process takes place more quickly and gelatin becomes permeable more rapidly. The temperature difference between the two should not be too marked and if the fixer is at too high a temperature, gelatin will swell too much and soften unduly, which may give rise to many difficulties.

d. Presence of Hardeners

Hardener usually shortens the drying time but lengthens the clearing time. In an automatic processor, a hardener is included in the fixing solution to shorten the drying time. The physical hardness of the emulsion does not have much effect on the fixing rate. Unhardened emulsion often offers less hindrance to diffusion.

e. Type of Film Material

The factors related to the film material also affect the rate of clearing and fixing the film:

- In silver halide films, silver bromide fixes more quickly than silver iodide.
- Smaller grains dissolve in less time than larger grains.
- Thinly coated emulsion layer clears more quickly.

f. Agitation of the Film

Agitation prevents the collection of a layer of exhausted fixer near the film surface. Fresh fixer approaches the film and the clearing time is decreased. Agitation in the early stage is important. If the film is agitated in the first few seconds of its arrival in the fixer-bath, any developer carried with it is neutralized.

g. Exhaustion of Fixing Bath

With the continuous use of fixer, the following changes occur in the composition of the fixing solution.

i. There is reduction in the concentration of hypo. This decreased concentration mainly affects the clearing rate.

ii. There is steady accumulation of soluble silver complex—the argento thiosulphate. The presence of this complex retards the chemical action.

iii. There occurs a steady accumulation of soluble halides—Bromides and iodides. Both these slow down the fixing action.

REPLACEMENT OF FIXING SOLUTION

The fixing bath becomes progressively weaker in its action as it works. Therefore, something is needed to maintain the efficiency of the fixing bath. The effects of the exhausted or nearly exhausted fixer are as follows:

• Long clearing time and inadequate fixing.
• The film may be inadequately hardened.
• Radiographs may be marked with deposits.

The duration of useful life of fixing bath depends upon the following factors:

• The number of films passing through the solution.
• Silver-halide content of the emulsion, which is processed.
• Amount of silver-halide, which is left on each radiograph to be removed in the fixing bath.
• The operator's skill.

Fixer is replenished by adding fresh fixer from time to time. In routine, the used solution continues to accumulate soluble silver complexes and soluble halides which result from the chemical reaction. It is suggested that the fixer should be discarded when it takes twice as long to clear the film as it did when fresh. Two fixer tanks can be used for better results. When the first tank is exhausted, the second is kept in the place of first. Fresh fixer is always kept in second position.

WASTE MANAGEMENT

The importance of recycling is well established in the 21st century. It applies to dental radiology also. From the waste in dental radiology operatory, lead foil and silver can be recovered from the film packets and the fixer respectively.

SILVER RECOVERY FROM FIXER

Silver can be recovered from the used fixer and the unused X-ray films. There are several methods of recovering silver from the fixer solution which are described here in brief.

a. **Electrolytic method:** By passing current, silver will be attracted to the cathode.

b. **Metallic replacement:** Metals such as copper, iron and zinc, when put into the solution replace silver.

c. **Chemical method:** Certain chemicals are added to precipitate silver in finely divided state.

d. **Galvanic method:** Dissimilar metals, in contact with each other, are immersed in the fixer. Silver is plated out on the immersed metal sheet.

WASHING OF X-RAY FILMS

The washing stage follows fixing. The films are thoroughly washed in running water or series of water chambers. If the films are not properly washed after fixing, it may result in:

i. Yellow brown stains because the argento-thiosulphate decomposes to form silver sulphide.

ii. The residual fixing agent decomposes to form silver sulphide and it may attack the image itself.

iii. All the residual salts crystallize on the film surface and make it difficult to view the radiograph.

Since all these substances are water soluble, they can be removed by water.

When the film comes out of fixing bath, it carries:

- Argento-thiosulphate that was formed as a result of the action of fixer
- Residual sodium thiosulphate
- Remaining salts which are the other constituents of the bath

All these can be removed by simply washing in water.

As soon as the film is put in water, the thiosulphate concentration is maximum in the emulsion, and zero in water, therefore diffusion starts. After sometime, water also contains thiosulphate, so the diffusion is retarded. To compensate for this, water is changed or continuous sprays are given. The frequency of changing water is more important than the volume of water in one wash. On an average film, negatives give up one half of their hypo in two minutes, i.e. the other half of hypo will be remaining; after 4 minutes one quarter, after 6 minutes one-eighth of the hypo remains and so on.

The rate at which thiosulphate is removed from the films in water bath is known as *washing-rate*. The washing rate depends upon following factors:

a. **Flow of water:** Change of water or rapid flow of water effectively removes the thiosulphate from the film emulsion. In automatic processor water is agitated continuously.

b. **Temperature of the water bath:** Washing rate increases if the temperature of water bath is raised, however, if the temperature is raised to more than 50°C, gelatin may be removed from the film base.

c. **Nature of fixing bath:** The hardening agent used in the fixer definitely affect the rate at which thiosulphate is removed. It has been seen that when potassium alum is used as hardening agent, the washing rate is slow. Chrome alum hardener has no effect on the subsequent washing. A slightly alkaline fixer promotes rapid washing.

d. **Agitation:** If water is continuously agitated, fresh water is brought against the films. In automatic processors water is agitated continuously. In manual processing, agitation is provided by a flow of water in the tank in which washing takes place.

In **automatic processors**, the temperature of the water bath is kept at 25–30°C whereas in manual processor cold tap water is used. Another difference is that in automatic processors, water is continuously changed and only 1–2 films are washed at a time, whereas in manual processors, many films are simultaneously washed in one tank. Therefore, washing may be carried out for lesser time, say 18–20 seconds in the automatic processor and approximately 10 minutes in the manual processor. Squeezing action of the automatic processor reduces the time of water bath (Fig. 7.2).

DRYING

It is essential to dry the films before they can be used conveniently. The purpose of drying is to remove water from the gelatin. Overdrying of the films should be avoided. The film must contain water to an extent not less than 10–15% of its weight; otherwise a fully dehydrated film will crack because of the brittle nature of the emulsion.

Factors Affecting Drying

The most usual method of drying photographic film is by air. Two important factors which affect drying are:

- Temperature of the air
- Flow of air passing along the emulsion

Raising the temperature of air increases the rate at which moisture evaporates from the gelatin, thereby shortening the drying time. In air automatic system, the period of drying is very short, and also, relatively little drying is needed because of the squeezing action of the rollers.

The humidity of air is also significant. The lower the humidity of air, the more rapid is the loss of moisture from the emulsion. The flow of air past the emulsion is important. Adequate flow of air, even cool, can dry the films quickly than static hot air. Continuous flow of air accelerates the drying process.

DARK ROOM AND ITS ACCESSORIES

The size of the dark room can vary depending upon the quantity and quality of the work which is to be carried out daily. The dental dark rooms can be of smaller size, since the developer and fixer tanks usually used is of small sizes. The average size requirement is 6 ft. × 8 ft. The ceiling should not be less than 2.7 metres high.

The floor should be made in such a way that it is non-slippery and resistant to staining. The ceiling and the walls should be well painted.

For protection from the ionizing radiations, the walls should have 2.0 mm equivalency of lead. 25 mm thick barium plaster can also be used. The area where films are stored should be covered well.

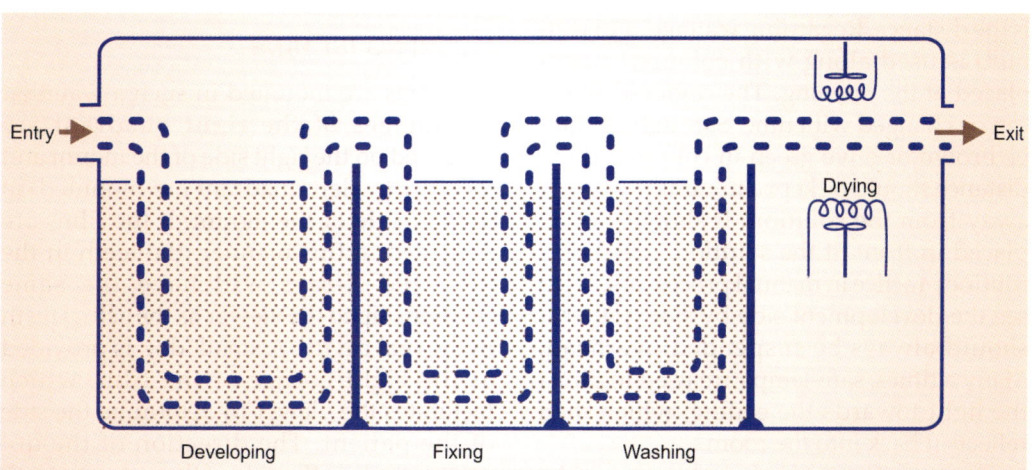

Fig. 7.2: Automatic processor

The main requirement of the dark room is that it should be light proof. The door should be light tight and with a proper lock to avoid accidental opening.

The room should be provided with comfortable ventilation to supply fresh air for the operator. The room is maintained at comfortable temperature. It becomes easy to maintain optimum temperature of the fixer and developer in such rooms.

The permissible temperature is 65–68°F and humidity 40–60%. Higher temperature or humidity may spoil the film.

SAFE LIGHTS

No emulsion is completely insensitive to light. The sensitivity of the emulsion depends upon:

- Colour
- Distance
- Intensity of light
- The duration of exposure

The dark room light provides a certain degree of safety, though not absolute.

Two factors are important as regard safety of light. One is the colour and second is the distance. Regarding wattage, a 15 watt bulb is used along with coloured filters placed at the opening. The coloured filters can be changed with time. Safe light should be brown or olive green in colour and the distance should be kept a minimum of 4 feet away from the solution. It should not be placed in front of the solution, which is a routine practice in manual processors, i.e. to see the development side by side; rather it should always be suspended overhead. Many a times, safe-lamps are used to direct the light towards the ceiling, which then reflects it back into the room.

The usefulness of safe lights should be tested from time to time. To determine safe distances, an X-ray film with two or three equidistant markings is taken. Keeping one portion naked and the other covered with lead sheet, it is opened at various distances, starting at one foot. Then the second portion of the film is opened at a distance of 1.5 feet and so on. Ultimately the film is developed to see which distance is absolutely safe.

One switch is usually employed to put off all the lights at once, except the safety light so as to prevent accidental exposure.

PROCESSING TANKS

In dental radiography development is usually undertaken in small tanks. The size of the tanks should be 8 × 10 inches. The smaller tanks usually contain one gallon of the developer and fixer and are placed in the master tank. The tanks should be of steel, so that the developer and fixer should not affect them and they should preferably be covered to avoid oxidation of the developer. This also minimizes the evaporation of the developer. Running water facility should be available near the tanks.

MOUNTING THE FILMS

The films are mounted in such a way that the images of the right quadrant are mounted on the right side of the mount and those of the left quadrant are mounted on the left side of the mount. If the films are arranged in this manner, the teeth in the mounted X-rays will have the same relationship to the viewer as the actual teeth in the oral cavity. A small 'dot' is provided at the right corner of the film, which facilitates the viewer to determine the side of the patient. The direction of the dot corresponds to the side of the patient's teeth in oral cavity (right or left).

FAULTS IN THE RADIOGRAPHS

Poor image in an X-ray film results in loss of diagnostic information and repetition of the entire procedure leads to loss of patient's time and energy. Many defects are commonly encountered in manual processing though automatic processing also produces certain faults.

Following is the list of faults mainly encountered with manual processing alongwith the possible causes thereof:

a. Light Radiographs

The radiographs appear light because of:
- Under exposure, which may be due to insufficient mA, kVp or time (Fig. 7.3A).
- Excessive film-source distance.
- Underdevelopment, which may be due to insufficient time, depleted developer, or excessive fixation (Fig. 7.3B).
- A complete white film is produced because of placing reverse side of the film during exposure or the X-radiations fail to fall, may be due to defect in the machine.

b. Dark Radiographs

Dark radiographs are produced because of the following reasons:
- Over exposure, which may be due to excessive mA, excessive kVp and/or excessive time (Fig. 7.4).
- Insufficient film source distance.
- Overdevelopment, which may be due to high temperature, and concentration of developing solution or inadequate fixation.
- Accidental exposure to light will also blacken the film.

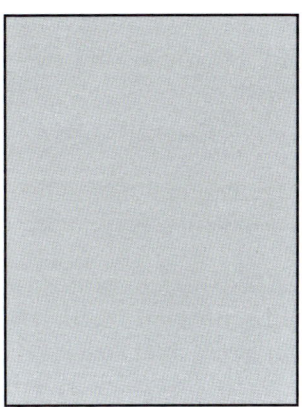

Fig. 7.3A: Under exposed film

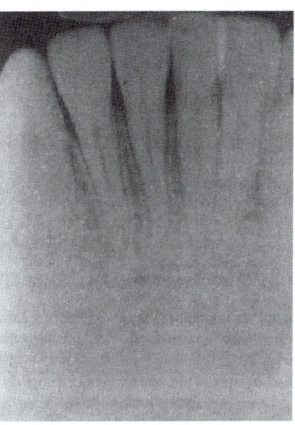

Fig. 7.3B: Under developed radiograph

c. Film Fog

Fog on the film is seen because of:
- Leaking light in darkrooms.
- Improper safelights and/or excessive wattage.
- Contaminated solutions.
- Deteriorated films or films stored at high temperature, light sensitivity of the films and even outdated films.
- Overdevelopment may also result in fog.

7

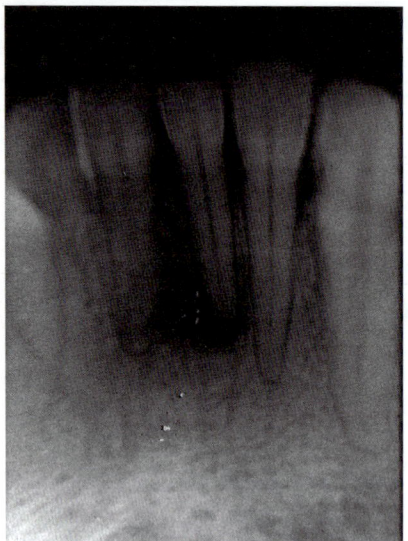

Fig. 7.4: Dark radiograph

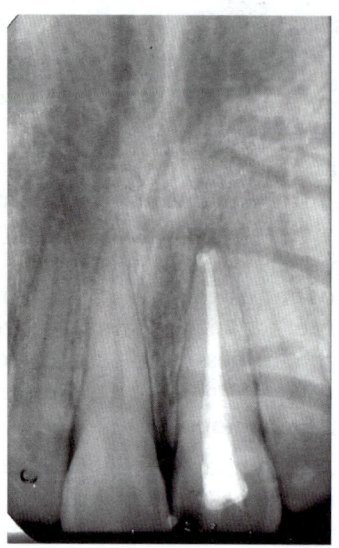

Fig. 7.5: Dark lines on the X-ray film

d. Dark Spots

The film shows dark spots because of various reasons such as:

- Fingerprints on the film where it is touched before development (Figs 7.6A, B).
- Black wrapper may stick to the film (Fig. 7.5).
- Excessive bending before development (Fig. 7.7).
- The film contacting with other films during fixation (Fig. 7.8A).
- Forceps touching the film during development (Figs 7.9A and B).

e. Light Spots/Water Spots

The reasons leading to light spots or water spots on the film are:

- Film contamination with fixer before processing (Fig. 7.8B).
- Film coming in contact with other films during development.
- Scratches over the film (Fig. 7.11).

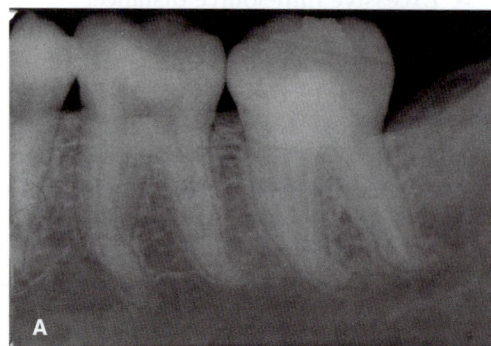

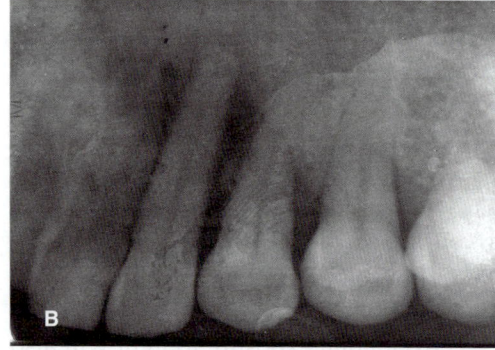

Figs 7.6A and B: Area of thumb impression

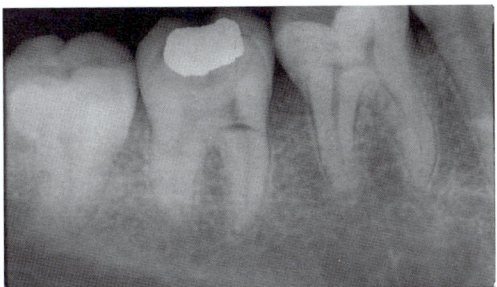

Fig. 7.7: Bending of film

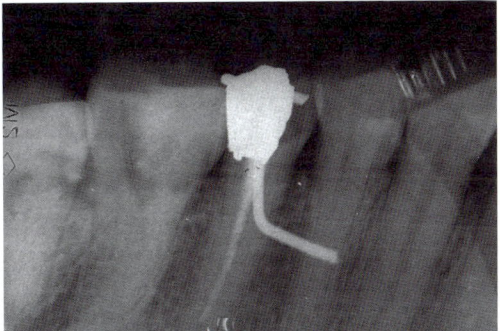

Fig. 7.9A: Mark of artery forceps

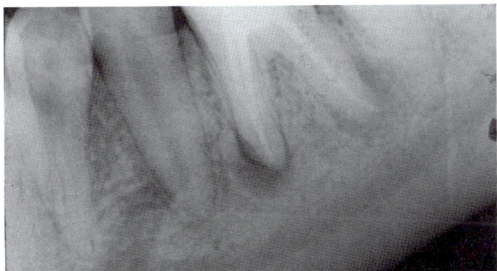

Fig. 7.8A: Two films join during processing

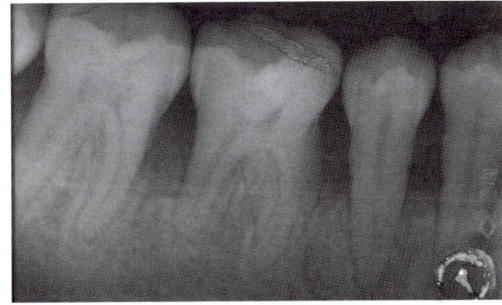

Fig. 7.9B: Forcep touching during exposure

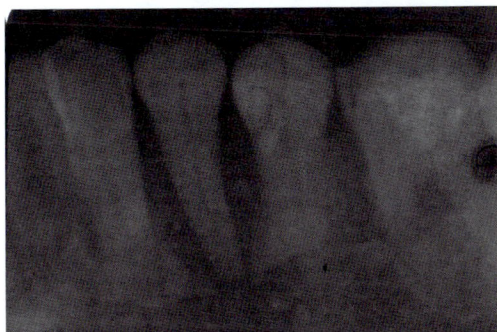

Fig. 7.8B: Fixer on film

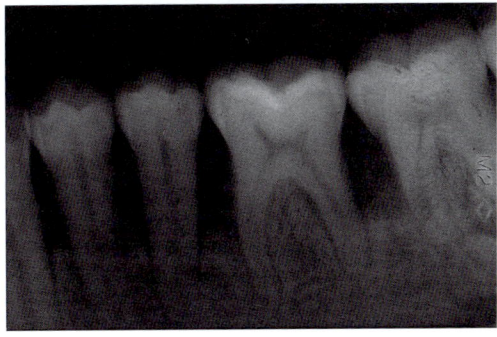

Fig. 7.10: Water spots over the film

f. Yellow/Brown Stains

The film shows yellow/brown stains due to:
- Contaminated solutions.
- Depleted developer or fixer.
- Inadequate rinsing after fixing.

g. Blurred Radiographs

The radiographs are blurred due to:

- Movement of the patient during exposure (Fig. 7.12A).
- Movement of the X-ray tube during exposure (Fig. 7.12B).
- Instability of the film during exposure.

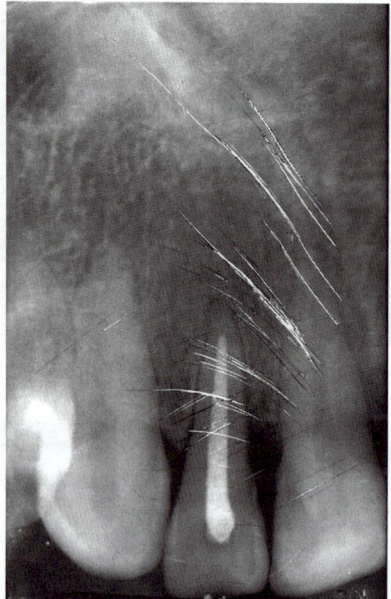

Fig. 7.11: Scratches on the film

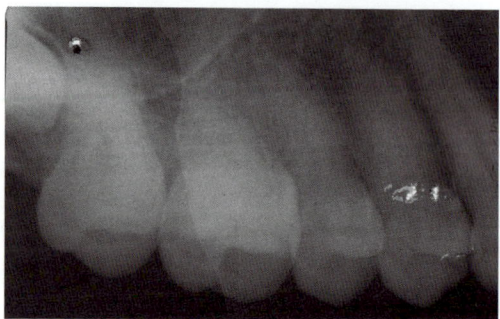

Fig. 7.12B: Distortion

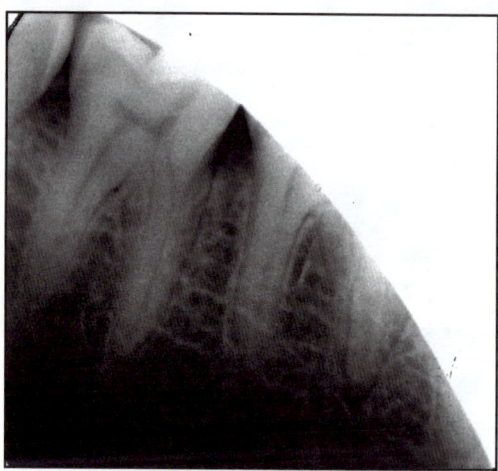

Fig. 7.13: Partial image

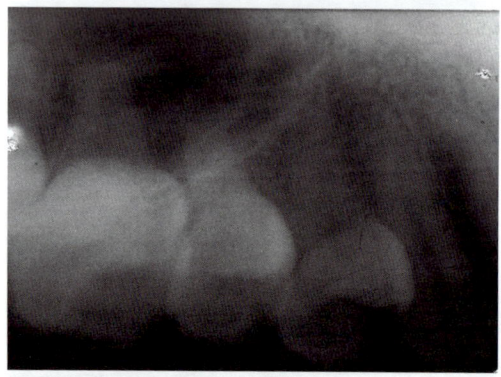

Fig. 7.12A: Blurred radiograph

h. Partial Images

The film exhibits partial images because of:
- Improper alignment of the X-ray tube or improper placement of the films (Fig. 7.13).

- A portion of film remaining outside the developing solution.

i. Double Image

Double image on the film is produced by:
- Exposure of the film twice (Figs 7.14A and B).

j. White Lines

The film exhibits white lines due to:
- Manufacturing defects in the film (Fig. 7.15).

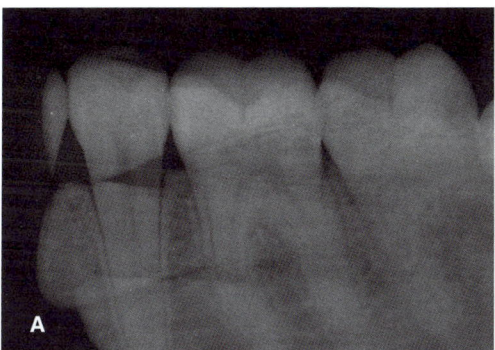

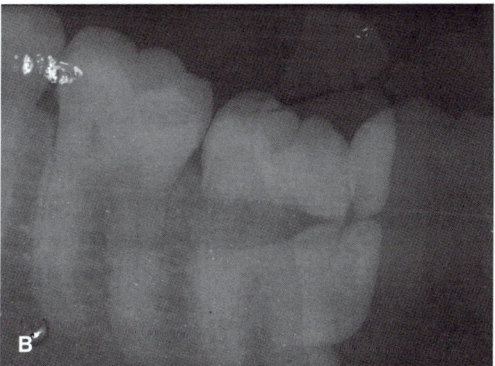

Figs 7.14A and B: Double images

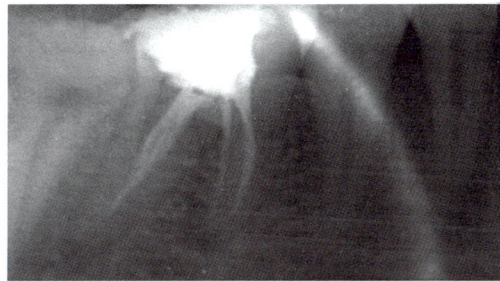

Fig. 7.15: Manufacturing defect in film (white lines)

In case of **automatic processors**, the various faults can be:

i. Pressure marks, because the roller springs may be too tight.

ii. Stripping of the emulsion, which may be because of defective rollers or defective chemical nature of the film.

iii. Streaks and mottles occur over the film because of faulty position of air driers, incorrectly positioned squeezers and even because of too high a temperature of the drier.

iv. Lengthwise scratches on the film because of too heavy finger pressure is put during opening the film in the processor. Any roller kept stationary for long can also lead to scratches over the film.

Bibliography

1. Anil AK, Jain K and Chen H: Matching of dental X-ray images for human identification. *Pattern Recognition* 2004;37:1519.
2. Chadwick BL and Dummer PH: Factors affecting the diagnostic quality of bitewing radiograph: A review. *BDJ*: 1998:80:184.
3. Farman AG: Fundamentals of Image acquisition and processing in the digital era. *Orthod Craniofacial Ras* 2003;6(Suppl. 1):17.
4. Grondel HG, Hollender L and Osvald O: Quality and quantity of dental X-ray examinations. *Dentomaxillofac Radiol* 1980;70:9.
5. Katsumata A, Hirukawa A, Fujishita M, Noujein M, Okumura S and Naitoh M: Image aretefacts in dental cone beam CT. *O Surg, O Med, O Path* 2006;101:652.
6. Katsmata A, Hirukawa A, Okumura S, Naitoh M, Fujishita M, Ariji E and Langlan R: Effect of image artefacts on grey nature dentistry in limited volume cone beam computerized tomography. *O Surg, O Med, O Path* 2007; 104: 829.
7. Mol A: Image processing tools for dental applications. *Dent Cl North Am.* 2000;44:299.
8. Watts DC and Mc Cabe JF: Aluminium radiopacity standards for dentistry: An international survey. *J Dent* 1999:27:73.
9. Watts DC, McCabe JF: Aluminium radiopacity standards for dentistry: An international survey. *J Dent* 1999;27:73.

7

Projection Geometry of Radiograph

One of the main objectives of radiography is to have an image as dimensionally accurate as the object be. The other features required are the visibility and readability of the various structures in one image. Projection geometry basically is the scientific mathematical method to achieve a perfect image. The area between the object and the film, the film and the X-ray source, effect of X-radiations and their quality and also the timings, etc. affect the quality of radiographic image. Projection geometry is the study of all these factors.

In dental radiology, the objective is to cast shadow of dental structures in such a way that the shadow of the object meet the requirement of being:

- Sharp
- Of the same size
- Of the same shape

In projection geometry, the sharpness of a shadow is determined by three factors. These factors deal with umbra (total shadow) and penumbra (partial shadow) of the object. Sharpness does vary with grain size of the film, use of screens and movement of the patient. Factors pertaining to umbra and penumbra are discussed here.

The *penumbra* is that part of shadow of any object that is larger than a point and yet represents a single point on the object. This is the amount of unsharpness of the image. The part of the object or shadow where all the light is absorbed is called *umbra*. The umbra is thus, the area of total shadow and the penumbra is the area of partial shadow.

First, the size of penumbra depends upon the tube-object distance (Fig. 8.1). As the distance is decreased, the penumbra is increased. The sources of radiation are always more than a point radiation, therefore, as large as the source of radiation as great as the penumbra.

Second, the film-object distance also affects the formation of penumbra. The effect of film-object distance is opposite to the effect of tube-object distance. Here, when the object is brought closer to the film the size of penumbra is reduced (Fig. 8.2).

The size of effective focal spot also affects the formation of penumbra. The angle of focal spot at which the target is placed with

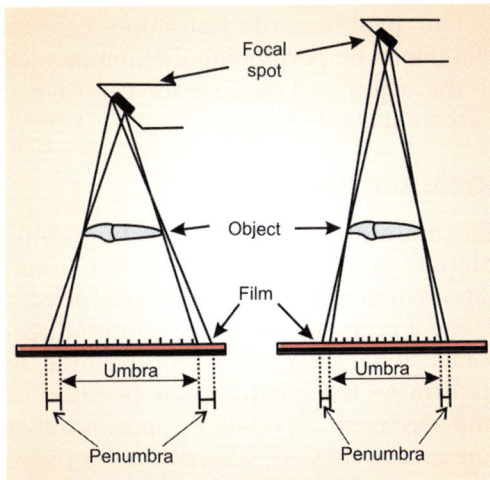

Fig. 8.1: Increase in source object distance

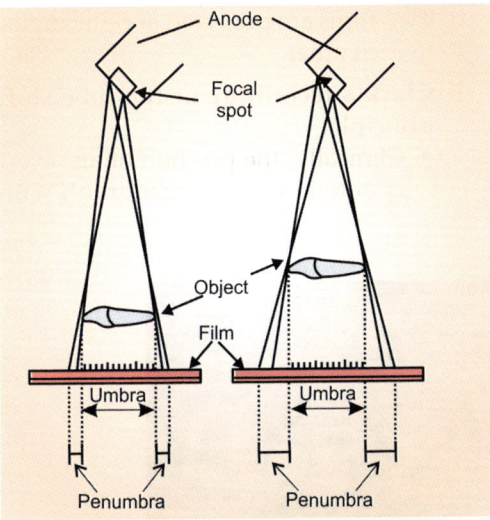

Fig. 8.2: Increase in object film distance

the long axis of the electron beam (angle is measured perpendicular to the long axis of the electron beam) is selected compromising between image quality and tube life. Decreasing the angle of target perpendicular to the long axis of electron beam decreases actual focal spot size and decreases heat

dissipation and thereby, tube life. This also decreases effective focal spot size and thus increases sharpness of image. A large angle will distribute the electron beam over a larger surface and decreases the heat generated per unit of target area, resulting in a larger effective focal spot and a larger edge gradient and loss of image clarity.

DISTORTION OF IMAGE

The X-ray image seems distorted in two ways:

a. Distortion of The Size

Distortion of the size implies increase or decrease in the size of the image on the film compared with the actual size of the object (Fig. 8.3). Distortion is dependent on relative focal spot to film distance and on object to film distance. Magnification of the object is minimized by increasing the focal spot to film distance and decreasing the object to film distance. These two methods of

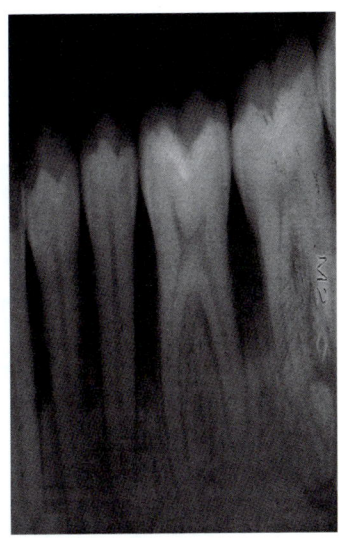

Fig. 8.3: Distortion of size

reducing magnification also increase image clarity; both sharpness and resolution. *Sharpness* is a measure of how well a boundary between two areas of contrasting radiodensities is delineated. *Image resolution* is a measure of visualization of relatively small objects that are close together.

b. Distortion of Shape

Distortion of shape is the result of unequal magnification of different parts of the same object (Fig. 8.4). Such a situation usually arises where the two parts of an object are at different distance from the focal spot. Shape distortion can be minimized by making an effort to carefully align tube, object and the film.

   i. The film should preferably be positioned parallel to the object.
  ii. The central ray should be perpendicular to the object and the film.

(Refer to bisecting and paralleling technique for further study).

The problem of distortion can be eliminated by positioning the film parallel to the object and passing the central ray perpendicular to both.

LOCALIZATION OF OBJECT

The main disadvantage of radiographic picture is its being two dimensional representation of three dimensional objects. Many a times, clinically we require three-dimensional information, for example, to determine the location and position of impacted teeth, especially canines and other foreign objects. Generally, two methods are employed to localize any object on the radiograph.

  a. Two films are projected at right angles to each other.

  b. **Clark's technique** or the tube shift principle.
     • Clinically, the position of an object is noted on each radiograph with

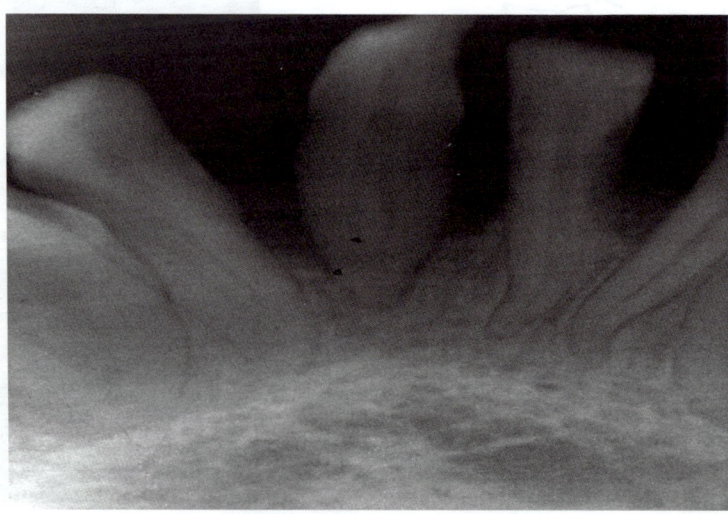

Fig. 8.4: Distortion of shape

8

reference to anatomic landmark. For example, if a pathology is suspected around the roots of mandibular molars, another occlusal X-ray will reveal the exact position of that pathology. This technique is better suited for mandibular teeth because in maxillary occlusal view, the superimposition of anterior part of the skull may obscure the area of interest.

- Second technique, which is more frequently used is the **Clark's technique** or the tube shift technique. The rationale for this procedure is demonstrated by the manner in which the relative position of radiographic image of two separate objects changes when the angle of projection is changed. Layman's explanation for this rule is that while travelling in a train, the trees or plants near to us move in opposite direction while the trees or plants far away from us move along the direction of the train.

What is important in this technique is the position of the object in question as compared with any reference point.

If the tube is shifted mesially (X-ray is taken from mesial angulation) and the object also moves mesially with respect to the reference point, then it is said that the object lie lingual to the reference object. Alternatively, if the object moves distally on moving the tube mesially then the object lies on the buccal side. In simple terms SLOB can be remembered; same lingual, opposite buccal. If the object in question does not move, it lies at the same plane.

This procedure assists in determining the position of impacted canines or other foreign bodies in the jaws.

Bibliography

1. Samfors KA, Welander U: Angle distortion in narrow beam rotation radiography. *Acta Radiol (Diagn.)* 1974;15:570.

8

Extraoral Radiography

Extraoral radiography, as the name suggests, includes all the views of orofacial region keeping the film outside the oral cavity. In many conditions, need of extraoral radiography arises, especially to visualize the structures not seen in intraoral radiography.

The other conditions where extraoral radiography is employed are:

- Patients unable to open the mouth
- Lesions of the temporomandibular joint
- Pathologies of sinuses
- Where gagging reflex is high
- Very young patients
- Where skull as a whole is to be radiographed

The radiographic techniques in extraoral radiography should be performed by the appropriate use of intensifying screens and the high-speed films. Sizes of the film vary from 5" × 7" to 10" × 12" depending upon the area to be included in the radiograph. It is wise to demarcate *R* and *L* on one corner of the cassette to indicate right and left of the patient's resultant radiograph. Conven-tional X-ray machines used for intraoral radiography can be used for extraoral techniques also. However, in few cases, cephalostat is used to position the patient's head accurately.

Various types of extraoral radiographic techniques are:

1. **Lateral oblique projections**
   a. Lateral body
   b. Lateral ramus
   c. Condyles

2. **Skull projections**
   a. Lateral skull projection
   b. Posteroanterior projection
   c. Projection for maxillary sinuses
   d. Reverse Towne's projection
   e. Submentovertex projection
   f. Tangential zygomatic arch

3. **Radiography of the temporomandibular joint**
   a. Transpharyngeal lateral temporomandibular
   b. Transcranial temporomandibular
   c. Transorbital anteroposterior temporomandibular

1. LATERAL OBLIQUE PROJECTIONS

Applied anatomy of the mandible as seen from the left side and the medial surface is depicted in Figs 9.1A and B.

In the lateral oblique view, different projections can be obtained by slightly varying the position of the patient to view either the body of the mandible alone or the body along with the ramus and condyles (Figs 9.2A and B, 9.3A and B).

a. For *lateral body*, the radiograph will show the body of the mandible from canine to the angle of jaw and also a part of the molar area. 5" × 7" films are usually used.

Position of the Patient

Teeth are kept in occlusion and the occlusal plane parallel to the floor. Head is tilted on one side. Cassette is placed on the side of the patient (Figs 9.3A and B).

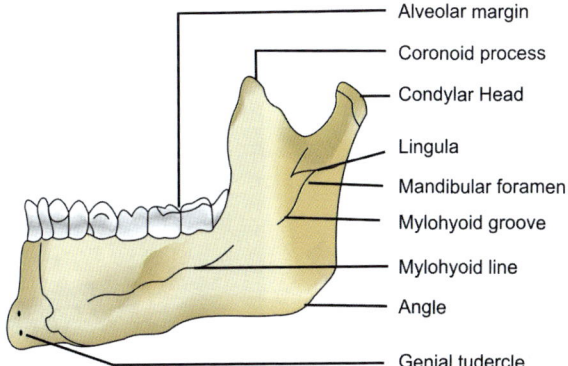

Fig. 9.1A: Medial surface of the mandible

Alveolar margin
Coronoid process
Condylar Head
Lingula
Mandibular foramen
Mylohyoid groove
Mylohyoid line
Angle
Genial tudercle

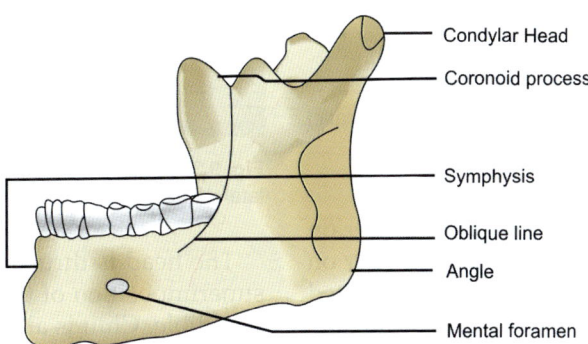

Fig. 9.1B: Mandible as seen from the left side

Condylar Head
Coronoid process
Symphysis
Oblique line
Angle
Mental foramen

9

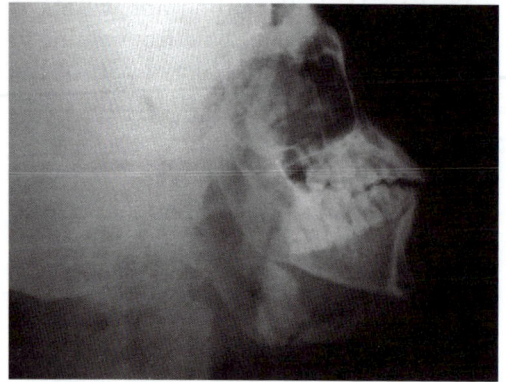

Fig. 9.2A: Lateral oblique view (mandible)

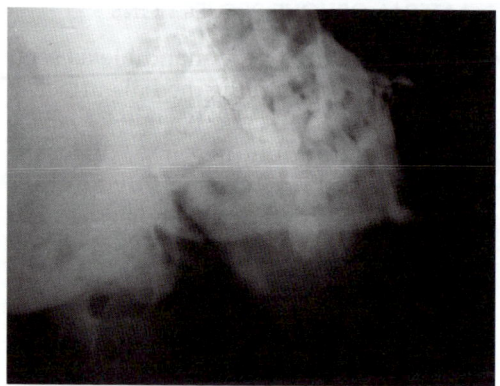

Fig. 9.2B: Lateral oblique view (mandible)

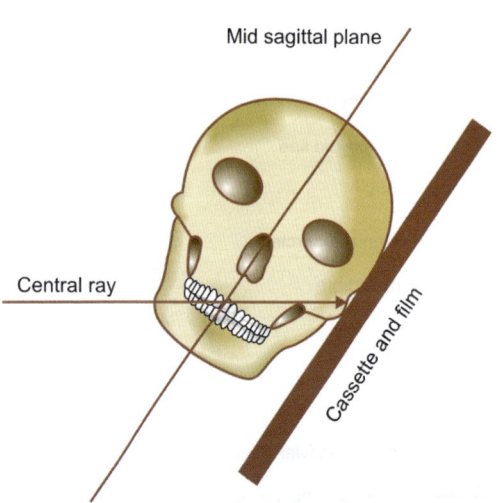

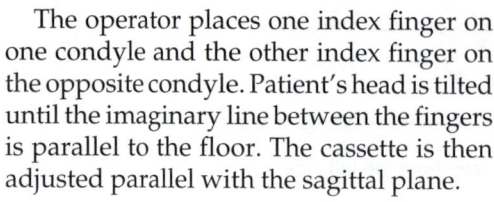

Fig. 9.3A: Lateral oblique projection (Diagrammatic)

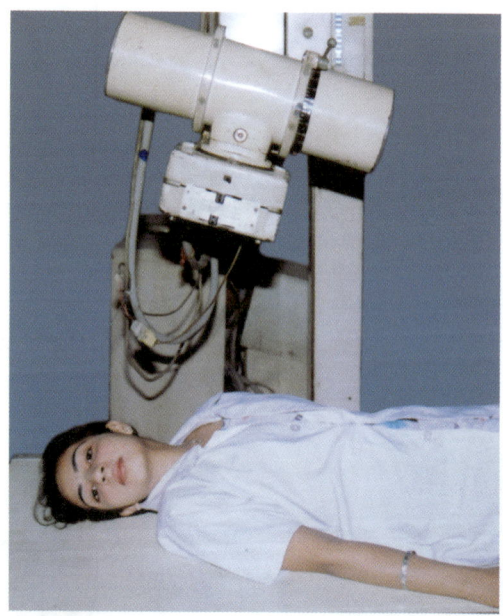

Fig. 9.3B: Position of patient and direction of tube for lateral oblique jaw projection

The operator places one index finger on one condyle and the other index finger on the opposite condyle. Patient's head is tilted until the imaginary line between the fingers is parallel to the floor. The cassette is then adjusted parallel with the sagittal plane.

The head is thrust forward to avoid superimposition of the vertebrae over the mandible. Chin is also projected forward. Head is rotated towards the film until the nose touches the plate. Head can be immobilized with the cassette with 2" gauge bandage.

The radiographs of posteroanterior view mandible are shown in Figs 9.4A, B.

Angulation and Projection of X-rays

The vertical angle of the tube is kept at 0° while the horizontal angle at 90°. The point of entry of the central ray is the angle of the jaw. The source to film distance usually taken is 24". Exposure parameters may vary but in routine 65 KV and 1/4 second exposure is given.

b. For *lateral ramus*, the technique is the same as for lateral body of the mandible, the only difference is that the patient's head is not tilted towards the film and the nose does not touch the film.

c. For *condyles*, mouth is kept open and the X-rays are passed through the sigmoid notch.

The anatomy of the maxilla and the lateral oblique view is depicted in Figs 9.5A, B.

2. SKULL PROJECTIONS

For skull radiography, proper position of the patient's head is very important.

Cephalostat is usually used to fix the patient's head at required level. Prior to patient's placement, two imaginary lines must be made clear.

- **Frankfurt line:** A line connecting the superior border of the external auditory meatus with the infraorbital rim.

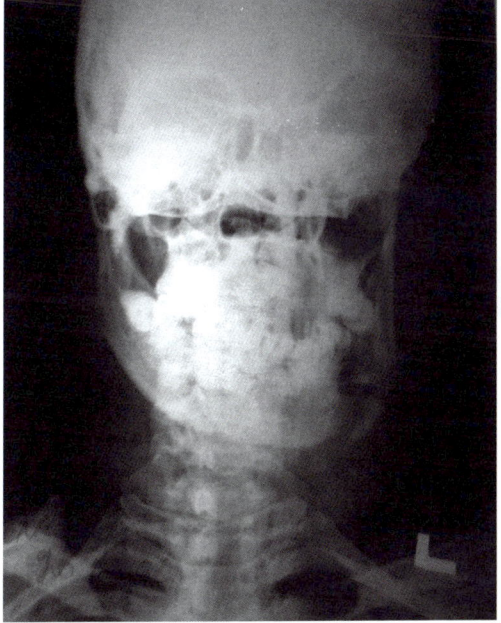

Fig. 9.4A: Posteroanterior view (mandible) showing fracture of left angle of mandible

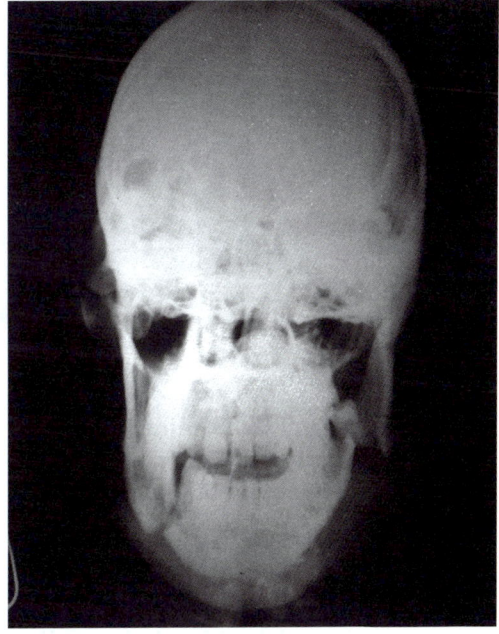

Fig. 9.4B: Posteroanterior view (mandible) showing fracture of body and condyle

9

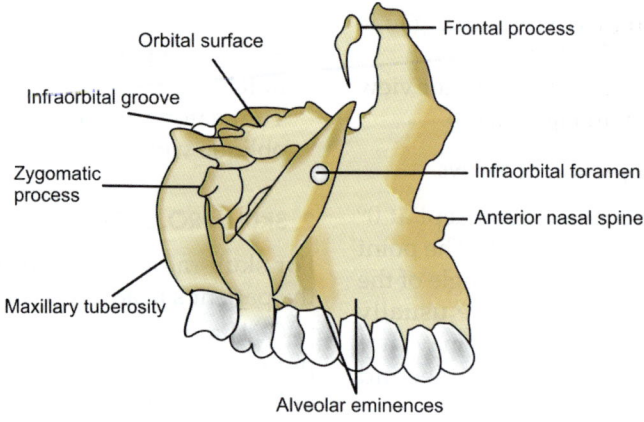

Orbital surface
Frontal process
Infraorbital groove
Zygomatic process
Infraorbital foramen
Anterior nasal spine
Maxillary tuberosity
Alveolar eminences

Fig. 9.5A: Right maxilla (diagrammatic)

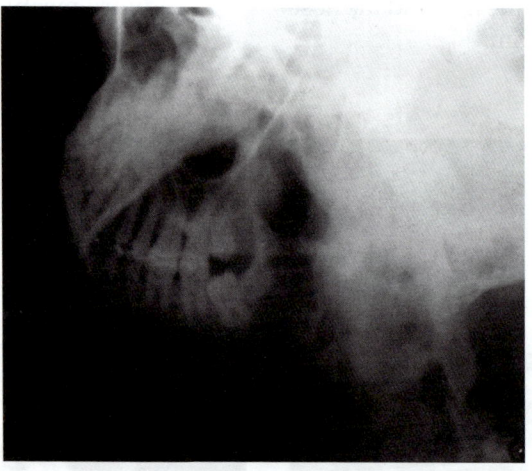

Fig. 9.5B: Lateral oblique view (maxilla)

- **Canthomeatal line:** A line joining the central point of the external auditory meatus to the outer canthus of the eye.

Skull projections can be lateral skull or posteroanterior projections. In both cases, the exposure parameters remain the same, i.e. 65–80 kVp and 10–15 mA depending upon the machine used. The source-film distance and the use of screen films are as usual. The skull anatomy is depicted in Fig. 9.6.

a. Lateral Skull Projection

These are basically used to survey the facial bones, pathologies along with sinuses. Facial growth can also be evaluated (Figs 9.7A to C).

9

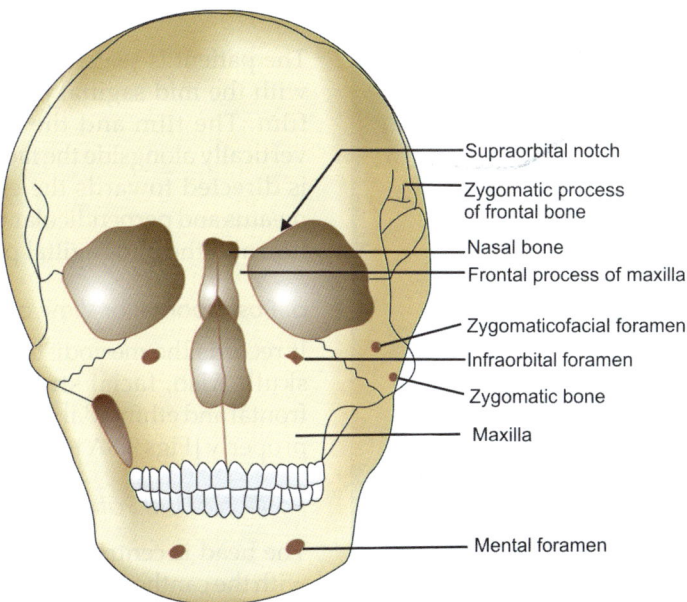

Fig. 9.6: Anterior view of skull (diagrammatic)

Supraorbital notch
Zygomatic process of frontal bone
Nasal bone
Frontal process of maxilla
Zygomaticofacial foramen
Infraorbital foramen
Zygomatic bone
Maxilla
Mental foramen

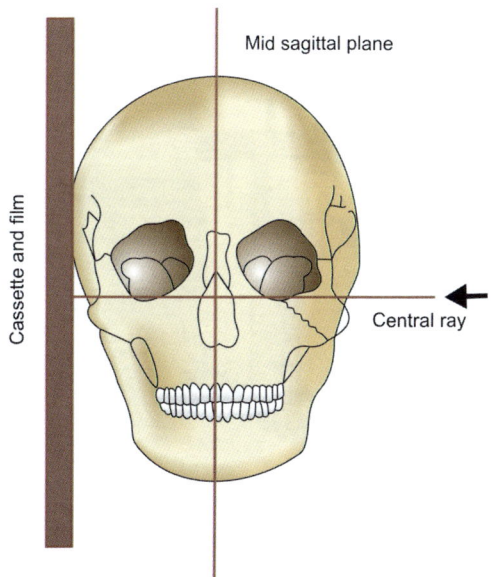

Mid sagittal plane

Cassette and film

Central ray

Fig. 9.7A: Lateral skull projection (diagrammatic)

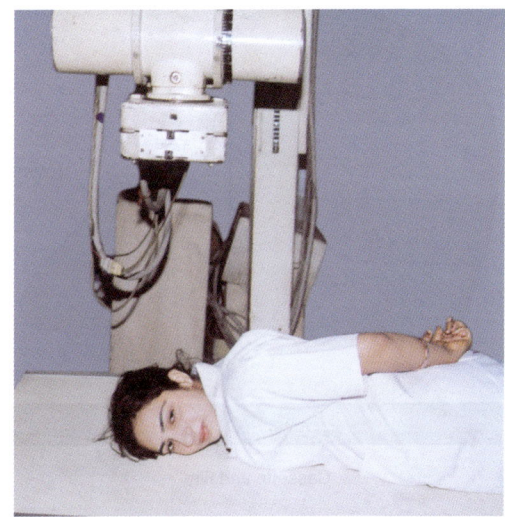

Fig. 9.7B: Position of patient and direction of tube for lateral skull projection

9

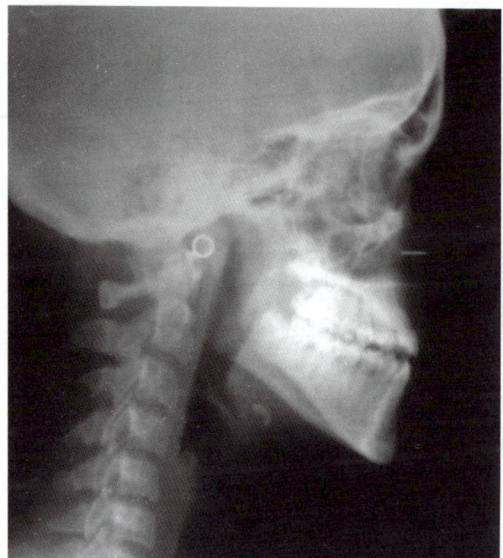

Fig. 9.7C: Lateral skull

Position of the Patient

The patient is seated upright or laid down with the mid sagittal plane parallel to the film. The film and the cassette are held vertically alongside the face. The central ray is directed towards the external auditory meatus and perpendicular to the plane of the film and the mid sagittal plane.

b. Posteroanterior View of Skull

It records the mesiodistal dimension of the skull. Also, facial structures along with frontal and ethmoidal sinuses can be viewed properly [Figs 9.8A to C and 9.9 (AP view)].

Position of the Patient

The head is centred in front of the cassette with the canthomeatal line perpendicular to the floor. The nose and the forehead should touch the film cassette. The central ray is

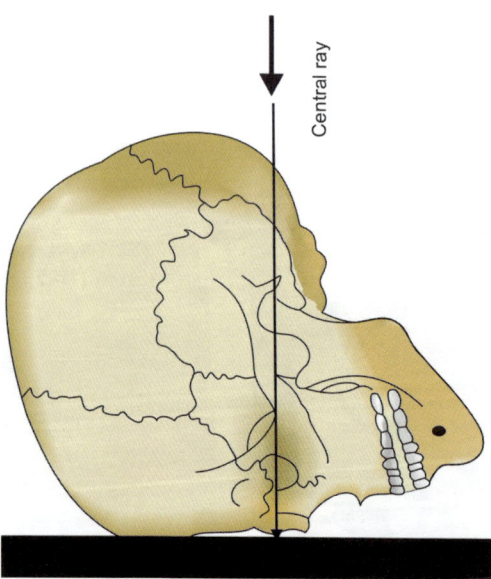

Fig. 9.8A: Posteroanterior (PA) skull projection (diagrammatic)

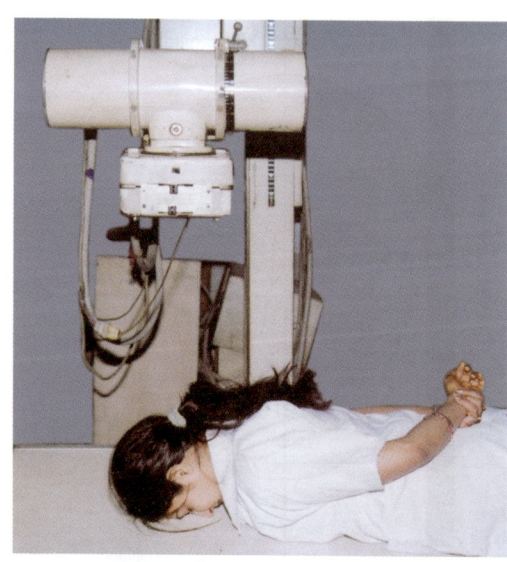

Fig. 9.8B: Position of patient and direction of tube for PA view skull

passed through the canthomeatal line perpendicular to the cassette.

60 inches source to the film distance is usually kept for cephalometric examination.

c. Projection for Maxillary Sinuses or Waters' position

It is a slight modification of the PA view skull and is also known as *occipitomental projections* (Figs 9.10A and B). Along with the maxillary sinuses, ethmoidal sinuses are visible and the zygomatic arch and the lower orbital rim can also be examined. The detail radiography of maxillary sinus is given on subsequent pages (Chapter 10).

Position of the Patient

The cassette is placed parallel to the floor and the patient's head is extended forward so that the chin touches the centre of the film. The adjustment is made so that the canthomeatal line forms an angle of 37° with the cassette.

The central ray is directed through the midsagittal plane directly over the maxillary sinuses.

Exposure parameters vary depending upon the kVp, X-ray machine used and the source to film distance. kVp used is 65–75.

d. Reverse Towne's Projection

These are used especially in cases of ramus fractures and condyle displacement. The posterolateral wall of the maxillary sinus is also visible (Figs 9.11A and B).

Position of the Patient

The film cassette is placed parallel to the floor and the patient's face and nose are made to touch the film. The central ray is then directed towards the frontal bone at an

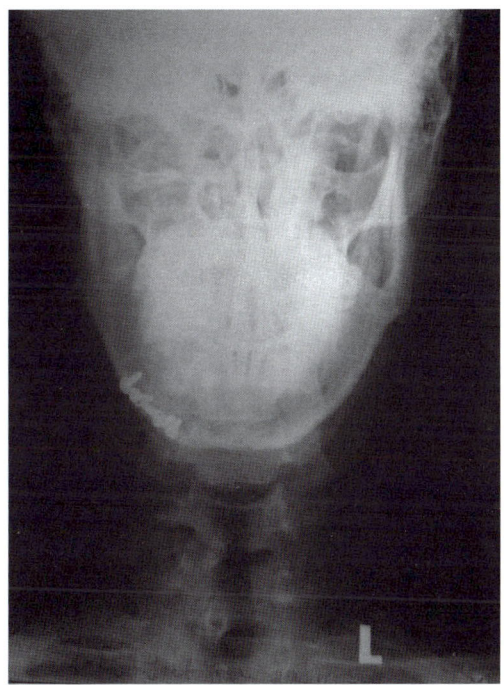

Fig. 9.8C: Posteroanterior view skull

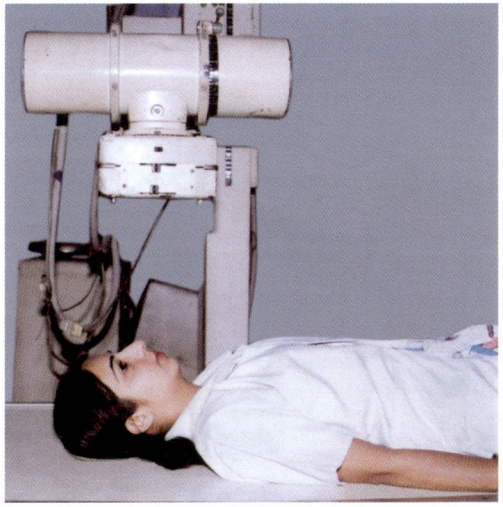

Fig. 9.9: Position of patient and direction of tube for AP view skull

9

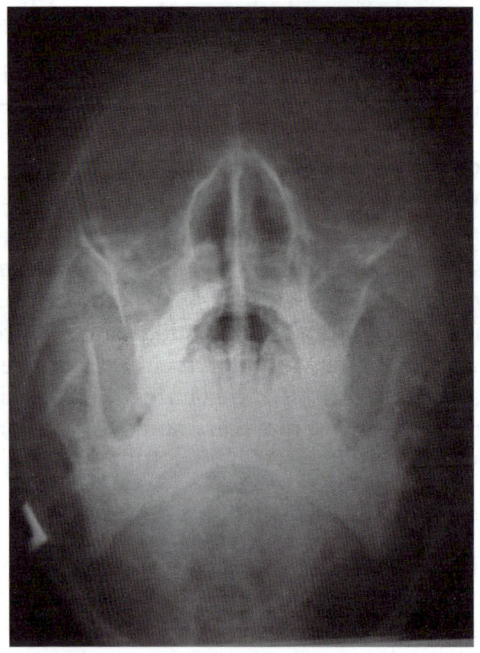

Fig. 9.10A: Occipitomental view (Waters' projection)

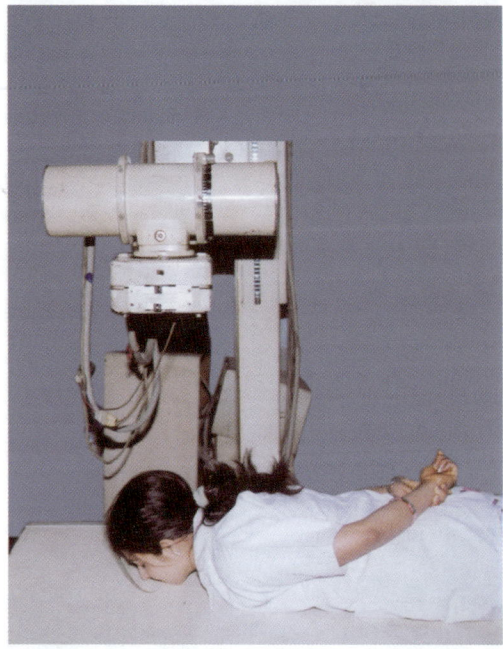

Fig. 9.10B: Position of patient and direction of tube for Waters' projection

Canthomeatal
line

Central ray

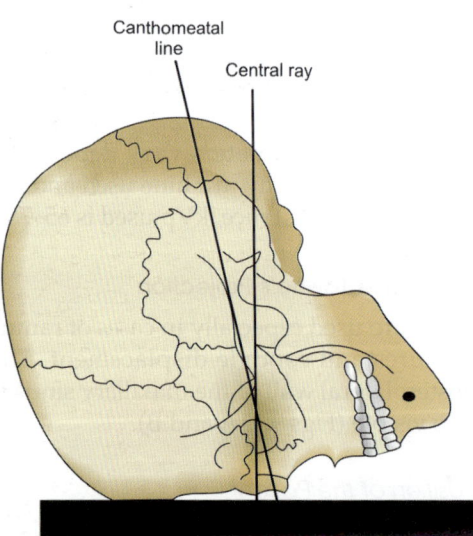

Cassette and film

Fig. 9.11A: Reverse Towne's projection (diagrammatic)

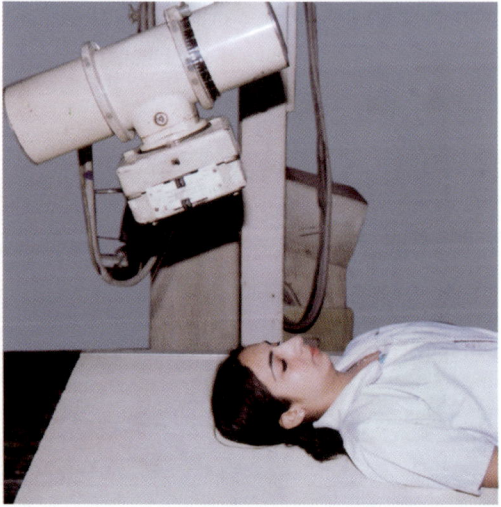

Fig. 9.11B: Position of patient and direction of tube for Reverse Towne's projection

angle of 30° to the canthomeatal line through the mid-sagittal plane. Exposure parameters vary and kVp used is 65–75.

e. Submentovertex Projection

This technique is employed to visualize the lateral movements of the condyles and the lateral displacement of the condyloid or coronoid processes, the sphenoidal sinuses and fractures of zygoma. The medial and lateral pterygoid plates and foramina in the base of the skull are often visible (Figs 9.12A to C).

Position of the Patient

The patient's head is extended well forward with the chin on the centre of the cassette. The midsagittal plane is kept perpendicular to the floor.

The central ray is directed from below the mandible upward towards the vertex of the

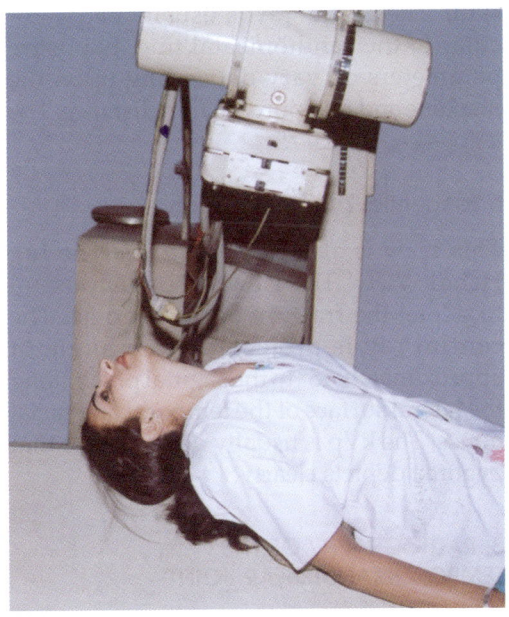

Fig. 9.12B: Position of patient and direction of tube for submentovertex projection

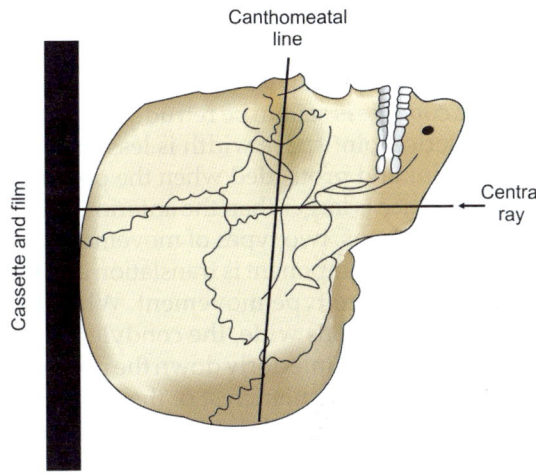

Fig. 9.12A: Submentovertex projection (diagrammatic)

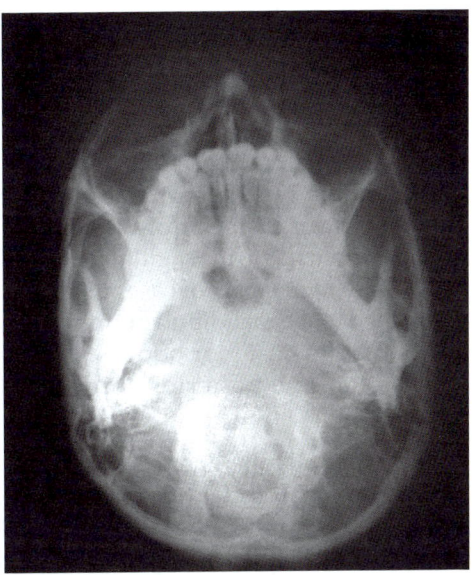

Fig. 9.12C: Submentovertex view (fracture zygoma)

9

skull. The central ray is usually perpendicular to the canthomeatal line. Exposure parameters do vary depending upon the machine and the source to film distance. The kVp is kept at 65–75.

f. Tangential Zygomatic Arch

This view is also referred to as 'The Jug Handle View'. This view is especially useful to depict the fracture of the zygoma. The central ray is projected at an angle of approximately 15° to the sagittal plane along the lateral surface of the temporal and facial bones. The kVp is usually decreased so that zygoma depicts clearly.

3. RADIOGRAPHY OF THE TEMPOROMANDIBULAR JOINT

Applied Anatomy

The temporomandibular joint is a very important joint in the body from the functional point of view. Disorders of the TM joint are also very common. Brief anatomy of the TM joint may be understood before getting radiographs from different angles.

The condyle is connected to the ramus of the mandible by a narrow isthmus. The anteroposterior diameter of the condyle is not perpendicular to the sagittal plane of the skull. In great majority of cases the condyle is attached to the mandibular ramus in such a way that its posterior border is a direct extension of the posterior border of the ramus.

The temporal component is comprised of the articular fossa and the articular eminence. The most lateral aspect of the eminence is occupied by a protuberance of

significantly increased convexity called the articular tubercle. The articular fossa is on the inferior side of the squamous part of the temporal bone that forms a small portion of the floor of middle cranial fossa.

The posterior limit of the joint is formed by the squamotympanic fissure and its medial extension, the petrotympanic fissure. Below the fissure, the tympanic portion of the temporal bone forms the major portion of the anterior wall of the external auditory canal.

The interarticular disc is a fibrous connective tissue filling most of the space between the condylar head and the articular fossa. The disc occupies anterior half of the joint space. The anterior border of the disc is attached to the superior head of the lateral pterygoid muscle. As the condyle translates forward, the disc also moves forward. As the disc moves forward tension is produced in the elastic posterior attachment. This tension is thought to be responsible for the smooth recoil of the disc posteriorly as the jaw closes.

Condylar concentricity is the term used for the condylar position around which the anterior and the posterior aspect of the radiolucent joint space are uniform in width. The condyle is said to be retruded when the posterior joint space width is less than the anterior and protruded when the posterior joint space is larger than the anterior. When the jaw opens, two types of movements are noted, one component is translation and the other is hinge type movement. When the lower jaw opens wide, the condyle moves anteriorly and inferiorly down the posterior slope of the articular crest of the eminence. On fully opening, the condyle position is usually at the height of the eminence or slightly anterior to it.

TM JOINT PROJECTIONS

a. Transpharyngeal Lateral Temporomandibular

To examine the TMJ of one side, the radiographs are taken in such a way that as the rays are passed from one side, it should not hinder different bony structures (Figs 9.13A, B and 9.14).

Position of the Patient

The patient is seated in an upright position with the midsagittal plane perpendicular to the floor. The patient is then asked to open the mouth wide. The cassette is placed along the side of head resting on the inner aspect of the patient's shoulder. The point of entry of central ray is sigmoid notch (sigmoid notch is just inferior to the zygomatic arch). From a point halfway between the external auditory meatus and the outer canthus of eye drop straight down to the ala tragus line.

The vertical angle is kept at –10°. Exposure parameters are 65–75 kVp and 20 mAs.

b. Transcranial Temporomandibular

The cassette and the film are placed perpendicular to the floor. The head is positioned in such a way that the ears, cheeks and temporal region are touching the cassette. This technique is same for both open and close mouth (Figs 9.15 and 9.16).

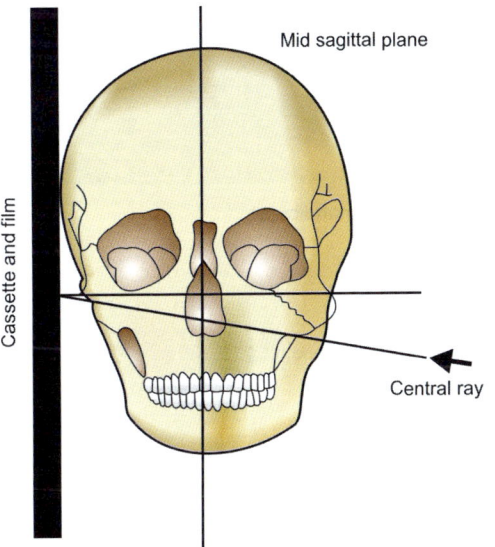

Cassette and film

Mid sagittal plane

Central ray

Fig. 9.13A: Lateral TM joint (–10° vertical angle) (diagrammatic)

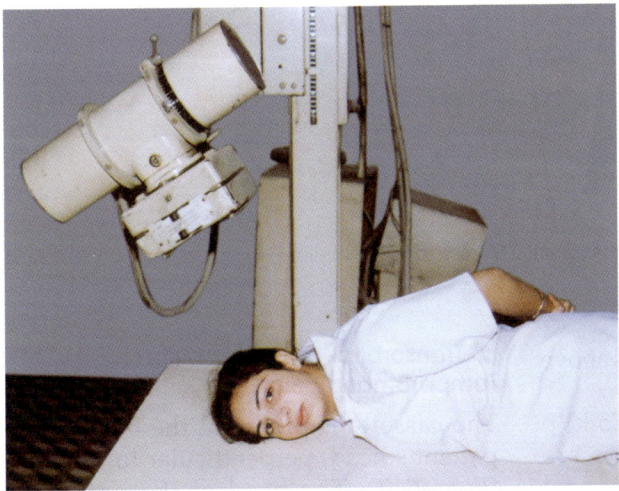

Fig. 9.13B: Position of patient and direction of tube for TM joint (closed mouth)

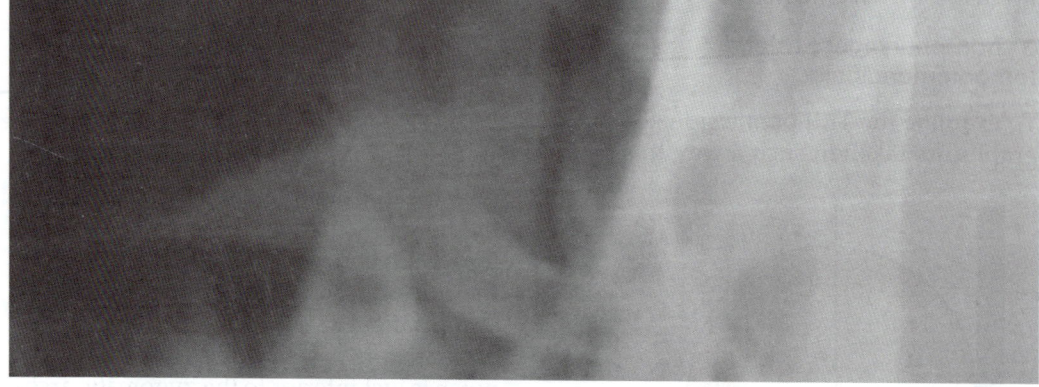

Fig. 9.14: Transpharyngeal lateral temporomandibular

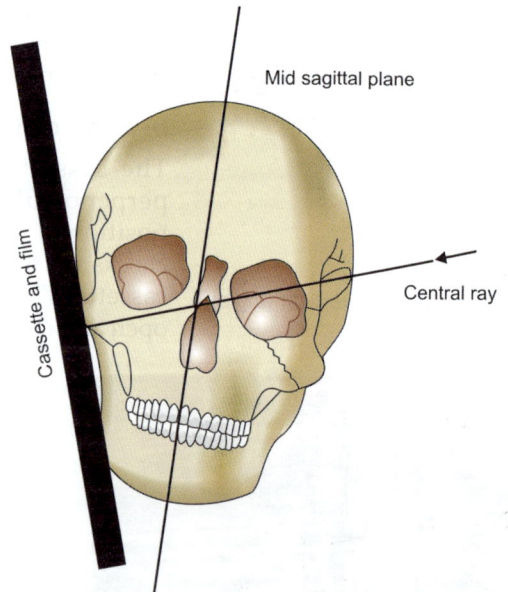

Fig. 9.15: Transcranial TM joint (diagrammatic)

The central ray is passed 2–5 inches above the external auditory meatus.

Vertical angle kept is 20–25°. 65–75 kVp and 20 mAs exposure parameters are used.

c. Transorbital Anteroposterior Temporomandibular

The cassette is placed at the back of the patient's head, perpendicular to the floor (Fig. 9.17). The head of the patient is

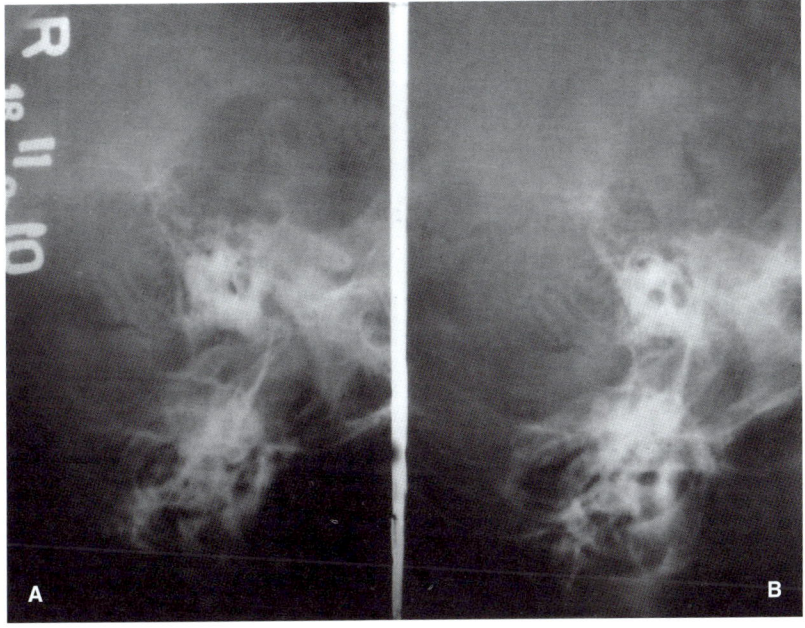

Fig. 9.16: Transcranial temporomandibular joint: (A) open mouth, (B) closed mouth

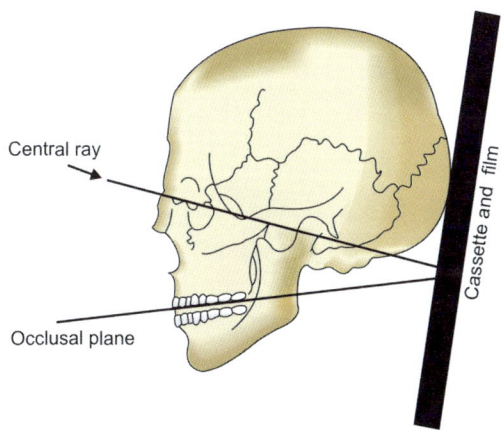

Fig. 9.17: Transorbital anteroposterior TM joint (diagrammatic)

positioned in an erect posture and, the occlusal plane is aligned parallel to the floor.

The patient is then asked to open the mouth. The central ray is passed through the orbits and a vertical angle of +30° is kept. Exposure parameters are 65–75 kVp and 20 mAs. This technique is also known as *orbitoramus technique*. The first two projections give a good image of the lateral aspect of the condyle while the transorbital projection gives a good view of the mesiolateral aspect of the condyle.

Bibliography

1. Akerman S, Jonsson K, Kopp S: Radiologic changes in temporomandibular hand and foot joints of patients with rheumatoid arthritis. *O Surg, O Med, O Path* 1991;72:245.
2. Baumrind S, Frantz RC: The reliability of head film measurements. I. Landmark Identification. *Am J Orthod* 1971;60:111.
3. Benson BW: Temporomandibular joint anthrography. *O Surg, O Med, O Path:* 1989; 67:600.

4. Benson BW, Langlain RP, Abramovitch K: Temporomandibular joint arthography: A study comparison between a fluoroscopic and non-fluoroscopic technique. *O Surg, O Med, O Path* 1989;67:600.

5. Cohen H, Ross S, Gordon R: Computerized tomography as a guide in the diagnosis of temporomandibular joint disease. *JADA:* 1985;110:57.

6. Dolowick MP, Riggs RR: Symposium on temporomandibular joint dysfunction and treatment. *Dent Clin North Am* 1983;27:561.

7. Holmund AB, Gynther G, Reinhold FP: Rheumatoid arthritis and disk derangement of the temporomandibular joint: A comparative arthoscopy study. *O Surg, O Med, O Path:* 1992; 73:273.

8. Huang CH and Hsu CY: Computer-assisted orientation of dental periapical radiographs to the occlusal plane. *O Surg, O Med, O Path* 2008;105:649.

9. Katzberg RW: TMJ Imaging. *Radiology* 1989;170:297.

10. Manson-Hing LR: Use of dental X-rays in roentgenography of the palatopharyngeal mechanism. *O Surg, O Med, O Path* 1960;13: 1085.

11. Samfors KP: Imaging of the Temporomandibular joint disorders. *Oral and Max Surg CNA:* 1989;1:13.

12. Weinberg LA, Chastain JK: New TMJ clinical data and the implications on diagnosis and treatment. *JADA:* 1990;120:305.

10

Imaging of Maxillary Sinuses

The maxilla and the maxillary antrum hold a key position in the mid-facial skeleton. Because of their anatomical location, relationship with contiguous structures and sutural contacts with other bones, they pose a great challenge to the dental surgeon in the interpretation and diagnostic evaluation of the diseases of the maxilla and the maxillary antrum.

The antrum of Highmore, an air-filled cavity lined by respiratory epithelium is occupying most of the maxilla and is like an inverted pyramid, with the superior aspect making the floor of the orbit, the medial wall coinciding with the lateral wall of the nose and the lateral wall bordering the infra-temporal surface of the maxilla. The floor of the sinus projects between the roots of the teeth (pneumatized maxilla) and the sinus itself is loculated.

The close proximity of the maxillary sinus to the teeth and maxillary alveolar bone makes it mandatory for the practitioner to recognize normal sinus anatomy on intraoral and extraoral radiography.

Besides, diseases of the sinus create symptoms that can be interpreted as of dental origin and vice versa. Hence, for an accurate diagnosis of the patient's problem, radiographic interpretation of the maxilla and the maxillary antrum is an essential requisite.

IMAGING MODALITIES

Intraoral Periapical Radiographs

These are of very limited value. Only a portion of the inferior aspect of the sinus is visible on the maxillary posterior periapical radiographs.

In these radiographs, the roots of the maxillary teeth may appear to project directly into the sinus and may produce conical elevations on the floor of the sinus, yet there is always a layer of bone and mucosa covering these roots (Figs 10.1A and B).

In a periapical radiograph one must remember that
• Most antral changes caused by pathosis are radiopaque.
• A radiopaque band of tissue following the contours of the sinus indicate generalized inflammatory reaction of the sinus mucosa leading to hyperplasia.

10

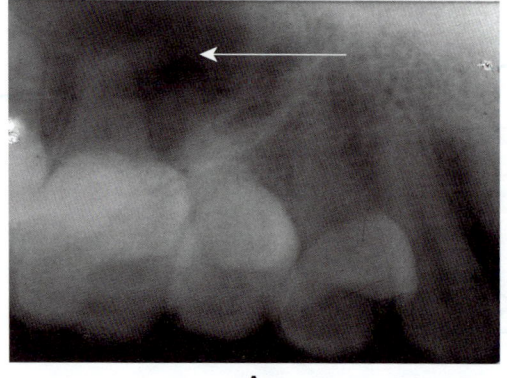
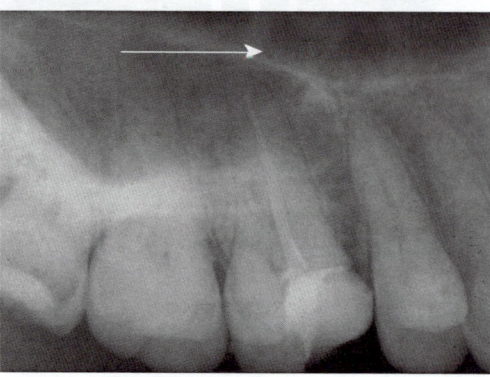

A **B**

Fig. 10.1: Shadow of maxillary sinus (radiolucent area over the roots)

- A localized opaque thickening adjacent to the source of inflammation as in severe periodontal disease indicates localized mucositis.
- A periapical radiolucency surrounded by a thin opaque line of bone indicates a periapical lesion and the radiographic appearance is called the *halo effect*.

Because of these limitations some type of extraoral projection is needed to image the maxilla and the maxillary sinus. The selected imaging technique must allow comparison of the contralateral sinus.

Occlusal Radiograph

The anterior maxillary occlusal projection, the cross-sectional maxillary anterior projection and lateral maxillary occlusal projection are excellent techniques to visualize maxilla from the palatal aspect (Fig. 10.2). By these techniques one can see the anterior maxilla and the dentition, palate, zygomatic processes of the maxilla, anterio-inferior aspect of each antrum, nasolacrimal canals, anterior floor of nasal fossa and the nasal septum.

Standard Radiograph

i. The Caldwell View (Occipitofrontal View)

This view provides the accurate view of the midline, posterior facial structures and the roof of the maxillary sinus.

Due to the superimposition of the petrous ridge, the lower half of the maxillary sinus cannot be viewed clearly.

When examining the sinuses, always remember that the sinus opacity may be unilateral. Thus, comparisons of the two sides may assist in demonstrating the abnormality.

ii. Waters' View (Occipitomental view)

This is a preferred visualization technique in which the lateral and the medial walls are optimally depicted. The roof of the sinus is seen as two parallel horizontal lines (Fig. 10.3).

Waters' projection is the most useful conventional radiographic technique to image the maxillary sinus. In this projection, the radiographic density of the normal maxillary sinus is same on both the sides and is equal to those of the orbits.

10

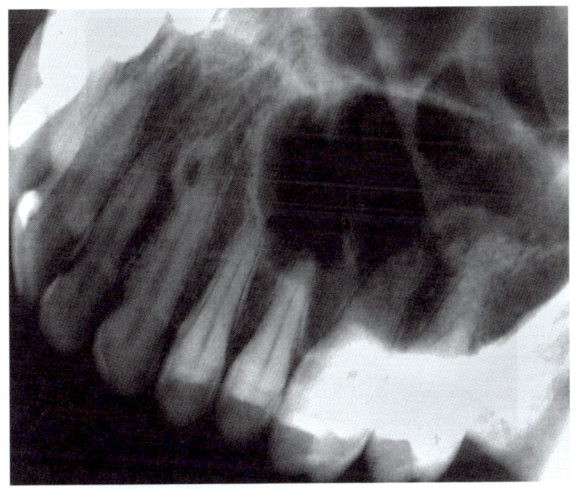

Fig. 10.2: Occlusal view of maxillary sinus

the maxilla. The floor and the alveolar recess of the maxillary sinus are seen as a curved line that dips below the straight line of the hard palate.

This is an ideal view when opaque foreign bodies are being looked for in the maxillary sinus.

iv. Submentovertex View

It is a good view to see the lateral and the medial walls of the maxillary sinus (Fig. 10.4).

Panoramic View (Orthopantomography)

An orthopantomogram gives a good view of the lower aspect of the antrum, which may be used to supplement the plain film depiction of the sinuses.

This view provides greater visualization of the sinuses than do periapical radiographs. It provides better information about the inferior, posterior, medio-superior and medio-inferior aspects of the sinus (Fig. 10.5). Regardless of the technique employed, the utility of plain radiography in the

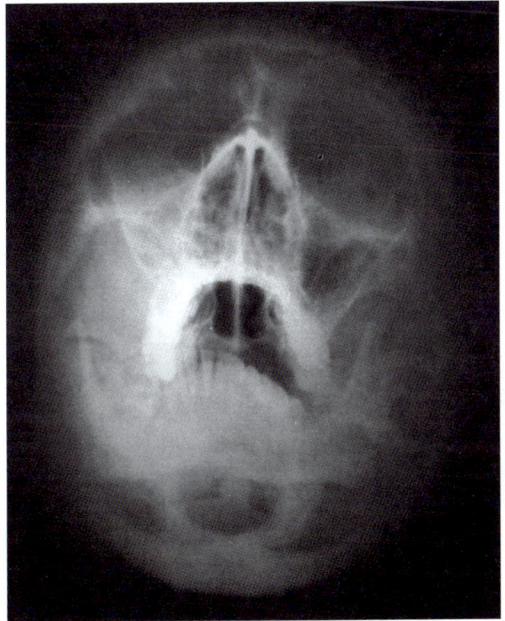

Fig. 10.3: Waters' view (maxillary sinus)

iii. Lateral View

In this view the paired sinuses are superimposed over each other along with

10

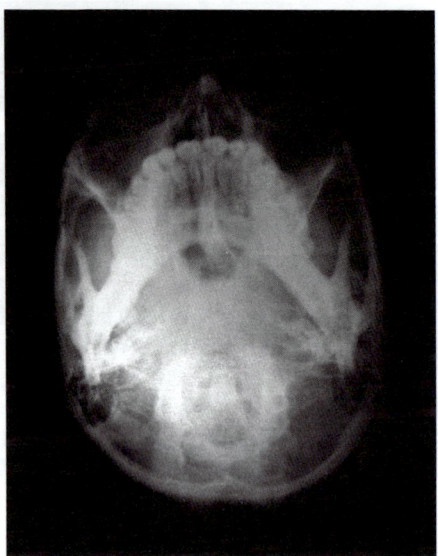

Fig. 10.4: Submentovertex view (maxillary sinus)

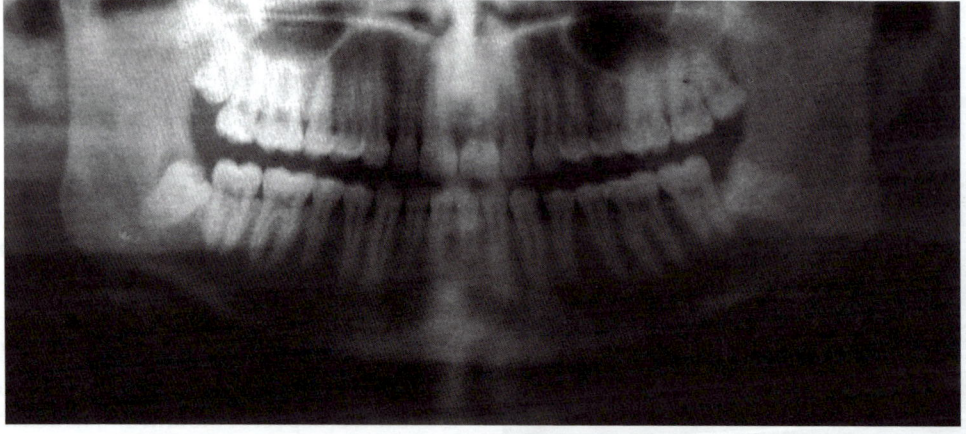

Fig. 10.5: Panoramic view (maxillary sinus)

evaluation of the maxilla and the paranasal sinuses is limited.

Computerized Tomography and Magnetic Resonance Imaging

The computed tomography and magnetic resonance imaging are regarded as a method of choice for detail imaging of the paranasal sinuses and the maxillofacial region.

In computerized tomography, the roof and the floor of the maxillary sinus are best evaluated on axial images. The lateral and the medial walls can be evaluated on both coronal and axial images (Figs 10.6A and B).

Magnetic resonance imaging (MRI) of the paranasal sinuses is a complementary imaging technique to CT. MRI can image intracranial complications of the inflammatory diseases. MRI can readily separate tissues of similar densities better than CT, which is useful to differentiate tumors from inflammatory disorders as well as haemorrhage and inflammatory secretions.

MRI is unable to image bone and air, so evaluation of bony anatomy and pathology is difficult. Hence, MRI is mainly useful to determine spread of disease, especially intracranially and intraorbitally. Distinguishing between neoplastic and inflammatory diseases is an additional advantage of MRI.

Dentascan

Dentascan is a CT dental reformatting program that allows reconstruction of the mandibular or the maxillary alveolar ridges in direct coronal and panoramic planes.

These images display the osseous anatomy of the jaw.

ANTRAL DISEASES AND THEIR RADIOGRAPHIC APPEARANCES

INFLAMMATORY DISEASES

Acute Sinusitis

Acute sinusitis can be caused by:

- Upper respiratory tract infections, e.g. common cold.
- Trauma, for example oroantral communication or a tooth fragment being pushed into the sinus.
- Periapical infection of posterior teeth. A single maxillary posterior tooth with chronic apical periodontitis may produce a localized inflammatory response. This response of the sinus mucosa to the odontogenic inflammation is known as *periapical mucositis*.

The **radiographic** picture would be:

10

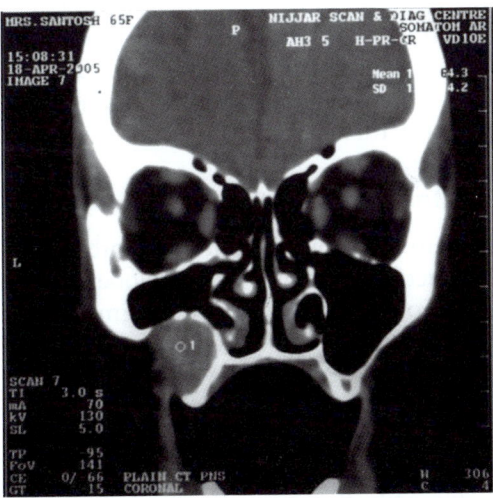

Fig. 10.6A: Coronal CT (haemorrhagic cyst left maxilla)

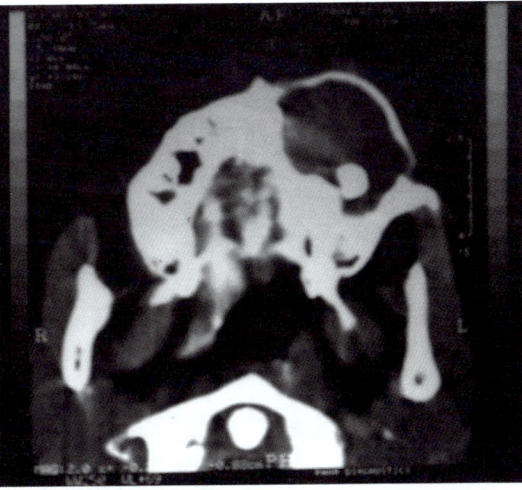

Fig. 10.6B: Axial CT (cystic expansion of buccal cortex)

10

- Periapical picture depicting antral halo because of resorption and remodelling of the antral floor. A periapical lesion that has resulted in an inward bulging of the sinus floor is characterized by a periapical radiolucency surrounded by a thin radiopaque line of bone. This radiographic appearance has been called the *halo effect* (Fig. 10.7).
- Opaque zone at the base of the sinus because of fluid collected in it.
- Total opacity of the sinus is because of mucosal hypertrophy and fluid in the sinus.
- Evidence of foreign body when applicable.

Chronic Sinusitis

Chronic sinusitis can be caused by
- Persistent infection of the sinus.
- Continued presence of a foreign body or communication.

  The **radiographic** changes would be:
- Irregular thickening of the radiopaque lining on the inner side of the sinus because of mucosal hypertrophy.

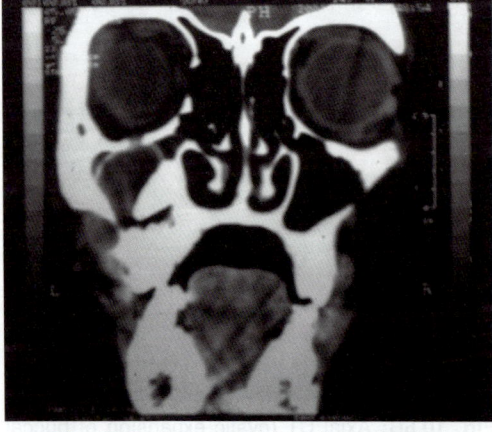

Fig. 10.7: Coronal CT (Maxillary sinusitis)

- Shrinkage of the radiolucent cavity of the sinus.
- Radiopacity at the base of the sinus cavity due to the collection of fluid (feature of liquids can be seen clearly in the radiographs).
- Round dome shaped radiopacity seen in the cavity may be because of a mucosal polyp. Appearance of multiple, smooth, rounded opacities on the sinus walls and floor is common with patients suffering from allergic sinusitis (Figs 10.8A and B).
- Increased thickness of the radiopaque lining of the sinus, i.e. thickness of the boundary walls.

TRAUMA

Fractures are commonly demonstrated by conventional radiographic techniques but CT is often necessary to show the fracture lines.

Nasal Fracture

Most injuries affect the paired nasal bones, which are best seen in the lateral skull view. An additional *soft tissue* (low kVp or filtered) lateral view may aid in depicting the nasal bone fracture (Fig. 10.9).

Orbital Blow Out Fracture

In pure 'blow out' fractures, the orbital rim is intact with no injury to the globe.

On plain films the bone fragments are displaced into the superior aspect of the maxillary sinus and/or one end of the single fragment may be in contact with the remaining walls, the so called *Trap door* appearance, which is represented by a linear radiopacity that extends into the superior aspect of the maxillary sinus. This 'trap door'

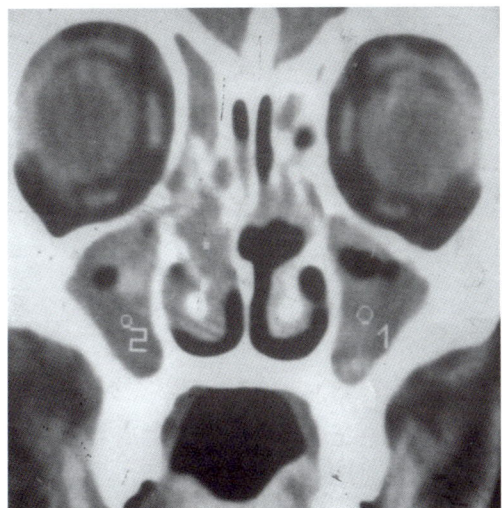

Fig. 10.8A: Coronal CT (Mucosal inflammation of maxillary sinuses. Area of calcification also visible)

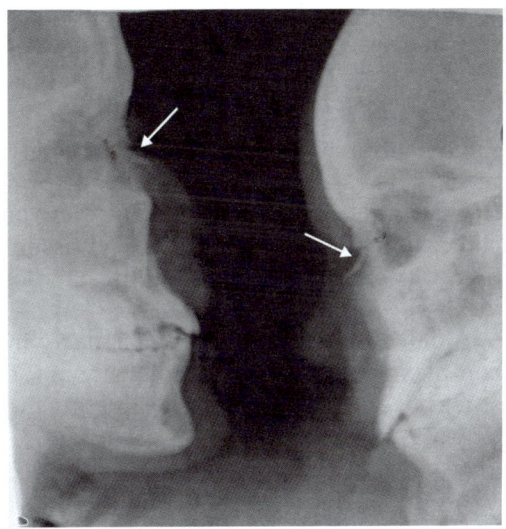

Fig. 10.9: Lateral skull views showing nasal bone fracture

10

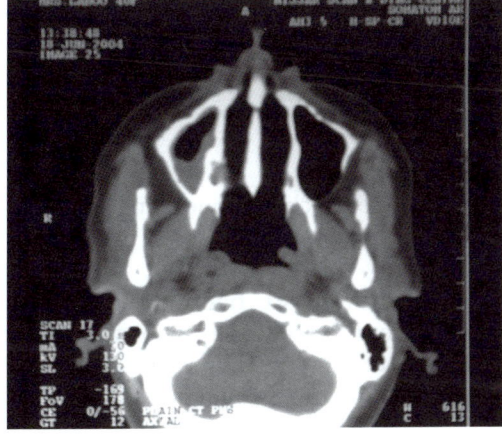

Fig. 10.8B: Axial CT showing fluid level in right maxillary sinus

is a hallmark feature of the orbital blow out fracture.

Subsequently, the soft tissue herniation, though the defect is identified as a rounded soft tissue density, the *hanging drop*, which may be confused with polyps and cysts within the tissue.

The Water's view best demonstrates the intact orbital rim together with herniation of the soft tissue contents into the maxillary sinus. Coronal CT scans are the most favoured imaging modality for identifying blow out fracture and for evaluating the involvement of adjacent tissues.

MRI has been found useful in differentiating the low signal of the muscle, fluid and blood from the high signal of herniated fat.

Orbital Rim Fractures

Isolated fractures of the orbital wall are rare. They are commonly associated with tripod fracture or Le fort II fracture. The Water's or Caldwell views are usually adequate to demonstrate the integrity of the orbital rims. Coronal CT may also be used, though the former can also be used to see the frontal sinuses. Besides, an axial CT may be used to evaluate the integrity of the anterior cranial fossa.

Zygomatic Arch Fractures

Zygomatic arch fractures may occur singly or may be associated with either tripod fracture or Le fort III fracture. The view of choice for studying them is the 'soft tissue' or low kVp submentovertex or 'Jug handle' view (Figs 10.10 and 10.11).

Axial CT may be of use particularly in complex fractures. Three-dimensional CT scans have proved helpful in evaluating the degrees of displacement.

Tripod Fractures or Zygomatic Maxillary Complex Fracture

In these fractures, the fracture segment usually moves as a unit and exhibits various degrees of displacement and rotation. It is established that the zygomatic fracture involves usually three sites viz. near

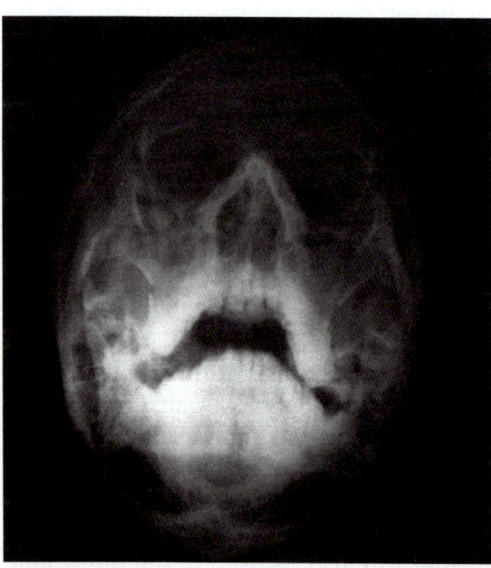

Fig. 10.10: PA view maxilla (fracture zygoma)

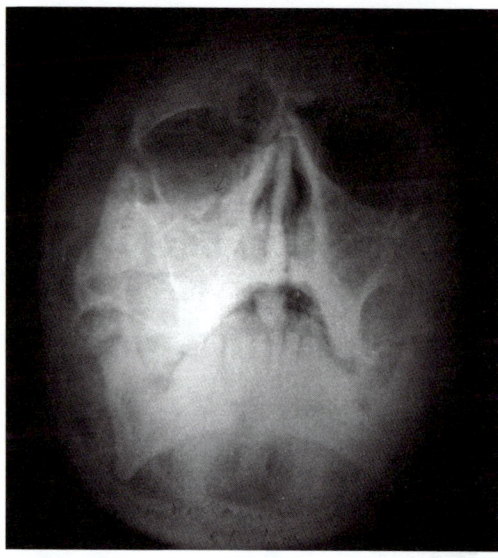

Fig. 10.11: PA view maxilla (Water's view) (fracture zygoma)

frontozygomatic suture, zygomatico maxillary suture and fracture of zygomatic arch (Fig. 10.12).

Clinically

- Depression of cheek bone along with step defect and tenderness at the site of fracture.
- Subconjunctival haemorrhage, the posterior limit of which is not seen.
- Paraesthesia in the region of area supplied by infraorbital nerve.

Radiologically

The fracture of suggestive bone usually results in radiopacity of the maxillary antrum because of the presence of blood.

Type I or non-displaced or minimally displaced fractures can be visualized in plain films or in Water's view.

Type II or segmented zygomatic arch or orbital rim fractures result in subtle rotation

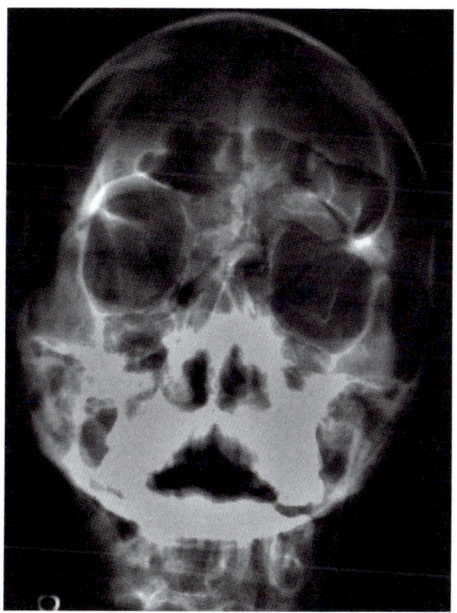

Fig. 10.12: Tripod malar fracture

10

of the fragment. The coronal CT is the radiographic technique of choice.

Type III or fractures with substantial rotation or displacement of the fracture fragment are best seen on a coronal CT scan.

Type IV or comminuted fracture with gross rotation or displacement is best seen on a coronal CT scan. Three-dimensional CT scans have proved helpful in evaluating the degrees of displacement.

Transfacial Fracture (Le Fort fracture)

Le Fort fractures are complex fractures that have in common the involvement of the pterygoid plate. Le Fort I and Le Fort II involve the maxillary sinus and Le Fort III is a craniofacial dysjunction. For such fractures, plain film radiograph is inadequate and scans are the modality of choice for evaluating all transfacial injury.

BENIGN LESIONS OF THE MAXILLARY SINUS (CYSTS AND TUMORS)

Cysts and tumors of the maxilla and the maxillary antrum are space occupying lesions which increase in size gradually to encroach on the contiguous structures such as walls of the sinus or the ostium. The signs and symptoms then follow.

Radiographic analysis provides an immense database to aid in the diagnosis of the sinus lesions. A panoramic radiograph is useful as a beginning investigation. Maxillary occlusal radiographs and periapical radiographs are also useful in addition to more sophisticated modalities such as CT and MRI.

Radiographically, it may be difficult to distinguish between an extrinsic and an intrinsic lesion. The presence of a cortical outline surrounding the sinus opacity suggests a process other than a mucous retention phenomenon.

A. CYSTS

a. Cysts of Intrinsic Origin

i. Mucous Retention Cyst or Antral Mucocele

The mucous retention cyst in the sinus is to be differentiated from mucocele. When the mucous retention phenomenon occurs in the oral cavity, it is usually referred to as mucocele. A mucocele in the sinus (antrum), however, is caused by blockage of the ostium with resulting accumulation of mucoid secretions. The antral mucocele sometimes causes destruction of the bony walls (Fig. 10.13). These cysts originate intrinsically. The radiographic features that characterize a mucous retention cyst or antral mucocele are its round to ovoid shape, its homogeneous opacity, its lack of surrounding cortical outline, and its usual

10

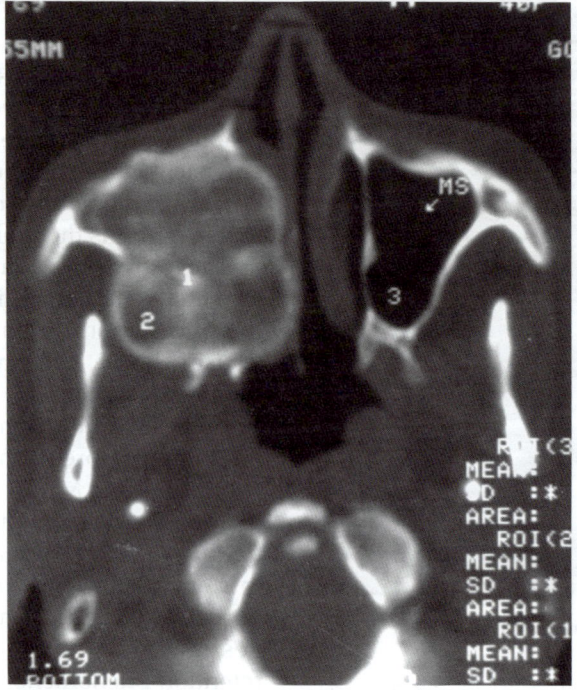

Fig. 10.13: Coronal CT (mucocele with pressure lesion)

location on the sinus floor. There appears to be a radiolucent *rim* because of air-soft tissue interface.

An antral mucocele in its early stages appears as a cloudy sinus and as the lesion grows the pressure increases and the sinus walls erode and may perforate.

b. Cysts of Extrinsic Origin

Cysts that develop outside the sinus may expand to produce a bowing inward of the sinus wall.

i. Radicular Cysts

The radicular cysts are most common of all cystic lesions and are most prevalent in the anterior maxilla and appear as a rounded or ovoid radiolucency at the root end of a tooth,

often demarcated by marginal bone sclerosis (Fig. 10.14).

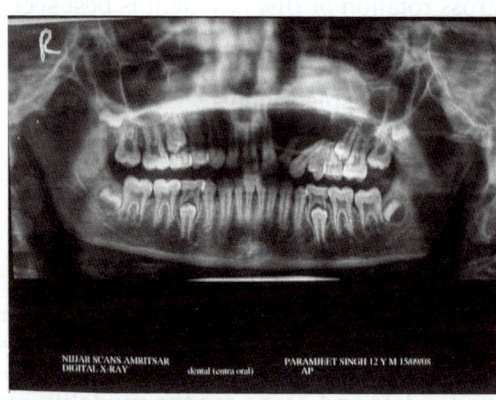

Fig. 10.14: OPG showing radicular cyst in relation to the upper left lateral incisor

ii. Odontogenic keratocyst

The odontogenic keratocyst radiographically presents as a well-circumscribed radiolucency with smooth margins and then radiopaque borders. Most of the lesions are unilocular, but larger lesions may be multilocular. They produce buccal expansion rather than palatal. Large maxillary lesions are destructive, may be expansile and usually involve the sinus (Fig. 10.15).

iii. Dentigerous Cysts

The dentigerous cyst appears as a well-corticated pericoronal radiolucency exceeding 3.0 mm. The margins are well-corticated, thin and smoothly curved. A tooth is an integral part of the dentigerous cyst (Figs 10.16 to 10.18).

iv. Calcifying Odontogenic Cyst (Gorlin cyst)

The most common radiologic appearance is a cystic radiolucency, which may be unilocular or multilocular. Expansion and perforation can be well-demarcated or irregular with characteristic calcifications. The radiopaque foci often are clustered around the occlusal or incisal surfaces of an impacted tooth.

CT and MRI complement conventional radiographs and show that calcifying odontogenic cyst originates as a unilocular lesion that may become multilocular with time, as CT and MRI display incomplete bony system.

v. Fibrous Dysplasia

It shows a typical ground-glass appearance (Figs 10.19A and B).

B. TUMORS

i. Ameloblastoma

Ninety percent of the maxillary lesions involve the premolar-molar region. On plain films and CT, the lesion appears as a multilocular (soap bubble) lytic lesion without mineralized components. Sometimes, the sinus wall may be destroyed.

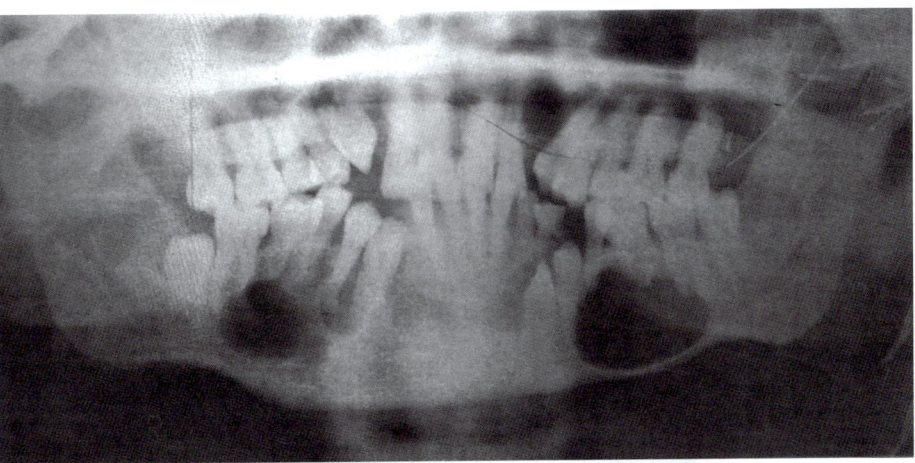

Fig. 10.15: Panoramic view. Multiple odontogenic keratocyst (mandible). Bilateral radiolucencies in body of mandible

10

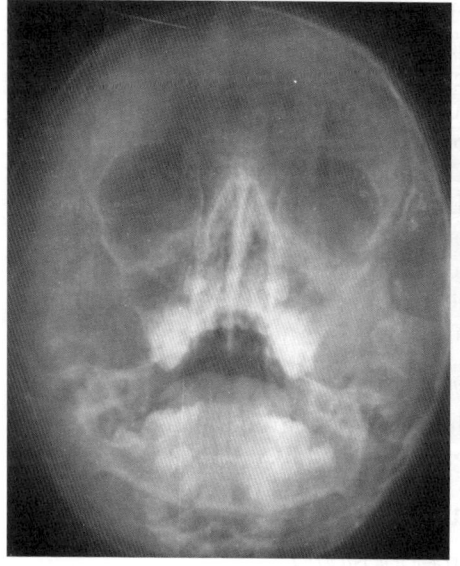

Fig. 10.16: Waters' view (bilateral dentigerous cyst)

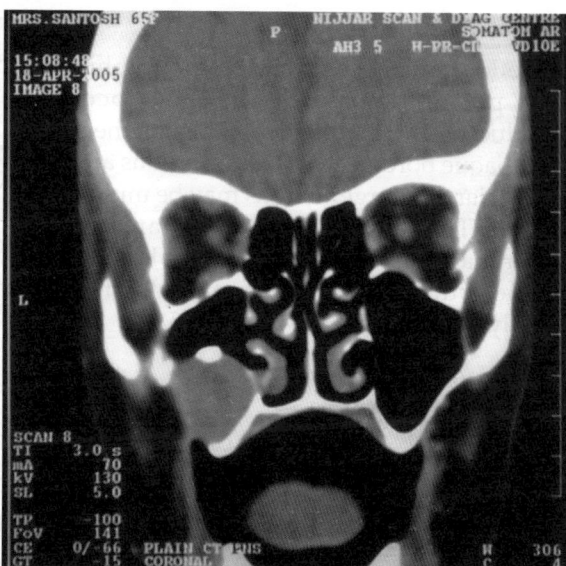

Fig. 10.17: Coronal CT (haemorrhagic cyst left maxilla)

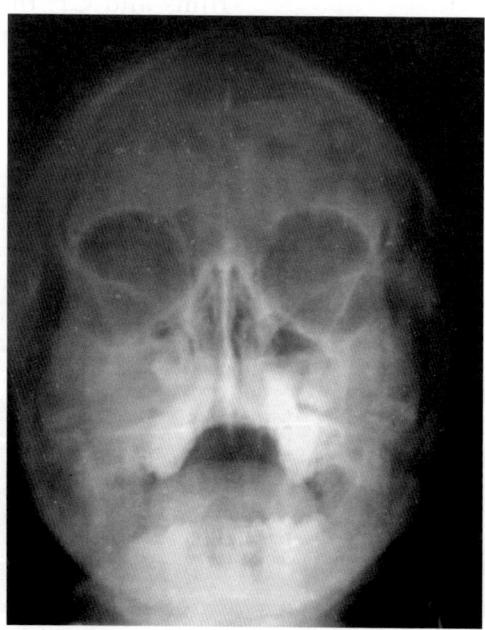

Fig. 10.18: PA view maxilla (bilateral dentigerous cyst with impacted teeth in both the sinuses)

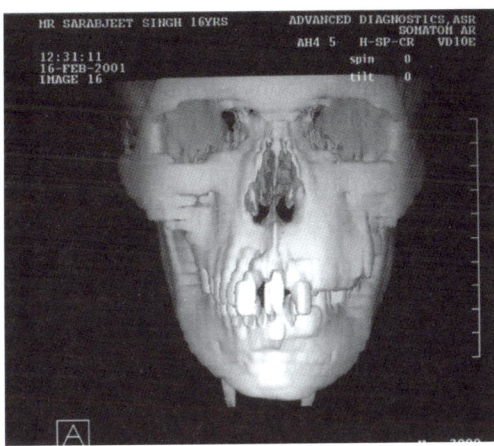

Fig. 10.19A: 3D CT showing fibrous dysplasia left maxilla and anterior mandible

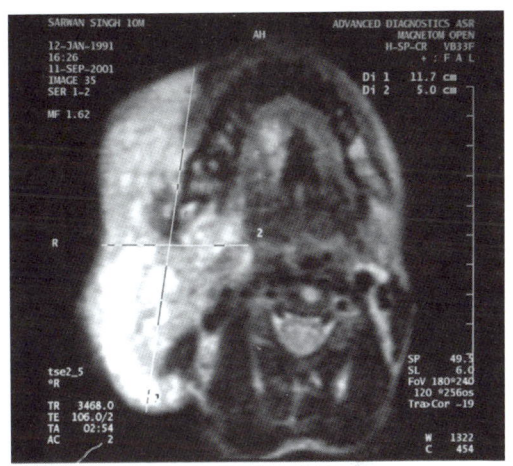

Fig. 10.20: MRI showing neurofibroma (right side maxilla)

10

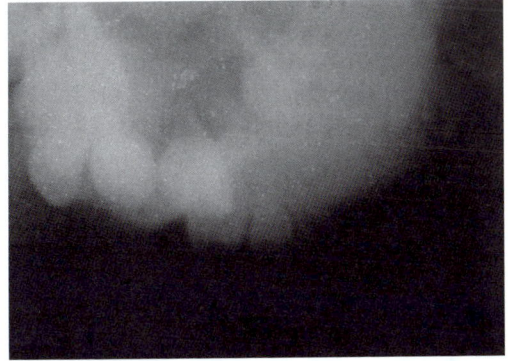

Fig. 10.19B: Occlusal view maxilla showing fibrous dysplasia (typical ground-glass appearance)

Figure 10.20 depicts neurofibroma of the right side of the maxilla.

ii. Odontoma

Two third of odontomas are found in the anterior and posterior aspects of the maxilla. Radiographically, the compound composite odontome resembles an accumulation of small, fully formed teeth where as the complex composite odontome appears as an amorphous radiopacity.

iii. Squamous Odontogenic Tumor (Benign Epithelial Odontogenic Tumor)

This rare, benign odontogenic tumor occurs more often in the maxillary lateral canine region, presenting as a triangular or semi-circular radiolucency within the alveolar bone between the roots of several teeth. Additionally, there is displacement of one or both the adjacent roots, destruction of crestal bone and a sclerotic rim at the margin of the lesion.

Squamous odontogenic tumor perforates through the cortices and extends to involve the palate, maxillary sinus, nasal floor and the nasal spine.

iv. Cementoma or Periapical Cemental Dysplasia

These are benign lesions that arise from the cementum that surrounds the tooth root.

Periapical cemental dysplasia begins as a radiolucent lesion but gradually calcifies to appear as a radiopaque mass separated from the tooth root by a radiolucent zone. The

10

gigantiform cementoma appears as a nodular, irregular shaped radiopacities in multiple locations.

v. Benign Cementoblastoma or True Cementoma

Radiographically, benign cementoblastoma appears as a well defined radiopacity attached to the tooth root with loss of outline of the affected root.

vi. Odontogenic Myxoma

The radiographic appearance of myxoma is variable. The lesion may have a *mottled* or a *honey comb* appearance, or it may present as an expanding radiolucency with an occasional multilocular pattern (Figs 10.21A and B).

Frequently, myxomas appear as multilocular with well developed locules, composed of trabeculae that tend to interact at right angles. In the maxilla, the septa may have a sunburst or hairbrush appearance, which represent bony septa being carried into the soft tissues with the tumor mass. Root resorption and tooth displacement are common. Anterior ethmoidal nerve syndrome is depicted in Fig. 10.22.

Malignancy of Maxillary Sinus

Squamous Cell Carcinoma

A sinus opacity and in most cases, antral wall destruction with adjacent bony involvement is pathognomic of maxillary sinus carcinoma.

Besides the conventional views, 3.0–5.0 mm contiguous section of CT scan permits an accurate evaluation of tumor extension. The primary pathologic and imaging feature of squamous cell carcinoma is the propensity to destroy bone even in the presence of a relatively small mass.

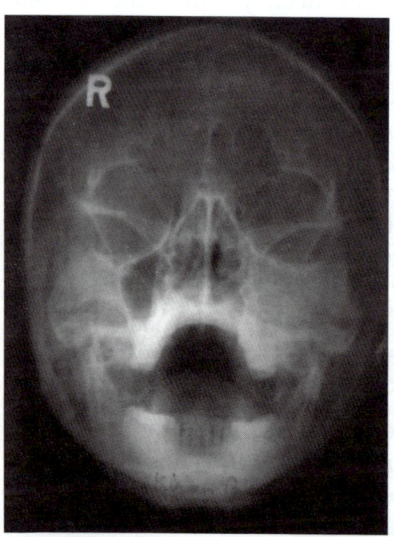

Fig. 10.21A: PA view maxilla in Waters' position (odontogenic myxoma left maxilla)

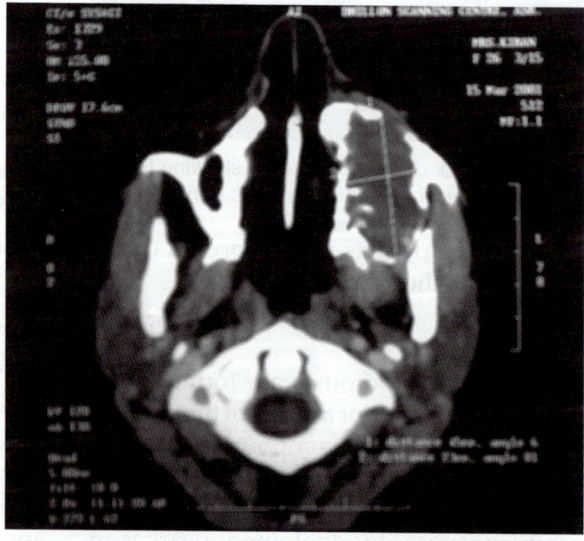

Fig. 10.21B: Axial CT (odontogenic myxoma – left maxilla)

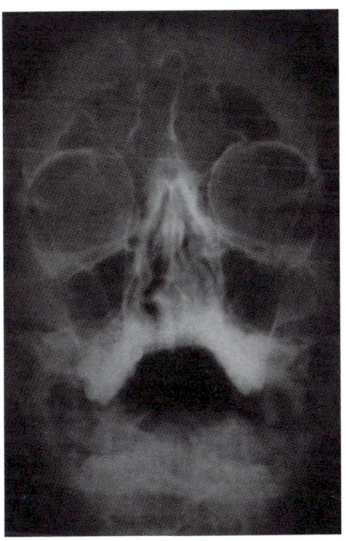

Fig. 10.22: Anterior ethmoidal nerve syndrome

ANTROLITHS

An antrolith is a calcified mass in the maxillary sinus or the antrum. It may be a sequelae of chronic inflammation with the presence of degenerative tissues or foreign bodies. In most of the instances, the patient is unaware of the presence of antrolith. The symptoms are same as those of chronic sinusitis.

Radiographic Features

These are small radiopaque bodies of varying sizes generally found in the base of the sinus. Generally, the antroliths are of homogeneous density, and rarely, they may have a more radiopaque area around. They usually have an irregular border (Figs 10.23A and B).

Bibliography

1. Allard RHB, Vander KW, Vander WI: Mucosal antral cysts. *O Surg, O Med, O Path* : 1981;2:51.
2. Blaschke DD, Brady FA: The maxillary antrolith. *O Surg, O Med, O Path* 1979;48:187.
3. Chaudhry AP, Gorlin RJ, Mosser DG: Carcinoma of the antrum. *Oral Surg* 1960;13: 269.
4. Gardner DG, Gullane PJ: Mucocoeles of the maxillary sinus. *O Surg, O Med, O Path* 1986;62: 538.

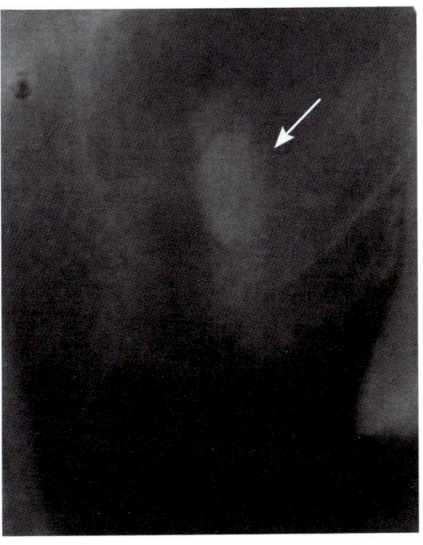

Fig. 10.23A: Root displaced into sinus

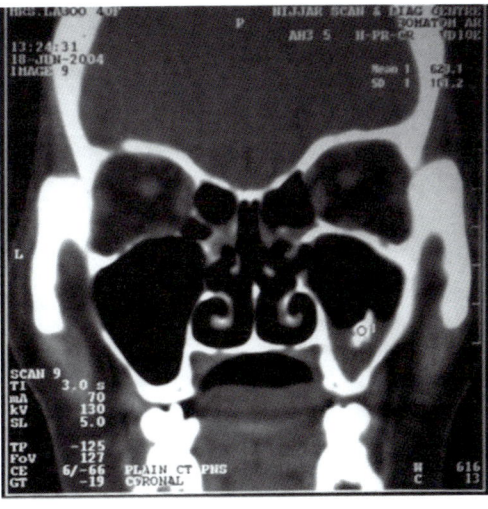

Fig. 10.23B: Coronal CT showing foreign body in right maxillary sinus

10

5. Lylon HE: Reliability of panoramic radiography in the diagnosis of maxillary sinus pathosis. *O Surg, O Med, O Path* 1973;35:124.

6. Miles DA, lass BJ, Langlain RP: Cyst of the maxillary antrum. *O Surg, O Med, O Path* 1984;57:225.

7. Mittila K: Roentgenological investigations into the relation between periapical lesion and condition of the mucous membrane of the maxillary sinus. *Acta Odont Scand*: 1965;23:1.

8. Ohba T, Cordero F, Preece JW : The posterior wall of the maxillary sinus as seen in panoramic radiography. *O Surg, O Med, O Path* 1991;72: 375.

9. Perez CA, Farman AG: Diagnostic radiology of maxillary sinus defects. *O Surg, O Med, O Path*: 1988;66:507.

Specialized Extraoral Techniques

Many a times, the routine extraoral techniques are not sufficient to diagnose various pathologies involving the maxilla and the mandible. Certain improved techniques are available, which can be utilized in required cases. Although general practitioners do not use these modalities in routine, they are used occasionally to aid in diagnosis. The basic principles of operation and clinical applications of these techniques are described for dental operators.

PANORAMIC RADIOGRAPHY

Panoramic radiography, conventionally known as rotational radiography, is the term applied to the radiographic technique which permits the recording of entire dental arches and contiguous structures on one extraoral film.

In conventional radiography, the object to be examined is placed between the X-ray tube and the film and all the three are held motionless. Movement of any of the three results in blurring of the image.

To understand the principles and working of panoramic radiography, let us first study laminagraphy/body section radiography/tomography.

These are terms applied to a technique by which the image of the selected segment of tissue is obtained and the structures on either side are kept blurred. The result can be obtained either by rotating the tube alone or both the film and the tube in opposite directions. Specific portions of the body can be radiographed following this principle. Fig. 11.1 clarifies this technique.

Plane O represents the points in the centre which is to be radiographed. X and Y are other molecular structures.

T_1 is the position of the tube in the beginning and T_2 is the position of the tube at the end. The arrow shows the rotation of the tube (Fig. 11.1).

The penetration power depends upon the following factors:
• Tube film distance
• Object film distance
• Angle of rotation
All these are kept at predetermined levels.

The movement of the tube will produce blurring of the image of the structures, which are not in the selected plane.

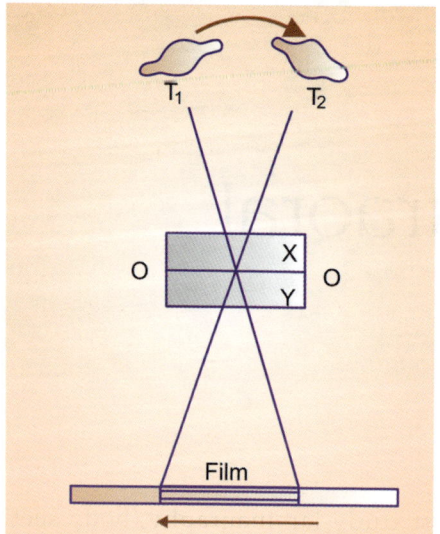

Fig. 11.1: Laminagraphy

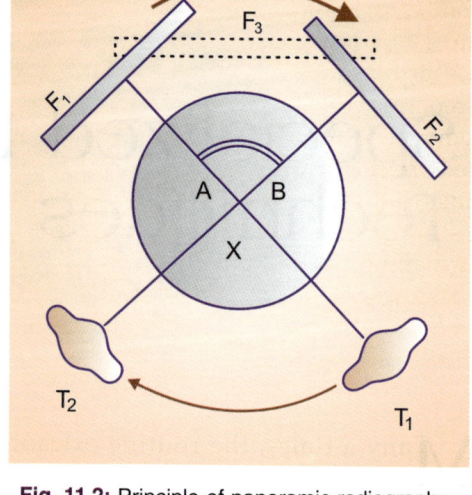

Fig. 11.2: Principle of panoramic radiography

Panoramic radiography is the modified form of tomography. Tomography is utilized in flat planes while panoramic radiography is utilized in curved planes. Since the dental arches are curved, the tube and the film are moved in opposite directions with an equal linear velocity (Fig. 11.2).

The panoramic unit enables us to flatten out the curved surfaces on one film. The principles of panoramic radiography were first described by Numata (1932).

Let us examine Figure 11.2. A radiograph of the curved plane A-B is to be taken. The film is kept at F_1 position while the tube T_1 is directed at right angles to the film. The point of entry of X-rays is through the point X. As the tube is moved towards the left, the film is moved towards the right with the same linear velocity. In the diagram, structures in the plane AB are examined, and other structures are blurred. Such an area

(AB in the picture, which is clearly visible in the radiograph) is known as *focal trough*.

Focal Trough

It is defined as *the three dimensional curved zone or layer where structures are reasonably defined on panoramic radiograph.* The shape and size of the focal trough and other areas are specified for particular panoramic machines. This can vary to some extent but is usually uniform for different systems. Objects in the focal trough can be revealed sharply, while the objects in front or behind are blurred, magnified or reduced in size or distorted to the extent of not being recognizable.

It is important to carefully align the patient's head, particularly the dental arches in the focal trough area. Image distortion will result if this is not followed properly.

When an object is displaced posteriorly from the X-ray film its image is elongated horizontally, whereas if it is displaced anteriorly towards the film, its image is compressed horizontally. Special attention must be paid to the proper positioning of the patient along the focal trough area. Preparation of the patient, as usual, requires removal of metallic objects in the head and neck region, for example ear rings, nose rings, necklaces, etc. The patient should be instructed to look straight and not follow the movements of the tube. He or she is positioned in such a way that the dental arches are located in the middle of the focal trough area. A device is available in the machine for this purpose. The mid-sagittal plane should also be adjusted properly. Failure to make these two adjustments may result in distortion of the image (Fig. 11.3).

The patient's back and spine is to be kept erect and the patient's chin and occlusal plane should be so adjusted that Frankfurt plane is parallel to the floor.

Left and right is marked on the film. Preferably, the patient's name and date are also indicated on the film. Intensifying screens are always used with panoramic films. Panoramic radiographs are depicted in Figs 11.4 to 11.6.

Advantages

a. **Wide coverage:** One of the major advantages of panoramic radiography is its scope of wide coverage on one film. It enables viewing the entire dentition, alveolar bone and also the contiguous structures. Temporomandibular joints are usually not clearly visible. With wide coverage, larger lesions can also be seen on the film.

b. **Simplicity of operation:** Technique of panoramic X-ray unit is comparatively simple. Almost in half an hour, a person could grasp the basic know-how of the machine and its working.

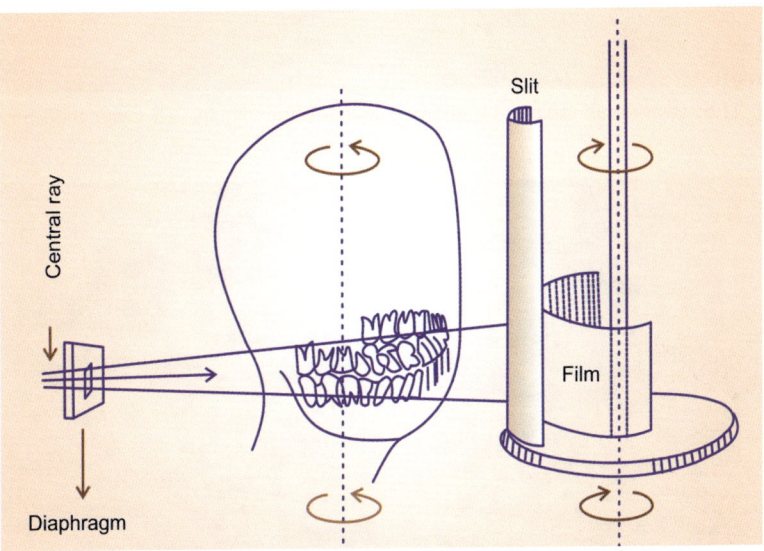

Fig. 11.3: Panoramic radiograph (diagrammatic)

11

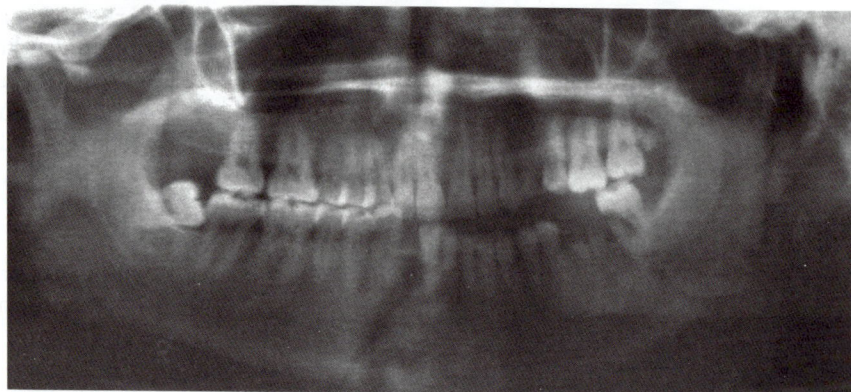

Fig. 11.4: Panoramic radiograph of both the arches showing fracture symphysis and left angle of mandible

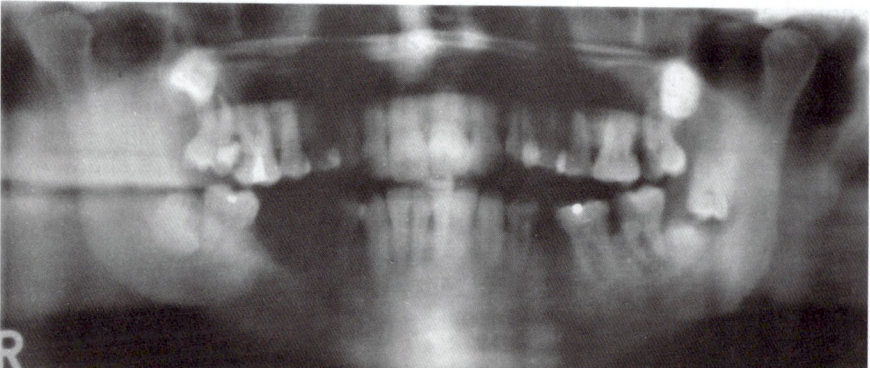

Fig. 11.5: Panoramic radiograph showing inverted mandibular left lower third molar

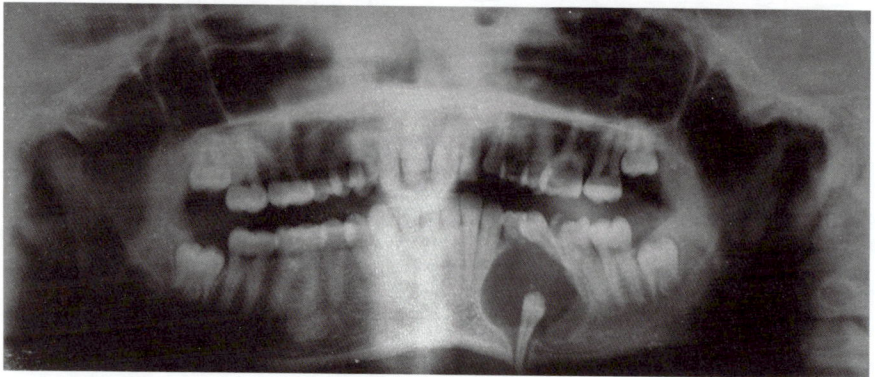

Fig. 11.6: Dentigerous cyst in relation to mandibular canine (panoramic view)

c. **Time saving:** Not more than 3–5 minutes are required for examining panoramic X-rays. Because of the less time consuming procedures, panoramic examinations are also used in screening procedures.

d. **Low radiation exposure:** The total radiation is less as compared to radiation in full mouth intraoral films. And also, there is lesser exposure to secondary radiations.

e. **In orthodontics:** Especially to see the growth and development of permanent teeth, and is also of importance in serial extractions. Panoramic radiographs are mandatory while planning serial extractions.

f. **Patient education:** Various pathological lesions are shown in one film, therefore, it is of importance for the education of patients. Patients can be made aware of further problems.

g. **Patient acceptance:** Patients, who gag easily, or those who do not tolerate intraoral films, mentally challenged or even young children accept panoramic radiographs easily.

h. **Panoramic** radiography is considered the technique of choice in patients suffering from trismus.

Disadvantages

a. **Image distortion:** Usually all panoramic radiographs produce magnified objects. Overlapping of structures is also evident many times. Exact tooth length, size and shape of the pathological lesion cannot be measured.

b. **Poorly defined images:** All panoramic radiographs lack sharpness, especially the posterior structures. Anteriorly they are bright. Use of intensifying screens, increased object film distance and movement of X-ray tube are some of the factors responsible for poor definition of films.

Tooth, alveolar bone, etc. are not very clear. Examination of obese patients also produce films of poor quality; this may be true with conventional radiography even.

c. **Cost:** The cost of a panoramic machine is quite high. In addition, the necessity for intraoral periapical radiographs is always there with panoramic radiographs. Since panoramic units do not or cannot eliminate the need for conventional intraoral units, the cost factor is considered to be of importance.

Keeping in view the advantages and disadvantages of panoramic radiography, the advantages certainly overweigh the disadvantages.

Panoramic Units

Different types of panoramic X-ray units are available. Each one has some distinctive features. A brief description of the three main units is given below:

1. **Panoramix:** In case of panoramix unit, the focal area of the X-ray tube is very small. It is 0.1 mm as compared to 1.0–2.0 mm in other conventional X-ray units. The small target is essential in maintaining satisfactory detail of the image, since the target object distance is very low.

   In performing the examination, the shield is placed over the lower portion of the arch when the maxillary arch is examined and on the upper portion, when the mandibular arch is examined. The unit is mobile and is mounted on a wheel.

2. **Panorex:** In this unit, the components are simple and conventional. The patient is positioned over a chair supported by a

11

11

platform, which moves when half the exposure is made.

The X-ray unit and the film are revolved around a single axis. Lateral shift of the chair midway during the exposure causes the second rotation. A brief suspension of exposure causes a central black line. The right and left sides of the film can be marked with a lead pencil.

3. **Orthopantomograph:** The components of this unit are essentially the same as the conventional ones. Patients may be seated or kept standing on a platform. The patient remains stationary while the X-ray tube head passes behind his neck from the right side to the left. While this is being carried out, the film rotates from the left side of the patient's face to the right side. In this case the change from one axis of rotation to another is automatic and requires interruption in the exposure cycle. Left and right, as usual, can be marked on the film.

PANORAMIC ZONOGRAPHY

In certain areas of examination of the skull and also in multiple fractures of the maxilla, panoramic radiography is not dependable. Other views are taken along with the panoramic one and the fragmented information is correlated to form the final diagnosis.

An advanced imaging modality called *panoramic zonography* has arisen out of the pressing need for high quality radiographs of cranial structures with little exposure.

The Zonarc system (Panoramic zono-graphy system) provides advancement over conventional radiographic units. Zonarc system is the combination of circular and linear X-ray tube movement and a cassette movement by the microprocessor. An important feature is that the larger shape can be adapted to the curvature of the surface being imaged.

The details provided by zonography are definitely superior to that of conventional technique for visualization of areas of alveolar processes, zygomatic corpus, and the lateral wall of both the orbits. The extent and orientation of fractures in some cases are apparent only on the zonograms. It is recommended in the diagnosis and post-treatment follow-up of fractures involving the mandible and the maxillofacial skeleton.

RADIOGRAPHY OF SALIVARY GLANDS

There are three pairs of salivary glands around our oral cavity; the parotid, submandibular and sublingual. All the three secrete saliva into the mouth and serve various purposes (Fig. 11.7).

Any obstruction in their respective ducts or in the intraglandular branches can be shown by injecting a contrast medium into the gland. This procedure is known as *sialography*.

Procedure for Parotid Glands

The parotid is the largest of the salivary glands, lying just below the zygomatic arch, in front and below the ear, and on the masseter muscle over the ramus of the mandible. The duct from the parotid gland (Stensen's duct) runs along the outer surface of the masseter to the buccal mucous membrane opposite the upper second molar. Stone formation is rare in the parotid gland as compared to other glands.

A cannula tip is inserted into the opening of the Stensen's duct opposite the second maxillary molar. Each gland is examined

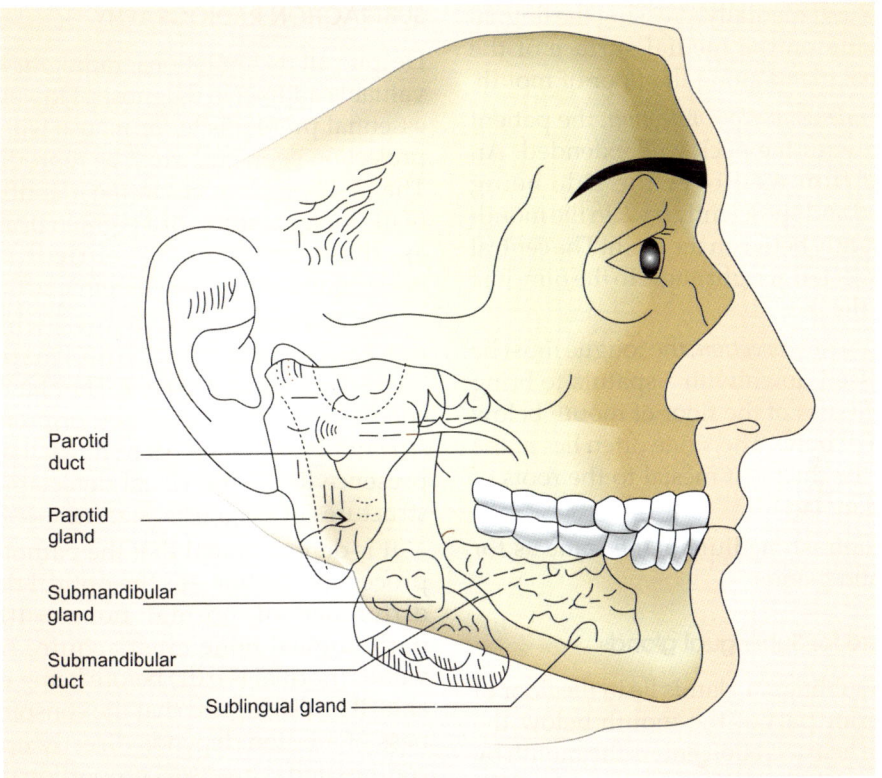

Fig. 11.7: Anatomy of salivary glands

Parotid duct

Parotid gland

Submandibular gland

Submandibular duct

Sublingual gland

11

turnwise. A small amount of contrast medium is injected.

The projections for parotid are the same as those for the ramus of the mandible.

In the *lateral positioning*, the head is in a true lateral position, with angles of the mandible overlapping each other. The central rays are passed over the angle of the mandible.

In the *lateral oblique view*, the head is straight almost similar to lateral view. The only difference is that the central rays are projected below and behind the angle of the mandible away from the film, at a 25° angle towards the head.

In the *frontal position (AP)*, the median plane is kept at right angle to the film. The head is slightly raised and the chin lowered towards the chest. In these cases, the main duct is well shown as it crosses the mandible, but the gland region is overexposed with intraglandular ducts largely obliterated.

Procedure for Submandibular Gland

The two submandibular glands lie on either side of the neck forming part of the soft tissues on the medial margin of the body of the mandible and between the mandible and the hyoid bone. Wharton's duct runs upwards and medially, crossing the lingual nerve lying on the medial surface of the sublingual gland along the floor of mouth.

In the inferosuperior projection, the patient is seated with the neck well extended. An occlusal film well over the side being examined and sufficiently back in the mouth is held lightly between the teeth. The central ray is projected at right angle to the film, just beneath the jaw.

In the lateral projection, the tongue must be well pressed down with a spatula to bring the soft tissues of the floor of mouth below the level of bone. The stone often lies at the head of the duct just mesial to the roots of the third molar.

The contrast medium is the same as for the parotid glands.

Procedure for Sublingual glands

The two sublingual glands lie in the floor of the anterior part of the mouth below the tongue. Their secretion enters the mouth by several small openings on either side of the frenulum and some may open into the submandibular duct. The projections are the same as for the submandibular glands.

Interpretation of Sialogram

The most meaningful information obtained from a sialogram is the distribution of ducts, the uniformity of ductal pattern, and filling or non-filling of regions.

On being injected, the dye will flow through the ducts into the glands and the passage of clearance will be seen in the radiograph. A number of pathologic processes change the normal sialographic appearance of the salivary glands viz. sialolithiasis, involvement of glands by tumors, autoimmune diseases and so on.

SUBTRACTION RADIOGRAPHY

Despite all its limitations, radiography is a valuable adjunct in diagnosis. However, an essential prerequisite for its use is that the projection geometry must be reproducible. The basic problem lies in the identification of the image features of a pathological state, as these are usually buried in the background of normal anatomic structures.

The radiographic structures, which do not contain diagnostic information of interest are labelled as *noise*. They have been collectively called *image noise* or preferably *structured noise*. It has been shown that their presence limits the visual detectability of structures of diagnostic significance.

It is demonstrated that the pathological process of the bone or the optical density difference of normal bone with the pathological bone must acquire higher values (normal is 0.01) before being detectable. It is also argued that the conspicuousness of a lesion depends directly upon its contrast and is inversely proportional to the complexity of the surrounding structures or the structured noise. Subtraction radiography is a technique by which *structured noise is reduced in order to enhance the detectable changes in the radiographic pattern occurring over a period of time.*

Technique

There are several methods of producing subtraction films, which include
a. photographic
b. colour
c. electronic
d. digital

Out of all these, photographic technique is the oldest and well accepted. This technique was first described by Zeides (1960). The

11

subtraction may involve a composite pair consisting of a positive transparent radiograph obtained initially, and an ordinary radiograph obtained after a period of time (Fig. 11.8). These can be studied with electronic superimposition also. It has been reported that in the diagnosis of periapical areas, the pathological lesions were detected six weeks before they were detected by conventional radiography. A prerequisite for subtraction radiography is that the projections must be identical or almost identical at the various times of examination. This photographic technique is lengthy and cumbersome. Consequently the digital method is usually employed in dentistry.

A high quality video camera is employed alongwith a computer and digital convertor. Two standardized radiographs produced with identical exposure geometry are used. The first one is the reference image and the subsequent image is superimposed. The reference image is displayed on a TV screen. Then the subsequent images are super-imposed on the reference image. Any difference between the original and the subsequent images will show up as dark or bright areas. The contrast can be adjusted to further enhance the difference. Practically, it is impossible to achieve perfect regis-tration of comparable structures so that some background structures always remain in the subtraction image. The smaller the lesion to be detected the higher the demand on the reproducibility of the radiographic technique and on the alignment procedure.

APPLICATION OF SUBTRACTION RADIOGRAPHY

- For detecting physiological and pathological changes affecting bone, especially in studies with longer follow-up periods. It is helpful in research projects aimed at studying the effect of various procedures affecting bone.
- Size of periapical lesions, their onset and progress can be evaluated.

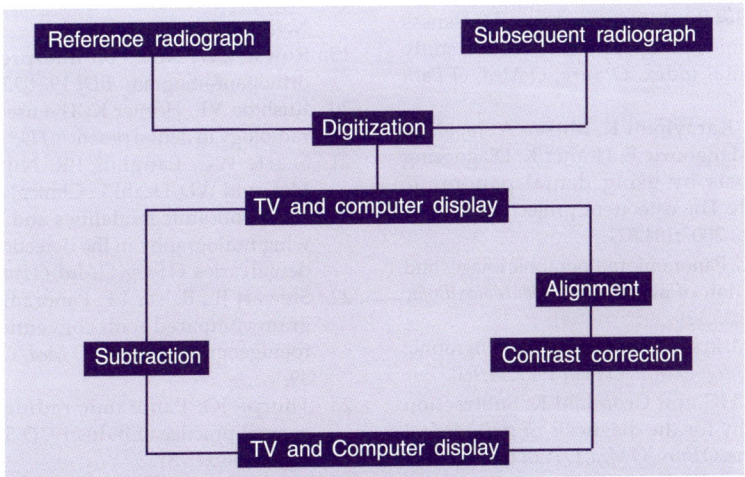

Fig. 11.8: Subtraction radiography

- In periodontology, for determining changes in the crest of the alveolar bone.
- For follow-up of periodontal and endodontal treatments. The radiographs will reveal the success or failure of the treatment.
- Beginning of caries or root resorption can also be noted.

In the **medical** field,
- Angiography
- Demonstration of chest, especially in pneumoconiosis
- Sialography
- Examination of small renal vessels during arteriography
- Investigation of neonatal cardiac diseases.

Bibliography

1. Akker HP: Diagnostic imaging in salivary gland diseases. *O Surg, O Med, O Path* 1986:66:625.
2. Bean LR, Akerman WY: Intra oral or panoramic radiography ? *Dent Clin North Am* 1984;28:47.
3. Christen AG, Segreto VA: Distortion and artifacts encountered in Panorex radiography. *JADA* 1968;77:1096.
4. Dutra V, Susin C, Dacosta NP, Veeck EB, Bahlis A, Fernandes RA: Measuring cortical thickness on panoramic radiograph : A validation study of the mental index. *O Surg, O Med, O Path* 2007;104:686.
5. Devlin H, Karayimni K, Mitsea A, Jacob R, Lindh C, Marjanovic E, Horner K: Diagnosing osteoporosis by using dental panoramic radiograph: The osteodent project. *O Surg, O Med, O Path* 2007;104:821.
6. Farman AG: Panoramic radiographic images and the prediction of asymmetry. *Dentomaxillofac Radiol* 2006;35:129.
7. Goebel WM: In vitro comparison of sialographic agents. *O Surg, O Med, O Path* 1977;44:960.
8. Grondahl HG and Grondahl K: Subtraction radiography for the diagnosis of periodontal bone lesions. *O Surg, O Med, O Path* 1983;55: 208.
9. Hartman LC, Wolfgang L: The application of panoramic zonography to the diagnosis of maxillofacial fractures. *O Surg, O Med, O Path* 1989;67:214.
10. Hurlburt CE, Wuerhman AH: Comparison of interproximal carious lesions detection in panoramic and standard intraoral radiography. *JADA* 1976;93:1154.
11. Langeland DE, Langlais RP, Morris CR: Principles and Practice of panoramic radiography. Philadelphia, W.B. Saunders, 1982;84.
12. Langland DE, Sippy FH: Anatomic structures as visualized on the orthopantomogram. *O Surg, O Med, O Path* 1968;26:475.
13. Leie Luis Weems AR, Richard LW, Greer FD: Evaluation of off-axis projection geometry in dental panoramic radiography. *O Surg, O Med, O Path* 1994;77:183.
14. Madden RP, Hodges JS, Salmen CW, Rindal DB, Michalowicz S, Ahmad M: Utility of panoramic relationships in detecting cervical calcified carotid atheroma. *O Surg, O Med, O Path* 2007;103:543.
15. McDavid WD, Welander U, Morris CR: Blurring effects in rotational panoramic radiography. *O Surg, O Med, O Path* 1982;53:111.
16. Mitchall LD: Panoramic roentgenography: A clinical evaluation. *JADA* 1963;66:777.
17. Mohammed AH, Manson-Hing CR: A comparison of panoramic and intraoral radiographic surveys in evaluating a dental clinical population. *O Surg, O Med, O Path* 1982;54:108.
18. Phillips JE: Panoramic radiography. *Dental Clin North America*, 1968;561.
19. Rowse CW: Notes on interpretation of the orthopantomogram. *BDJ* 1971;130;425.
20. Rushton VE, Horner K: The use of panoramic radiology in dental practice. *J Dent*: 1996;24;185.
21. Scarfe WC, Langlais PR, Nummikoski P, McDavid WD, Deahl T : Clinical comparison of two panoramic modalities and posterior bite wing radiography in the detection of proximal dental caries. *O Surg, O Med, O Path* 1994;77: 195.
22. Stewart JL, Beiser LF: Panoramic roentgenogram compared with conventional intraoral roentgeogram. *O Surg, O Med, O Path* 1968;26: 39.
23. Thorpe JO: Panoramic radiography in the general practice of industry. *O Surg, O Med, O Path* 1966;24:781.
24. Treasure P, Chandler NP, Wilson CG: Image shift of intracoronal pins viewed on bite wing

and panoramic radiographs. *O Surg, O Med, O Path* 1994;77:80.

25. Tronje G: Image distortion in rotational panoramic radiography. V: Object morphology; inner structures. *Acta Radiol* 1982;23:59.

26. Turner KC: Limitations of panoramic radiography. *O Surg, O Med, O Path* 1968;26:312.

27. Turp JC, Vach W, Harbish K, Alt KW, Sturb JR: Determining mandibular condyle and ramus height with the help of an orthopantomogram a valid method ? *J Oral Rehab* 1996;23:395.

28. Updegrave WJ: Seminar on panoramic radiography. *O Surg, O Med, O Path* 1967;24: 38.

29. Updegreve WJ: The role of panoramic radiology in diagnosis. *O Surg, O Med, O Path* 1966;22:49.

30. Valachovic R: The use of panoramic radiography in the evaluation of asymptomatic adult dental patients. *O Surg, O Med, O Path*: 1986;61:289.

31. Webber RL, Wenn RA, Greer DF, Charleston SC: Evaluation of off-axis projection geometry in dental panoramic radiography. *O Surg, O Med, O Path* 1994;77:183.

32. White SC, Forsythe AB: Patient selection criteria for panoramic radiography. *O Surg, O Med, O Path* 1984;57:681.

33. Tsesis I, Katz A, Tamse A and Kafir A: Comparison of digital with conventional radiography in detection of vertical root fractures in endodontically treated maxillary premolars: an ex vivo study. *O Surg, O Med, O Path* 2008;106:124.

11

Advances in Radiological Techniques

The extraoral radiological techniques along with specialized techniques do have certain limitations. The basic problem of exposure to the patient and its related implications, led the researchers to evolve newer techniques where exposure can be minimized without affecting the quality of interpretation, and subsequently diagnostic value. Some of the techniques are described below.

XERORADIOGRAPHY

This is a relatively new method of recording images where the usual silver halide films are not utilized. No chemical developer, fixer, etc. are used and no dark room is necessary for this technique. This method is based on the electrostatic process similar to that used in photocopying device.

Technique

The image is first recorded on a plate, which is made up of aluminium and is coated with a layer of vitreous selenium. This plate possesses certain characteristics viz.:

- It is an insulator in the dark, but may become conductive when exposed to light.
- If given an electrostatic charge, it is capable of retaining the charge for hours together.
- X-rays or light affect conduction in the charged plate.

Before being put to use, selenium particles are given a uniform electrostatic charge and are stored in a unit called *conditioner*. After the plate is charged and ready to use, it is placed in light-tight and air-tight cassettes. Air-tight cassettes are required because air may distort the image.

When X-rays fall on the film they cause selective discharge of the selenium particles, depending upon the amount of radiation used and the relative density of the object.

The pattern of electric discharge on the plate is referred to as *latent image*, and is analogous to the image produced by reduction of silver bromide molecules to free silver.

The latent image is then converted into a visible image by a process called *development* in a unit called *processor*. In the processor the plate is exposed to charged particles called the *toner*. A unique feature of xeroradio-graphic technique is that both positive and negative images are obtained. When a positive current is applied to the processor, negative toner particles are attracted to the plate and vice versa (Fig. 12.1).

Two thumbwheel switches are provided in the processor unit:
- The first allows the operator to select whether the final image will be a positive or negative one.
- The other switch alters the length of the developing cycle, and thus controls image density. After the charged particles are attracted towards the pattern of the

surface, the image is transferred to a special kind of paper known as *Xerox opaque paper*. Once a fixed record is obtained, the selenium plate can be discharged, cleaned and with proper care, used again. It is established that a selenium plate can be reused upto 1000 times.

Gratt et al, in their various studies, have explained xeroradiography in detail. They obtained high quality, low dose dental xeroradiograph images with the use of Xerox 125 medical system. They also

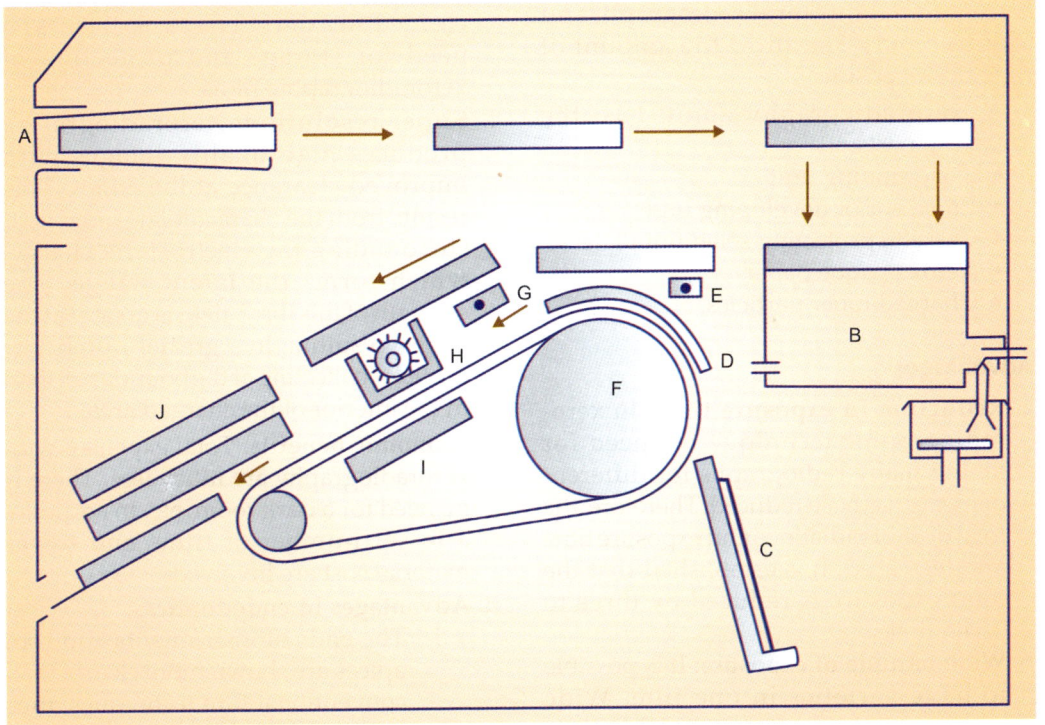

Fig. 12.1: Diagrammatic representation of xeroradiographic technique. A, Cassette containing exposed xerographic plate is inserted in the slot; B, Developing chamber where toner powder is sprayed on the surface; C, Removal of film from the tray; D, Contact with the powdered plate; E, Ion-emitting device, effect is to loosen the powder; F, Another ionizing device for charging opposite polarity; G, Third ionizing device, which loosens the remaining powder; H, Brush, which cleans the plate; I, Paper passes through an oven; J, Proper xeroradiograph image

investigated the clinical feasibility of using xeroradiographic cassettes extraorally, which were thicker and less flexible than film packets used intraorally, and observed no difference between the two as far as quality and patient's acceptance were concerned.

After construction of a prototype intraoral dental xeroradiographic system, which is considered different from the Xerox 125 medical system, they initiated clinical studies evaluating the utility of xeroradiographs in dentistry. The resultant dental images were superior in quality to conventional intraoral radiograph, and required only one-third the amount of radiation exposure.

A xeroradiographic unit has the following parts:
- Conditioning unit
- Processor or developing unit
- Cassette protecting selenium plate
- Xerox opaque paper
- Charged toner particles.

Advantages

a. **Reduction in exposure time:** In xeroradiographic technique the need for taking many radiographs for different densities has been reduced. Therefore, the total dose of radiations and exposure time are decreased. It is established that the total exposure is reduced by three to seven times.

b. **Wide latitude of exposure:** It is possible to have varieties in one film. Wide variation in kilovoltage results in little change in image quality. It also reduces the chances for repeating the X-rays and obtaining incorrect exposures.

c. **Ease in manipulation:** Manipulation of xeroradiographic technique is simple.

There is no need for complex dark rooms and accessories. Chemicals as developer and fixer are also not required.

d. **Ease of viewing:** A xeroradiograph is viewed in ordinary light. This causes less fatigue to the observer's eyes. For viewing xeroradiographs, transillumination is not required. An X-ray image on the other hand should be placed either on a bakelite plastic sheet or opaque paper for viewing.

e. **Elimination of accidental film exposure:** It is because the light intensity necessary for photoconduction is comparatively large and even if the plate is exposed, the charged area can be erased. So there is no need for storage and protection of xeroradiographic films.

f. **Super resolution:** Xeroradiography produces high quality images with improved clearance at the edges. This results from the characteristic force-field surrounding the electrostatic charge, which forms the latent image. The strength of this force-field is greater at the edges, resulting in a greater number of particles collecting at the boundaries than in the interior of the charged area.

g. **Economic benefits:** Total expenses with xeroradiography are much less. There is no need for a dark room, etc. In addition, a lesser number of films and lower material cost are involved.

h. **Advantages in endodontics:**
   i. The ends of instruments and root apices are shown more clearly than conventional film techniques, thus facilitating accurate root length measurement.
   ii. Superior imaging system for evaluating the density and compactness of root canal filling materials.

iii. Facilitates the detection of multiple roots in cases of morphological surveys.

iv. Tooth, root or bone fractures, which are not easily detectable with conventional radiography, are clearly visible on xeroradiographs.

v. Three fold reduction in radiation exposure as compared to conventional films, especially significant when multiple radiograph of a single region is required for thorough evaluation of an endodontic case.

Uses in Medical Field

Uses of xeroradiography in the medical field include:

i. *Mammography:* Minute specks of calcifications are not visible on a conventional radiograph. The breast are better seen with xeroradiography.

ii. *In angiography*: Because of the better edge effect, the quantity of contrast medium required is much less as compared to conventional radiograph.

iii. Demonstration of soft tissue tumors.

iv. Demonstration of calcification of soft tissues.

v. Localization of non-metallic foreign bodies, etc.

Disadvantages

a. **Patient discomfort:** Since the plate is electrically charged, its placement in the oral cavity with a humid environment causes discomfort to some patients.

b. **Fragility of the photoconductor:** Although the selenium layer is electrically stable, it can be scratched easily. Some authors, however, have contradicted this

saying that the selenium surfaces show good resistance to scratching, chipping and abrasion. Placement and retention on the film in the confined area is difficult.

c. **Temporary image retention:** An exposed plate is to be developed quickly. Since this technique involves residual charge patterns, it is necessary to complete the imaging process as soon as possible. The film should be developed within 2–3 minutes, or a maximum of 15 minutes, otherwise black spots appear on the image. Few authors overweigh this limitation saying that the multiple copies can be obtained as long as charge pattern is retained.

d. **Manipulative difficulties:** Exposure time depends upon the thickness of the selenium plate, which some manufacturers do not clarify. Manipulation of exposure time becomes difficult when the exact thickness is not known.

e. **Slower speed:** Speed of the xeroradiographic films is slower than conventional silver halide films. All research is centred on this disadvantage, so as to improve upon the speed, and completely utilize the benefits of xeroradiography.

Keeping in view the vast advantage of xeroradiography and its future prospects, which are no doubt bright; if only film speed is increased, the advantages would far overweigh the disadvantages and this technique could well be employed in diagnosing various dental ailments.

ZEUGMATOGRAPHY

Zeugmatography or nuclear magnetic resonance (NMR) imaging is a newer system in scan radiology. It has many advantages over other systems and the potential of diagnosing tumors is maximum with this technique. It is completely safe, has no radiation effect, and the equipment has no moving parts. NMR, which is still under the budding stage will definitely be a major scanning modality in future.

Principle

Protons have two fundamental properties, which are made use of in NMR

- Spin
- Small magnetic movement

Protons of hydrogen ions, which is a constituent of water (water being the major component of body) are utilized in NMR. Protons behave as small spinning magnets and when placed in a magnetic field, they tend to move parallel to the field. Because of their spin, the protons respond differently with their axis precessing about the direction of the magnetic field. If a coil is now wound around a volume of protons, the tube can be adjusted to turn the magnetization through 90°. This is called 90° pulse. The protons now precess at 90° around the magnetic field at the same frequency, and induce a minute current in the coil, which, when amplified, can be displayed over an oscilloscope. This is known as *Free Induction Decay (FID)* and lasts for some seconds. This energy is utilized in scanning procedures. There are a number of different combinations possible to produce NMR scans. No single method has been established.

Advantages

- NMR images appear to be without any detectable hazard, since it uses non-ionising electromagnetic radiations.

- Anatomical images, as good as CT scans, usually have the possibility of greater tissue characterization.
- Imaging of blood vessels, their blood flow and even thrombi can be visualized.
- NMR equipment contains no moving parts and is not that expensive.
- To enhance the future prospects of NMR, contrast agents can be developed giving more useful information.

Disadvantages

- The technique is time consuming, therefore, there is a greater likelihood of the appearance of artefacts.
- It is contraindicated in patients with cardiac pacemakers.
- Due to non-visualization of bone, diffuse bone diseases are likely to be non-informative.

A bright future awaits NMR technology especially because of non-ionising electromagnetic radiation used in it.

RADIOVISIOGRAPHY

The routinely used radiographic films have halide emulsions. These emulsions have two major disadvantages:
- Usually a high radiation dose is required
- Film processing interrupts treatment.

A system called radiovisiography, claims to minimize these problems. By means of a solid state radiation detector, which is more sensitive than conventional silver halide films, the system presents intraoral radiographic images immediately after exposure (Fig. 12.2).

The radiovisiography unit consists of three components:
  a. Radio
  b. Visio
  c. Graphy

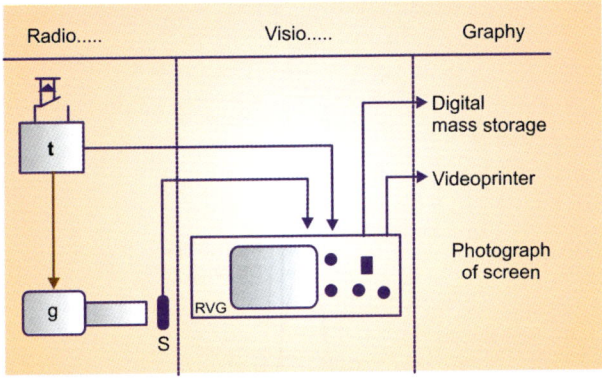

Fig. 12.2: Diagrammatic representation of radiovisiography

a. Radio

The radio part consists of a conventional X-ray generator (g) connected to a highly precise timer (t) for very short exposure. This is also connected to a sensor. The system has a sensitive area consisting of a scintillating screen, a fiberoptic and a miniature charged couple device imaging system.

b. Visio

The Visio part stores the incoming signals during exposure and then converts them into several gray levels.

Since the image is stored point by point, further treatment viz., enhancement and negative to positive conversion, is possible.

The mode is to be activated before exposure. It also improves resolution.

c. Graphy

The graphy part consists of digital mass storage units that can be connected to various video printout devices. Direct photographs of the screens may provide an opportunity to access the radiographic feature.

The RVG system provides the necessary magnification which is required in ordinary films and can be viewed only with magnifying glasses. Resolving ability of human eye depends upon the base intensity of illumination. RVG provides a wide variety of electronic means to adapt to a given situation.

STEREORADIOGRAPHY

If two radiographs are taken sequentially with a change in the position of the tube but no change in the position of the subject or the two cassettes, then a three-dimensional view can be acquired giving the appearance of depth of that object.

The two radiographs are reviewed after superimposition producing an impression of depth (Fig. 12.3).

Technique

The patient is immobilized and the first exposure is made in the usual way. The film is changed and the tube is shifted 2½ inches laterally and the exposure is repeated without any change in the position of the

12

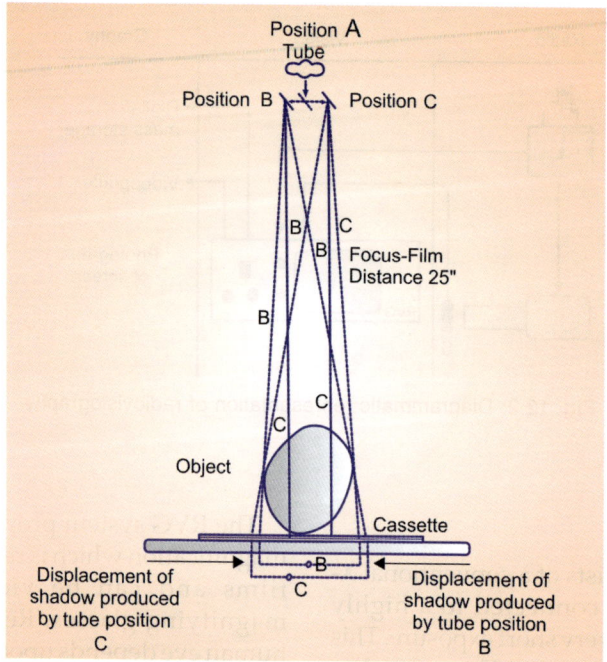

Fig. 12.3: Stereoradiography

patient. Two exposures can be taken in the frontal position by shifting the tube on the side by 1¼ inches and again on contralateral side by 1¼ inches. The focus-film distance should be 10 times the distance of total shift that is 25 inches.

The exposure should be along anatomical lines and films should be processed in the same environment. The patient must be sufficiently immobilized to allow time to move the tube by hand and change the cassette.

To determine the correct method of viewing, a pair of stereoscopic films is used. Indicating R (right) or L (left) of the patient, the films are placed edge to edge and the image is slightly out of alignment. The image projected towards the left would be produced by the right tube shift and vice versa.

The in-depth view can be seen from the side opposite to the one that is radiographed and then the sides are reversed. Faults in labelling and viewing should be carefully checked.

Stereobinoculars with which one can view the films are available. However, with experience one can optimally view an image even with the naked eye. The films are placed side by side in a rectangular illuminator with the right stereo film to the right and the left stereo film to the left. With proper adjustments, the two images are merged into a single three-dimensional view. A dual stereoscope permits viewing by two observers simultaneously.

THERMOGRAPHY

Principle

The variation in the amount of heat emitted by infrared radiations from different structures or parts of the body is recorded, so as to produce a visual image.

Body heat is produced by cellular metabolism and is lost by radiation, evaporation and convection. Heat lost by evaporation and convection cannot be measured; however, heat lost by radiation can be measured.

Malignant cells, because of their increased cellular metabolism, produce a rise in temperature in the overlying skin. Increased blood supply is responsible for a rise in temperature and correspondingly, an increased loss of heat from the overlying tissues.

Uses

Most of the uses of thermagraphy are in the medical field. Its use in dentistry is yet to be investigated. Its application includes

- Early detection of malignant diseases of the breast.
- Investigation of arterial disease—this is used to evaluate narrowing of carotid vessels.
- Demonstration of deep vein thrombosis.
- To differentiate between full thickness burns and partial thickness burns.
- In abdominal conditions, as in acute appendicitis, cholecystitis, etc.

Bibliography

1. Benz C, Mouyen F: Evaluation of the new radiovisiography system image quality. *O Surg, O Med, O Path* 1991;72:627.
2. Benz C: Evaluation of the new radiovisiography system image quality. *O Surg, O Med, O Path* 1991;72:627.
3. Campbell JA: Advances in dental radiology. *Canad J*, 1986;14.
4. Chen SK, Hollender L: Detector response and exposure control of the Radio Visiography System (RVG 32000 ZHR). *O Surg, O Med, O Path* 1993;76;104.
5. Gratt BM, Sickles EA, Lacy AM: Dental xero-radiography for imaging biomaterials: A comparison with conventional radiography. *JPD*: 1980;44, 567.
6. Gratt BM, Sickles EA: Use of dental xero-radiographs in periodontics in comparison with conventional radiographs. *J. Periodontol* 1980;51:1.
7. Gratt BM, Sickles OA: Electronic thermography of normal facial structures: A pilot study. *O Surg, O Med, O Path* 1989;68(3):346.
8. Gratt BM, White SC, Bauer JG: A clinical comparison between xeroradiography and film radiography for the detection of recurrent caries. *O Surg, O Med, O Path* 1988;65(4):483.
9. Gratt BM, White SC, Sickles EA, Jeromin LS: Imaging properties of intraoral dental xeroradiography. *JADA* 1979;90;805.
10. Gratt DM, Sickles EA, Nguyen NT: Dental xero-radiography for endodontic: A rapid X-ray system producing high quality images. *J Endo* 1979;5:266.
11. Guerrero ME, Jacobs R, Loubele M, Schufyser F, Suetens P State of the art on cone-beam CT imaging for pre-operative planning of implant placement. *Clin Oral Invest* 2006;10:1.
12. Hashimoto K, Arai Y, Iwai K, Araki M, Kawashimo S, Terakodo M: A comparison of a new limited cone beam computed tomography machine for dental use with a multidetector row helical CT machine. *O Surg, O Med, O Path*: 2005;95:371.
13. Hintze H, Wenzel A: *In vitro* comparison of D and E speed film radiography and RVG and visualix digital radiography for the detection of enamel approximal and dentinal occlusal caries lesions. *Caries Res* 1994;29;363.
14. Horner K, Shearer AC, Walker A. *et al.*: Radiovisiography: An initial evaluation. *BDJ* 1990;168:244.
15. Jeromin L, Geddes G, White S, Gratt B: Xeroradiography for intraoral radiology. *O Surg, O Med, O Path* 1980;49:178.
16. Kalathingal SM, Tyndall DA, Caplan DJ: *In vitro* assessment of cone beam local computed

12

tomography for proximal caries detection. *O Surg, O Med, O Path*, 2007;104:699.

17. Katsmata A, Hirukawa A, Okumura S, Naitoh M, Fujishita M, Ariji E, Langlan R: Effect of image artefacts on grey nature dentistry in limited volume cone beam computerized tomography. *O Surg, O Med, O Path* 2007;104: 829.

18. Katsumata A, Hirukawa A, Fujishita M, Noujein M, Okumura S, Naitoh M. Image artefacts in dental cone beam CT. *O Surg, O Med, O Path*: 2006;101:652.

19. Kau CH, Richmond S, Palomo JM, Hans MG: Three dimensional cone beam computed tomography in orthodontics. *J Ortho* 2005;32: 282.

20. Ludlow JB, Laster WS, Bailey LT, Hershey GH : Accuracy of measurements of mandibular anatomy in cone beam computed tomography images. *O Surg, O Med, O Path* 2007;103:534.

21. Ludlow JB, Mol A: Digital imaging; In: White SC, Pharoah MJ. Oral Radiology, *Principles and Interpretation*. 5th Ed: Mosby 2004;225.

22. Misch KA, Yi ES, Sarment DP: Accuracy of cone beam computed tomography for periodontal defect measurements. *J Periodontol* 2006;77:1261.

23. Mischkowski RA, Pulsfort R, Ritter L, Zoller JE, Keeve E, Brochhagen GH, Neugebauer J: Geometric accuracy of a newly developed cone-beam device for maxillofacial imaging. *O Surg, O Med, O Path* 2006;101:652.

24. Mouyen F, Benz C, Sonnabend E, Lodter JP: Presentation and physical evaluation of Radiovisiography. *O Surg, O Med, O Path* 1989; 68:238.

25. Mozzo P, Procacci C, Taccom A, Martini PY, Andreis IA: A new volumetric CT machine for dental imaging based on the cone beam technique: Preliminary result. *Eur Radiology* 1998;8: 1558.

26. Nair MK and Nair VP: Digital and advanced imaging in endodontics: A review. *J Endo* 2007;33:1.

27. Rawls RH, Owen DW: The dental prognosis for xeroradiography. *O Surg, O Med, O Path* 1972;33:476.

28. Richards AG: New concepts in dental X-ray machine. *JADA* 1966;73:69.

29. Richards AG: Trends in dental radiography. *O Surg, O Med, O Path* 1977;44:807.

30. Sanderimk GCH: Imaging: New versus traditional technological aids. *Int Dent J*: 1993;43: 335.

31. Scarfe WC, Farman AG, Sukovic P. Clinical applications of cone-beam computer tomography in dental practice. *J Can Dent Assoc* 2006;72:75.

32. Shearer AC, Horner K, Wilson NHF. Radiovisiography for imaging root canals: An *in vitro* comparison with conventional radiography. *Quint Int* 1990;21:789.

33. Shearer AC, Horner K, Wilson NHF. Radiovisiography for length estimation in root canal treatment: An in vitro comparison with conventional radiography. *Int Endod J*: 1991;24; 233.

34. Terakado M, Hashimoto K, Arai Y, Honda K, Sekiwa T, Sato H: Diagnostic imaging with newly developed ortho super high resolution computed tomography (ortho CT) *O Surg, O Med, O Path* 2000;89:509.

35. Tsiklakis K, Syriopoulos K, Stamatakis HC: Radiographic examination of the temporomandibular joint using cone-beam computed tomography. *Dentomaxillofac Radiol* 2004;33:196.

36. Vandenberghe B, Jacob R, Yang J: Diagnostic validity (acuity) of 2D CCD versus 3D CBCT images for assessing periodontal breakdown. *O Surg, O Med, O Path* 2007;104, 395.

37. Wenzel A, Hintze H, Mikkelsen L, Mouyen F: Radiographic detection of occlusal caries in non-cavitated teeth. A comparison of conventional film radiographs digitized film radiographs and radiovisiography. *O Surg, O Med, O Path* 1991;72:621.

38. Wenzel A, Larsen MJ, Fejerskov O: Detection of occlusal caries without cavitation by visual inspection, film radiographs, xeroradiographs and digitized radiographs. *Caries Res* 1991;25: 365.

39. White SC, Gratt BM: Clinical trials of intraoral dental xeroradiography. *JADA* 1979;99:810.

40. White SC, Hollander L, Gratt BM: Comparison of xeroradiograph and film for detection of proximal surface caries. *JADA* 1984;108:755.

41. White SC, Hollander L, Gratt BM: Comparison of xeroradiograph and film for detection of periapical lesions. *JDR* 1984;63:910.

42. White SC, Stafford ML, beeninga LR: Intraoral xeroradiography. *O Surg, O Med, O Path* 1978;46:62.

43. White SC: Caries detection with xeroradiograph. The influence of observer experience. *O Surg, O Med, O Path*: 1987;64:118.

13

Advanced Imaging Modalities

A correct diagnosis has ever been the aim of the operator. The use of advanced imaging modalities in making diagnosis presents new opportunities as well as challenges for the clinician. The proper use and interpretation of these readily available diagnostic modalities require a clear understanding of their respective limitations and capabilities.

The images provide information regarding calcified tissues, soft tissues or their metabolism that is otherwise not accessible to the human eye. Clinical correlation among history, clinical signs, laboratory tests and the results of the imaging examination helps to achieve accurate diagnosis.

With the advent of digital radiography, computer assisted images detect even minute changes in hard tissues. The availability of numerous imaging modalities places a responsibility on the clinician to opt for these modalities after a careful assessment of the patient.

Various advanced imaging modalities currently in use are discussed.

ULTRASONOGRAPHY

Ultrasonography is one of the non-invasive diagnostic modalities in the field of medicine. It is derived from the Latin word ULTRA, which means beyond or excess and SONOGRAPHY a technique for recording and interpreting sound.

In ultrasonography, high frequency ultrasound (20KHz) beyond the human audible range is utilized as an imaging tool by virtue of the beam-like radiation of sound energy with appropriate equipment. The equipment is capable of detecting echoes returning from soft tissue interfaces and is used to scan tissues of the body (Fig. 13.1).

Evolution

The origin of ultrasonography dates back to the early 17th century when pulse echo method was used for the detection of submarines and other objects as SONAR during the world war. This forms the basis for medical ultrasonography. Various authors have used this modality in different forms.

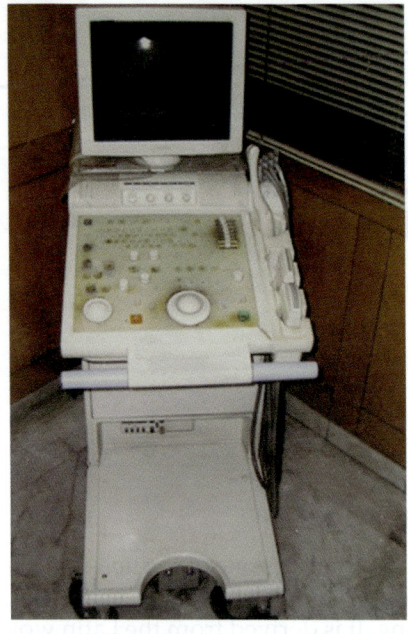

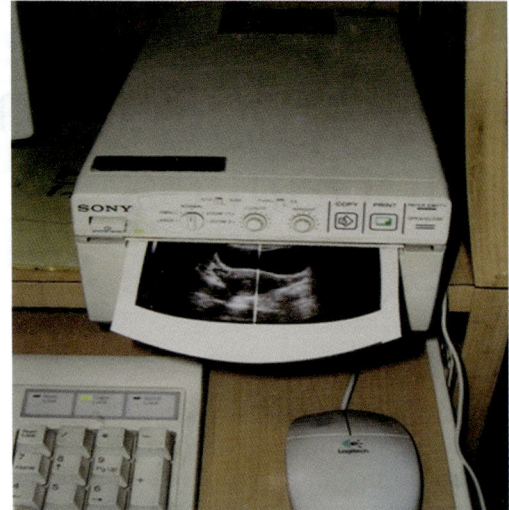

Fig. 13.1: Ultrasound machine and printer. [*Courtesy:* Kannan Diagnostics, Mysore]

13

Physical Basis

Diagnostic ultrasound utilizes the piezoelectric effect. When a voltage is applied to certain materials they expand or contract depending on the polarity. Alternatively, on application of mechanical pressure to these materials such as by a reflected ultrasound wave returning from the body, voltage is produced across them. This phenomenon is known as the *piezoelectric effect*.

Transducers (Scanning Probes)

A transducer is any device that converts energy from one form to another. An ultrasound transducer converts electrical energy into ultrasound energy and ultrasound energy back into electric energy (Fig.13.2).

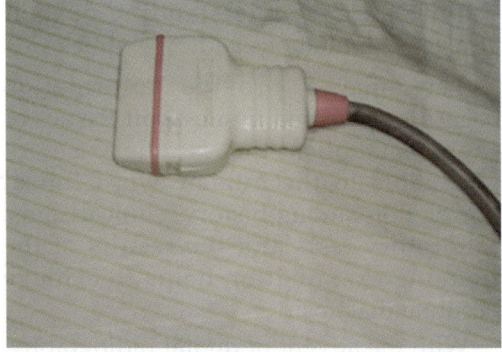

Fig. 13.2: Transducer/scanning probe. [*Courtesy:* Kannan Diagnostics, Mysore]

Diagnostic ultrasounds are produced by a transducer, which contain a piezoelectric material in the range of 1 to 10 megahertz. These sound waves are directed in a narrow beam at the body tissues. When ultrasonic radiation passes through matter, its intensity and size decrease with increasing distance from the emitting transducer due to interactions with matter such as reflection, scattering, refraction and diffraction. The reflection of the ultrasonic wave is the most important interaction phenomenon from the point of view of clinical application. The reflection of any beam depends on the acoustic impedances of the tissues concerned. The reflected ultrasound waves that reach the transducer induce varying voltages across it depending on the contour and size of the body tissue on which they are applied. These voltages may be amplified and measured. The amount and pattern of reflected sound waves indicate the density and uniformity of the tissues examined. This constitutes the usual method of detecting and measuring ultrasonic radiations. So the same transducer can be used to both generate and detect ultrasonic radiations but not simultaneously.

The scanning probe is the most expensive part of any ultrasound unit. It contains one or more transducers that transmit the ultrasound pulses and receive back the echoes during scanning. Each transducer is focused at a particular depth. The beam of an emitted ultrasound varies in shape depending on the type of transducer and the generator.

Properties of Ultrasound Waves

i. *Wave propagation*: It describes the transmission and spread of ultrasound waves to different tissues. Ultrasound waves propagate as longitudinal waves in soft tissues. The molecules vibrate and deliver energy to each other so that ultrasound energy propagates through the body. The average speed for soft tissues is 1540 meters per second.

ii. *Wavelength*: It is inversely proportional to frequency. Higher the frequency, shorter the wavelength. The shorter the wavelength, better the resolution, giving a clearer image and greater detail on the screen.

iii. *Focusing*: Ultrasound waves can be focused either by lenses or mirrors or electronically in composite transducers. In the same way that a thin beam of light shows an object more clearly than a widely scattered, unfocused beam, so also with focused ultrasound, a narrow acoustic beam images a thin section of tissues and thus gives a better resolution of details.

For best results it is necessary to focus at the depth in the body that is of the greatest relevance to the particular clinical problem. For general purpose scanners, this usually means using different transducers for different purposes and adjusting the focal zone on the unit as necessary.

Many transducers have a fixed focus. Composite transducers such as linear and convex array and annular sector transducers have an electronically variable focal length, which can be adjusted to the required depth.

iv. *Attenuation*: Higher frequencies are more readily absorbed and scattered (attenuated) than lower frequencies. Thus, to reach deeper tissues, it is necessary to use lower frequencies because the waves are likely to be diverted as they traverse intervening structures. In practice, it is better to use about 3.5 MHz for deep tissue scanning in adults and 5 MHz or higher if available for scanning the thinner bodies of children. 5 MHz or greater

13

frequencies are also best suited for scanning superficial organs in adults.

v. *Amplification*: The echoes that return from deeper structures are not as strong as those that come from tissues nearer the surface. They must be amplified, so a *time-gain-compensation (TGC)* amplifier is used in ultrasonography. This improves the quality of the final image.

vi. *Boundaries*: Ultrasound may be reflected or refracted when it meets the boundary between different types of tissues. Tissues vary greatly in their effect on ultrasound. For example, the skeleton and gas in the bowel or chest behave very differently from soft tissues. When ultrasound waves meet bone or gas in the body, they are significantly reflected or refracted. Thus, it is usually impossible to use ultrasound effectively when there is a lot of gas in the bowel.

The skeleton reflects ultrasound so strongly that the architecture within a bone or heavily calcified tissue cannot be seen and there is an acoustic shadow behind it. As a result, imaging through an adult skull or other bone is not possible.

Interpretation of Ultrasound Images

Sonographic images are identified in terms of echoes as *hypoechoic, hyperechoic* and *anechoic* images. A mass is hypoechoic if it has an intensity lower than that of adjacent tissue. The term hyperechoic is used for masses of higher intensity and isoechoic for masses with an intensity similar to that of adjacent tissues. The appearance of hypoechoic masses is darker whereas the hyperechoic masses appear rather bright, and the isoechoic ones have a similar appearance (Figs 13.3 to 13.5).

A calcified mass appears hyperechoic and a clear fluid or blood appears anechoic.

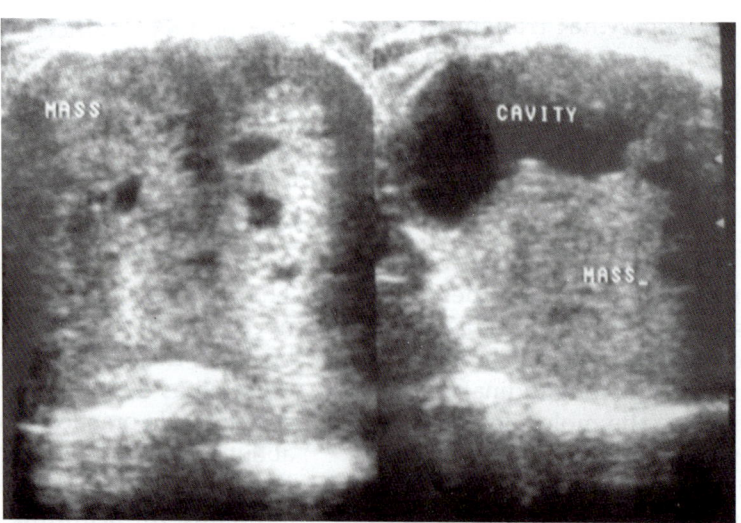

Fig. 13.3: Ultrasound showing cystic areas (plexiform ameloblastoma)

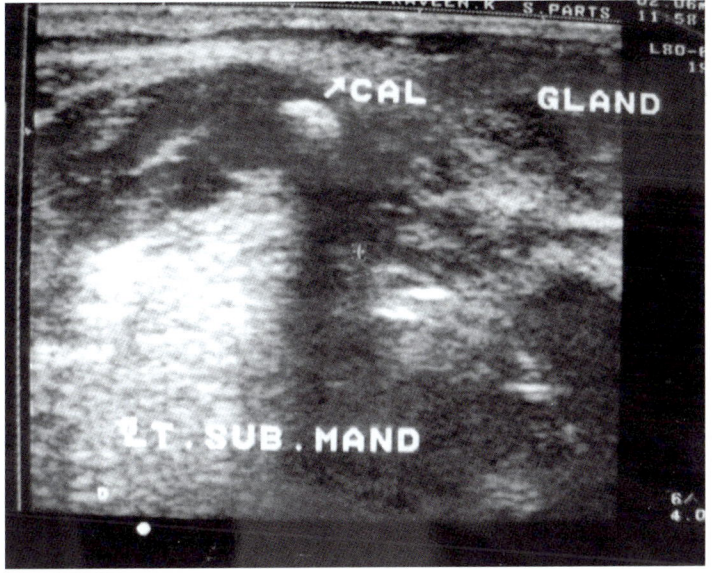

Fig. 13.4: Ultrasound showing sialolith

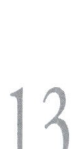

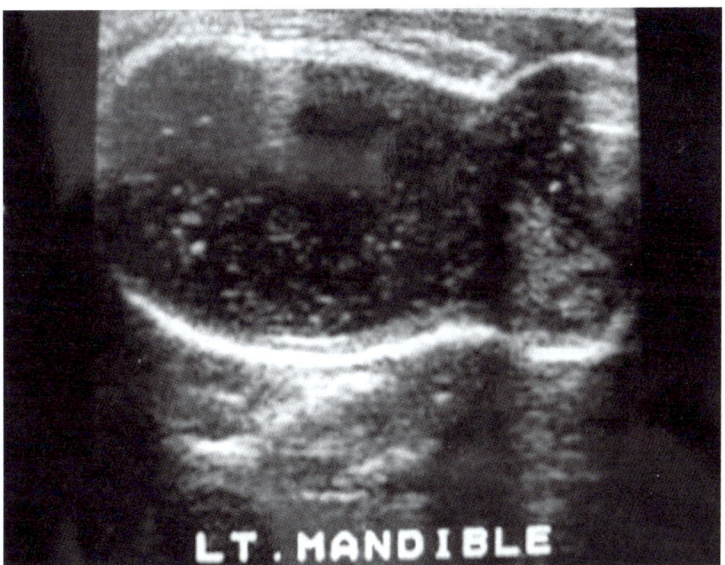

Fig. 13.5: Ultrasound of the mandible showing cystic lesion (unicystic ameloblastoma)

[Figs. 13.3 to 13.5—*Courtesy:* JSS Dental College and Hospital, Mysore]

13

Advantages of Ultrasonography

- Widely available
- Relatively inexpensive
- Non- invasive
- Easily reproducible

Techniques of Diagnostic Ultrasound

The diagnostic ultrasound techniques can be utilized in the following ways:

A. THE PULSE-ECHO SYSTEMS

The use of pulse-echo technique is basic to diagnostic ultrasound. In this system the pulse generator produces a brief electric pulse that is sent to a transducer containing a piezoelectric material, which converts the electrical pulse to a sound pulse. This sound pulse is transmitted into the tissues being examined by a transducer. The echoes that return to the transducer from the interfaces between structures of differing acoustic impedances are converted to electrical impulses and are displayed on the oscilloscope.

A and B scanning are the basic pulse-echo techniques on which the other techniques are developed.

B. GRAY-SCALE ULTRASONOGRAPHY

Gray-scale ultrasonography provides a much more detailed analysis of the internal architecture of various structures than the A and B scanning. Here, the scan converter is used to obtain images that permit information to be displayed in eight to ten shades of gray. This technique is widely used in the diagnosis of soft tissue lesions. It provides information regarding organ boundaries, tissue interfaces and the internal structure of soft tissues as well.

C. REAL-TIME ULTRASONOGRAPHY

Real-time ultrasonography consists of a continuous display of B-mode images. It has the capability of showing physiological movements within the tissues (e.g. swallowing), which is possible because more than 30 images are composed within one second.

D. THREE-DIMENSIONAL ULTRASONIC SCANNING

This provides a 3-D scan presentation. It has the capacity to measure accurately the volume of regions of interest and ensures excellent visualization of the structures examined.

E. M-MODE SCANNING (MOTION MODE)

It consists of:

  i. TM-mode (time-motion mode)
 ii. PM-mode (position-motion mode)
iii. UCH (ultrasonic cardiography)

The principal application of M-mode scanning is to monitor the heart. It uses either A-scan or B-scan display.

If A-scan display is used, motionless clips indicate motionless interfaces and back and forth vibrating clips indicate interfaces that are in motion. The magnitude of each clip represents the degree of movement of the tissue interface.

If B-scan display is used, fixed dots indicate a motionless tissue interface and moving dots are related to a moving tissue interface.

An advanced feature of M-mode display allows it to be synchronized with the electrocardiogram tracing for better evaluation of cardiac function.

F. DOPPLER-SHIFT SYSTEMS

In these systems the change of frequency of radiation reflected by a moving surface or object is measured. This is achieved by comparing the frequency of the original and reflected radiations and generating (electronically) a new signal whose frequency is equal to the difference between the original and reflected frequencies, i.e. the Doppler shift.

COLOR DOPPLER ULTRASONOGRAPHY

This provides a color display of blood flow along with the standard gray scale image so that the evaluation of vascularity of the tissues is possible.

General Diagnostic Applications

- *Mass detection:* Gray scale ultrasound is the method of choice for initial evaluation of most palpable or clinically suspected masses. Clinically occult or non-palpable lesions, whether intra-organ or extra-organ in location, can be detected and relations and displacement of adjacent viscera assessed.
- *Consistency evaluation:* Three main sonographic texture patterns of lesions are recognized, namely cystic, solid and complex, which is mainly a fluid pattern but contains solid components such as pus, debris, blood or neoplastic excrescences. The minimal detectable size of a cyst is in the range of 0.5 to 1.0 cm for superficially located lesions, and 1.0 to 2.0 cm for deeper lesions.
- *Mensuration and volume determination:* The common applications include diagnosis and monitoring of arterial aneurysms, fetal cephalometry and calculation of mass and organ volumes.

- *Needle biopsy and radiotherapy localization:* An ultrasonograph displays accurately the size, position, and depth data for internal organs and masses, and relates this information to skin surfaces. This ability makes it very useful for guided needle aspiration biopsy and radiation therapy portal delineation.

Head and Neck Applications

- Ultrasonography is one of the special diagnostic methods of choice for head and neck tumors and detection of recurrence or lymph node metastasis at an early stage (Figs 13.3 to 13.5).
- It can be used as an adjunct to clinical examination in inflammatory soft tissue swellings of head and neck and can be used to monitor the course of the disease as well.
- This method is efficient and effective in determining the type and vascularity of vascular lesions and plays a crucial role in their management.
- Imaging of the maxillary sinus has little value due to its bony walls. Acute maxillary sinusitis cases can be monitored successfully during treatment for residual fluid. However, mucosal swellings, polyps and cysts are poorly demonstrated.
- In fracture cases, it is used to reveal the nature, and aids in their reduction since it can overcome the disadvantages of palpation and radiography.
- Real time ultrasonography of the TMJ is found to be an ideal means of confirming the position of the condyle within the glenoid fossa.
- Salivary gland imaging by ultrasonography is encouraging due to its ability to detect masses in the gland (Fig. 13.4). It

13

can differentiate between extrinsic and intrinsic masses and between different inflammatory lesions and autoimmune diseases. Ultrasonographic imaging of the lymph nodes provides valuable information regarding anatomic location, nature, volumetric evaluation and determination of their vascular connections. It contributes significantly to the detection, treatment planning, and follow up of lymph node involvement in malignancies.

Intraoral Applications

- Ultrasonography provides excellent differentiation between solid, cystic and vascular lesions of the floor of the mouth and aids in diagnosis of developmental cysts of the floor of the mouth.
- Lingual abscesses can be effectively detected by this imaging technique. Malignant involvement of the tongue can be investigated regarding its extent better than by any other imaging method.
- Ultrasonographic studies of human teeth have revealed that it is possible to differentiate between healthy and demineralized enamel and the degree of demineralization may be assessed from relative echo-amplitude changes.
- Ultrasonography of the periodontium needs further improvement in technology to assess bone loss.

DIGITAL RADIOGRAPHY

Electronic dental imaging or filmless radiography has had a tremendous impact on clinical practice in dentistry. Since the use of dental digital imaging results in reduction of patient-absorbed dose, it was accepted quickly into dental practice.

A digital radiograph produces a dynamic image in which visual characteristics of density and contrast can be manipulated to meet the specific diagnostic requirements or to correct exposure technique errors.

Computer technology in the field of radiography has made image acquisition, manipulation, storage, retrieval, and transmission to remote sites in digital forms possible.

Several techniques record images in a digitized form, such as intraoral and extra oral radiography, computed tomography and magnetic resonance imaging.

Principle

The word 'digital' refers to the numeric format of the image content as well as its discreteness. Digital images are numeric and discrete in two ways:
  i. Spatial distribution of picture elements or pixels.
  ii. Different shades of gray for each pixel.

Analog and Digital Images

The electric signal that is produced by the sensor is a voltage that varies as a function of time. This is an analog signal, which in principle can have any value between the maximum and minimum voltages. The sensor is connected to a special board in the computer called the frame grabber. The frame grabber samples the signals at short intervals. This process is called sampling. This converts the analog image to a digital signal.

Once sampled, the signal is assigned a value, a step called quantization. These values are stored in the computer and represent the image.

Thus, a digital image consists of a large collection of individual pixels organized in a matrix of rows and columns. Each pixel has a row and column coordinate that uniquely identifies its location in the matrix. These numbers have discrete values ranging from 0–255. Completely black is represented by 0 and white by 255, with other shades of gray having values between 0 and 255.

In order to see the images, the computer organizes the pixels in their proper locations and gives them a shade of gray that corresponds to the number that was assigned during the quantization step.

Digital Detector Characteristics

a. Image acquisition

Several methods of image acquisition exist. These are:

i. Conventional radiograph digitized using a flat bed scanner and transparency adapter.
ii. Conventional radiograph digitized using a charge-coupled device camera.
iii. Semi-direct digital image, acquired using photostimulable phosphor plates.
iv. Direct digital image, acquired using a charge-coupled device, complementary metal oxide semiconductor or other electronic devices.

b. Image characteristics

i. *Contrast resolution*: It is the ability to distinguish different densities in the radiographic image.

Theoretically, the detector can capture 256 (2^8) to 65,536 (2^{16}) different densities. However, a monitor can only display 242 gray levels. A further limitation is the human visual system that is capable of detecting only about 60 gray levels at any time under ideal viewing conditions. Under viewing conditions in a dental operatory, human eyes can detect only about 30 gray levels.

ii. *Spatial resolution:* It is the capacity for distinguishing fine details. For digital imaging systems, the theoretical limit of resolution is a function of picture elements or pixel size. Resolution is often measured and reported in terms of line pairs per millimeters. Test objects consisting of sets of very fine radiopaque lines separated from each other by spaces equal to the width of the line are constructed with a variety of line widths. At least two pixels are required to resolve a line pair, one for the line and one for the space.

Charge-coupled devices used in digital imaging can resolve seven line pairs per millimeter, whereas conventional intraoral films can resolve up to 20 line pairs per millimeter.

iii. *Detector latitude*: The ability of the imaging receptor to capture a range of X-ray exposures is termed latitude. An intraoral image receptor should record the full range of tissue densities from gingiva to enamel and it should also record the subtle differences in densities within these tissues. The useful range of densities in film radiography is from 0.5 to 2.5. The latitudes of CCD and CMOS detectors are similar to the film and can be extended with digital enhancement of contrast and brightness. PSP receptors enjoy larger latitudes and have a linear response to five orders of magnitude of X-ray exposure.

iv. *Detector sensitivity*: It is the ability to respond to small amounts of radiation. Intraoral film sensitivity is classified according to speed group criteria developed by ISO. Currently, no standard classification for digital image receptors exists. Current PSP systems

13

for intraoral use require about 50 percent of the dose needed for F speed film.

A number of factors such as detector efficiency, pixel size, and system noise affect the sensitivity of digital image receptors.

Advantages

- Lower radiation dose.
- Computer manipulation of characteristics such as:
  - Contrast
  - Resolution
  - Image enhancement
- Instant image display.
- No need for conventional processing thus avoiding processing errors and hazards of handling processing chemicals.
- Automated image analysis.
- Storage and archiving of patient information.
- Teleradiology—transfer of images to remote places.
- Patient education and interaction.
- Digital subtraction eliminates distracting background images and offers the option of gray scale visualization in reverse, i.e. radiolucent structures appear white and radiopaque structures appear dark.

Disadvantages

- Expensive, especially the panoramic systems.
- Large disc space required to store images.
- In direct digital radiography, the sensor and computer are connected directly, which makes intraoral placement of the sensor difficult.
- Loss of image definition and resolution compared to conventional film both on the monitor and printout.

- Image manipulation may be misleading to new users.
- Difficult for some intraoral systems to view multiple images at the same time. (full mouth survey).
- Printout may fade with time and pose problems.
- Legal issues—it is questionable whether digital images could be used as evidence in lawsuits because images can be manipulated.

IMAGE DETECTORS

1. Charge-Coupled Device (CCD)

The CCD was the first digital image receptor to be adapted for intraoral imaging.

CCD is a light or X-ray sensitive array of semiconductors on a silicon chip. Charge coupling is a process by which accumulated light or X-ray photons are transferred from one electron-well to the next in a sequential manner and finally to a read-out amplifier. When the CCD is exposed to radiation, the covalent bonds between the silicon crystals are broken, producing electron hole-pairs. The number of electron hole-pairs is proportional to the amount of radiation the area receives. The electrons are then attracted to the most positive potential in the device where they form *charge-packets*. Each packet corresponds to a pixel and this represents the latent image.

The image is read in a *bucket-brigade* fashion by transferring each row of pixel charges from one pixel to the next. At the end of the row, the charge is transferred to a read-out amplifier and then to an analog-to-digital converter located within or connected to a computer.

The two main sensor arrays are:

a. *Linear array:* useful in cephalometric and panoramic imaging.
b. *Area or two-dimensional array:* These are of two types:
  i. Fibro-optically coupled sensors, which use scintillation screens made of gadolinium oxybromide or cesium iodide coupled to a CCD. This works similar to the conventional screen film combinations.
  ii. Direct sensors, where the CCD array captures the image directly.

Advantages

- Low radiation dose
- Instant image
- Image manipulation

Disadvantages

- Smaller receptor size of most systems makes only single tooth imaging possible.
- Bulky sensor with cable connected to computer.
- Relatively short lifespan of CCD due to deterioration by X-ray bombardment.
- Narrow exposure latitude due to burnout of structures when overexposed.
- Storage of the image is a tough task due to the need for special archiving equipment (optical disk, CD, large memory hard disk).
- Blooming: It is similar to allowing too much light through a view box, blinding the operator, and washing out the radiographic information in excessively bright image. This occurs in CCDs due to excess charge leakage to other pixels.
- High cost.

Types of Charge-Coupled Device Systems

a. Combination of rare earth intensifying screen as the primary receptor, fibro-optical coupling to transmit the fluorescence, and conventional light sensitive CCD to receive it, e.g. Radiovisiography.

b. A 'hardened' X-ray sensitive CCD as primary receptor. e.g. Sens-a-ray, Sidexis.

c. Similar to (a), but uses lenses instead of fiberoptics, e.g. Flashdent.

d. A combination of an intensifying screen and a hardened CCD, e.g. Visualix.

2. Photostimulable Phosphor (PSP)

Luminous substances have long been used for various purposes. In the early 70's it was considered a good method to use scanning optics to release the energy from a storage phosphor, and to convert the information pattern into digital form. Such a system is definitely sensitive to X-rays. Since then, there have been numerous improvements in phosphors and imaging systems (Fig. 13.6).

a. The PSP plate is flooded with white light to return all electrons to the valence band (Fig. 13.7).

b. Exposure to impart energy to europium valence electrons results in their movement into the conduction band. Some electrons become trapped at F centers.

c. A red scanning laser imparts energy to electrons at the F centers promoting them to the conduction band from which they return to the valence band. With the electrons returned to the valence band, energy is released in the form of light photons in the green spectrum. This light is detected by a photomultiplier tube or diode using a red filter to screen out scanning laser light (Figs 13.8A and B).
  Several attributes are required of a storage phosphor material.

13

i. The compound must create and store a latent image without appreciable degradation until it is ready to be scanned.

ii. It must be possible to stimulate efficiently the phosphor with light, so that the energy stored in the latent image can be released.

iii. The released energy must have a wavelength that can be readily detected in the presence of stimulating light.

The photostimulable phosphor used for radiographic imaging is a Europium–doped barium fluorohalide. Barium in combination with iodide, chloride or bromide forms a crystal lattice. Europium is added as an impurity, acting as an activator to create luminescence centers (holes). The barium fluorohalide is mixed with a polymer which binds the storage phosphor crystals to a base. The storage phosphor is covered with a protective coating which helps prevent physical and atmospheric damage to the storage phosphor. The combination of storage phosphor, base and protective coating is referred to as a *storage phosphor plate*.

When the storage phosphor is exposed to X-rays, an electron of the Eu^{2+} ion is excited to the conduction band creating an electron vacancy at the trivalent europium site (Eu^{3+}). This electron is then trapped in the halogen valency or the F center in the crystalline lattice of the storage phosphor. About half the valencies and trapped electrons recombine spontaneously and cause luminescence. The other half forms metastable states, the local concentration of vacancies and trapped electrons being proportional to the X-ray exposure.

13

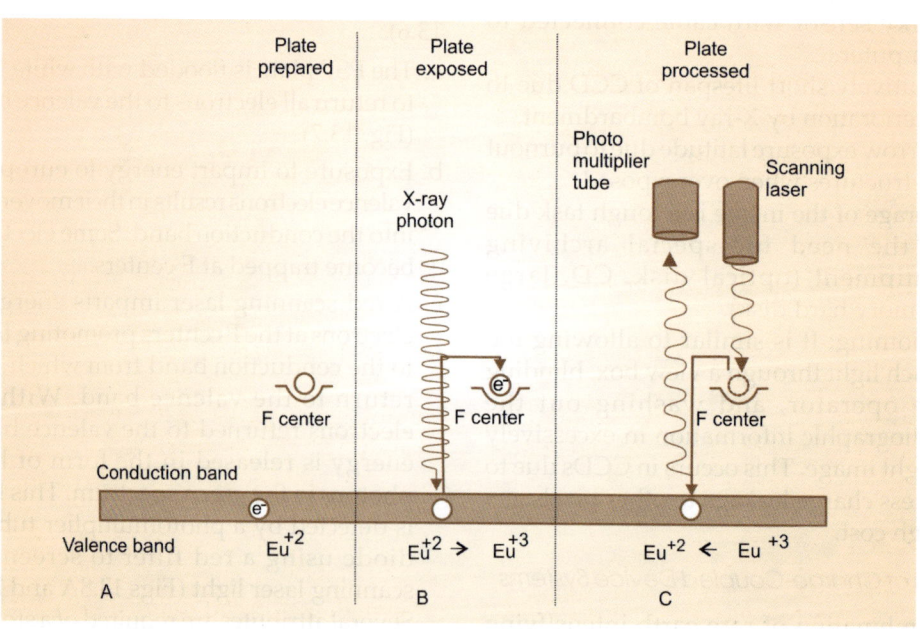

Fig. 13.6: PSP image formation

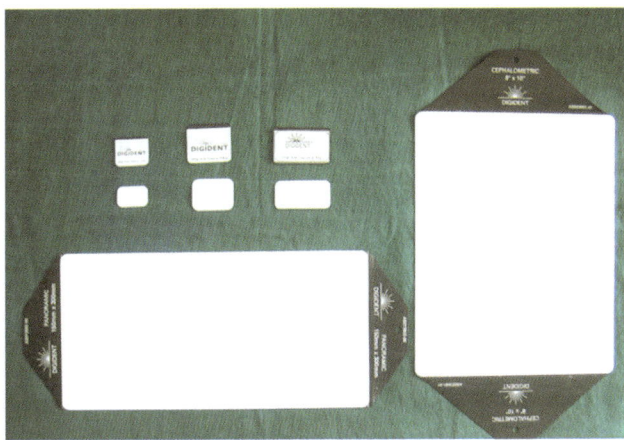

Fig. 13.7: Photostimulable phosphor plates

13

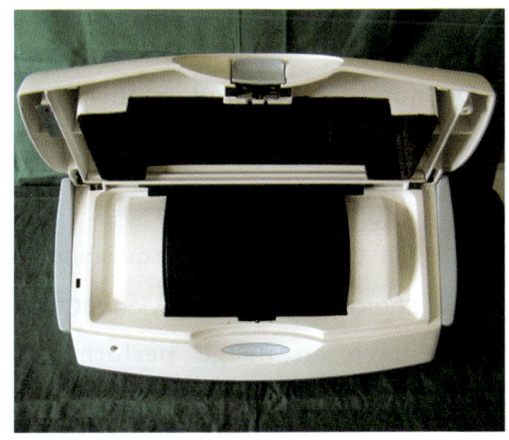

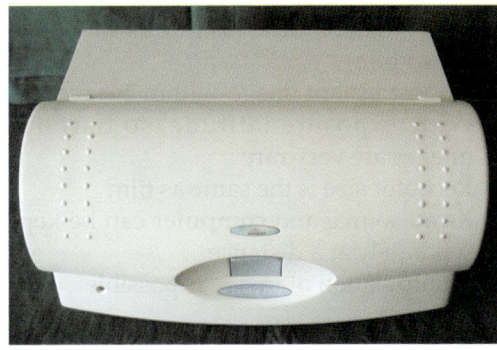

A   B

Figs 13.8A and B: Different views of PSP laser scanner

A lower level of radiation is required by this system compared to non-screen dental films because storage phosphor absorbs much more radiation and latent image formation is more efficient.

The excited barium fluorohalide complex has a rather wide absorption band centered at 600 nm. Red light from helium neon laser (wavelength 633 nm) or semiconductor (diode) laser (wavelength 680 nm) is used for stimulation. Current dental PSP systems have a resolution of 6 to 8 line pairs per millimeters.

A number of approaches have been adopted for reading the latent images on the PSP plates. One technique employs a rapidly rotating multifaceted mirror that reflects a beam of red laser light. As the mirror

13

revolves the laser light sweeps across the plate. The plate is advanced and the adjacent line of phosphor is scanned. The direction of the laser scanning the plate is termed the fast scan direction, while the direction of plate advancement is the slow scan direction.

This is used by Soredex in its Digora system and Air Techniques in its Scan X system.

An alternate approach to plate reading involves a rapidly rotating drum that holds the plate. The rotation of the drum past a fixed laser provides a rapid scan. Incremental movement of the laser in the slow scan direction allows image data to be acquired line by line. This is used by Gendex in the Dentopix system and by Orex in the Panorama Xi system.

Advantages

- Less radiation dose (as low as 10% of E-speed film)
- Almost instant image-within 20 seconds
- Wide exposure latitude, so burnout images are very rare
- Receptor size is the same as film
- X-ray source and computer can be kept separately at a distance
- Manipulation of image is possible

Disadvantages

- High cost
- Problem of image storage as with CCD
- Minor inconvenience due to protective bags

3. Complementary Metal Oxide Semiconductors (CMOS)

These are silicon-based semiconductors and are different from charge-coupled devices in the way the pixels are read. Each pixel is isolated from its neighboring pixel and is directly connected to a transistor. The process of image formation is similar to that of CCD. However, the charge is directly transferred to the transistor as a small voltage. Then it is addressed separately and read by a frame grabber, stored, and displayed as a digital gray value.

Advantages

- Integration
- Low power usage
- Manufacturability
- Low cost
- CMOS technology is already in use in computer chips and this high volume manufacturing capacity can be benefited from.

Disadvantages

- Do not perform well in low light conditions.
- Cannot withstand the regional demands of medical imaging systems.
- More fixed pattern noise.
- Less active area for image acquisition.

4. Bulk Charge Modulated Device (BCMD)

These have an image performance comparable to charge-coupled devices and the advantage of improved price and performance over existing CCD sensors. They also have high sensitivity and low noise. A low cost production process and low power usage are other advantages.

5. Amorphous Selenium

This type of sensor was first tried in xeroradiography but due to toner readout it was not widely accepted. Recent advances in this technology make use of a thin layer of amorphous selenium on an aluminum support. The selenium is rendered sensitive to X-rays by charging its surface to a high potential. When X-rays hit the charged surface, electron-hole pairs are created in the selenium and freed electrons migrate to the surface, which results in a latent image charge. This detector with latent image charge is passed under an array of electrometers, which scan the image and read it into a computer. This is currently used in chest radiography only and is yet to be adopted for oral radiography.

6. Charge Injection Device (CID)

These sensors exhibit high sensitivity and low noise comparable to CCD sensors. They have the advantages of a low cost production process and lower power usage similar to CMOS.

7. Flat Panel Detectors

These are used in medical imaging and also in prototypes of extraoral imaging devices. They can provide relatively large matrix areas with pixel sizes less than 100 microns.

Two approaches have been taken in selecting X-ray sensitive materials for flat panel detectors. The first approach utilizes indirect detectors which are sensitive to visible light, and intensifying screens made of gadolinium oxysulphide or cesium iodide to convert X-ray energy into light. These devices are limited by the thickness of intensifying screens. Thicker screens although efficient, produce greater diffusion of light photons leading to reduced image sharpness.

The second approach involves direct detectors which use a photoconductor material such as selenium with properties similar to silicon but with a higher atomic number that permits more efficient absorption of X-rays. The electron freed during X-ray exposure of selenium is conducted in a direct line to an underlying thin film transistor (TFT) under the influence of an applied electric field. Direct detectors provide higher resolution but lower efficiency in comparison with indirect detectors. Energy is released and read out by applying appropriate row and column voltages to a particular pixel's transistor. Currently flat panel detectors are expensive and likely to be limited to specialized imaging techniques like cone beam computed tomography.

DIGITAL IMAGE DISPLAY

1. Cathode Ray Tube (CRT)

Conventional computer monitors use cathode ray tube designs. High quality monitors are able to display 256 different gray values or a combination of gray and color values. CRT displays involve conversion of digital information into analog voltages which are supplied to electronic guns. The beam of electrons emanating from the electronic gun rapidly scans the phosphor-coated screens and builds up an image line by line. The image is refreshed at the rate of 60 times/second or more to avoid the appearance of a flicker. Color monitors utilize 3 electron guns, 1 each for red, blue and green phosphors.

2. Thin Film Transistor (TFT)

The TFT technology is used in laptop and flat panel computer displays in addition to being used in flat panel detectors. The output of laptop display is limited in intensity and does not have the dynamic range or contrast found in conventional desktop displays. Desktop versions of TFT LCD displays have overcome brightness and viewing angle problems but consume

13

more power and thus are not suited for laptop configurations.

IMAGE PROCESSING

Image processing involves steps that improve, restore, analyze or in some ways change a digital image. The objective of image processing is to make relevant information more evident by creating images that are better suited for human visual perception or to gather data by analyzing the image content. Its primary goal is to improve diagnostic accuracy by using image information more effectively. The digital image processing operations can be grouped into five fundamental classes: image enhancement, restoration, analysis, compression and synthesis.

i. Image Enhancement

It implies that the adjusted image is an improved version of the original one. This application can be accomplished by increasing contrast, optimizing brightness or reducing sharpness and noise. Image enhancement can be subjective or objective. Subjective enhancement involves making the image visually more appealing and objective image enhancements are closely linked with image restoration operations.

Filters can be applied to digital images to improve image quality by removing some forms of noise. Noise refers to any aspect of the image that degrades features of interest. Noise may be high frequency noise or speckling and low frequency noise or gradual intensity changes. Also, it can be random or periodic.

Filters can be spatial domain filters or frequency domain filters.

Digital subtraction radiography is also an image enhancement operation. However, it affects the diagnostic image chain at the image formation level.

The use of color in digital imaging is controversial. However, conversion of gray scale images to color is possible with newer digital imaging systems called pseudo color. Pseudo color may be used as a segmentation tool. It may also be used to highlight parts of an image after segmentation operation has been applied. The use of color has also been advocated to encode multidimensional information.

ii. Image Restoration

It involves undoing known or estimated degradations introduced during image formation. The image is restored by substituting the gray values of defective pixels with some weighted average of gray values from the surrounding pixels. Most of the preprocessing operations are set by the manufacturer and cannot be changed.

iii. Image Analysis

It is designed to extract non pictorial information from the image that is diagnostically important. Such information can range from measurements to fully automated classification. Digital rulers, densitometers and a variety of other tools are available for measurement. Tools are being developed for measuring the complexities of trabecular bone pattern.

The three basic steps of image analysis are *segmentation, feature extraction* and *object classification.*

Segmentation is the most critical step in the process of image analysis. It is done to simplify the image and reduce it to its basic components. It subdivides the image by separating the foreground from the background. After segmentation of objects in the image a variety of features can be measured that assist in determining to what class each object belongs. In dental radiography, *features of interest* include measures of size and shape, relative location, average density, homogeneity and texture.

To complete the image analysis process the object should be *classified* relevant to the diagnostic task.

iv. Image Compression

It is done to reduce the size of the digital image files for storage or transmission. Image compression can be of two types. *Reversible compression* also called image coding is used when the exact data of the original image needs to be preserved. The maximum compression rate for reversible compression is usually less than 3:1.

Irreversible compression algorithms are developed to achieve high levels of compression while retaining subjective image quality. Compression rates of 12:1 to 14:1 can be achieved.

v. Image Synthesis

New images can be synthesized based on the image data acquired from multiple projections. The main purpose of these modalities is to access information about the object of interest in three dimensions. CT, MR Imaging and Positron Emission Tomography scanners are the most well known and sophisticated image synthesis modalities in medical and maxillofacial imaging.

SUBTRACTION RADIOLOGY

Image subtraction was originally tried in medical radiology. It was done with positive and negative photographic prints of the radiographs which were then compared. Early studies used photographic subtraction to study the arterial vasculature of the mandible.

Subtraction imaging with photographic methods has major limitations such as the inability to correct projection geometry, density and contrast of the radiograph.

Digital Subtraction Radiography

In recent days, the development and application of digital techniques have made subtraction radiography overcome the drawbacks associated with the photographic method, digital subtraction radiography (DSR) can now be considered a practical approach to the comparison of dental radiographs by electronic manipulation of the images.

Technically it is an image enhancement method that removes the structure noise from images.

DSR is sensitive to the extent that it can detect a 0.12 mm change in the thickness of cortical bone as opposed to visual examination of radiographs, which can only detect a 0.85 mm change in the thickness of bone.

DSR requires two identical images to produce another image representing only the density difference between these two. The sensitivity of digital subtraction to record minute differences depends on the degree to which the two images match in overall density, contrast, projection geometry and hardening of the X-ray beam. Techniques have been developed to correct the differences in these characteristics.

However, DSR is difficult to use in day-to-day practice because it requires reproducible alignment of the central ray of the X-ray beam, the teeth and the film each time.

13

Methods to Obtain Identical Radiographs

For Radiographs with Identical Projection

- Use of bite registration geometry and film holders attached to the radiation source.
- Extraoral stabilization of the patient and a long source to object distance to minimize magnification.
- A stored video image of the patients face taken during the first radiographic examination to align the patient for subsequent exposures.

For Radiographs with Identical Overall Density and Contrast

The change in overall density or contrast may occur in serial radiographic images. These changes are caused by fluctuation in line voltage, variations of exposure parameters, films or processing. The matching of the overall density and contrast of two films to be subtracted is commonly done by employing a contrast correction algorithm. This programme matches the gray level distribution of subsequent images to gray levels found in the original reference image. In this way small changes in density and contrast over time may be corrected retrospectively using digital image processing.

Procedure/Technique

The digital in DSR refers to the use of a computer to manipulate the image. A conventional radiograph is considered an analog image due to spatial and gray scale resolution. The digitization process converts the conventional radiographic image to a digital image by taking a picture of the radiograph using a high-resolution black and white video camera and these video signals are transferred to a computer-imaging device called digitizer. The digitizer places a grid over the original radiograph and creates small squares or picture elements (pixels). Each pixel is converted to a number corresponding to its gray level. The process of digitization decreases the information but converts the image into a form that can be read and analyzed by the computer.

To produce a subtraction image, a perfect set of radiographs and special computer software are used. The first radiograph among the perfect set is digitized and converted into a positive image in the computer. The software then allows the operator to align the second radiograph under the video camera. When the alignment is complete, the second radiograph is digitized. The computer then subtracts the digitized gray scale value at each pixel to obtain the subtracted image. A perfect subtraction with no differences between images will have a value of zero (black) at all pixel locations. To facilitate visualization, an offset gray value of 128 is added to produce a gray background against which any superimposed change or lesion is more readily visible. In a perfectly subtracted image, teeth and other anatomical features are not visible. So color can be added to the subtracted image and can be superimposed on the original radiograph to facilitate interpretation.

In case of minor discrepancies in pairs of images, an image-processing computer can manipulate the images and correct them using custom algorithms or rules. In spite of the power of the computer, it is advisable to use high quality films with nearly identical projection geometry.

Clinical Applications

- Progress of alveolar bone loss.
- Advancement of caries from an incipient lesion through the dentinoenamel junction.
- Assessment of a healing or an expanding periapical lesion after root canal therapy.
- Detection of initial saucerization or formation of an angular defect around implants.
- Assessment of spread of bone loss along the threads of root-form implants (often obscured by the sharp contrast between the bone and the implant surface).
- TMJ-Evaluation of minute changes in the position of the condyle, integrity of the articular surfaces and assessment of the remodelling of bone around granular hydroxyapatite implants.

TELERADIOLOGY

Teleradiology is defined as *the electronic transmission of radiologic images from one location to another for the purpose of interpretation, consultation or both.*

Teleradiology systems allow direct digital or digitized film images to be transmitted to distant locations where they can be observed and stored as hard copies for interpretation.

The first transmission of a dental radiograph over a long distance was experimented in the early 20's. However, in the 1950s, the first transmission of a radiograph over a telephone line was successfully carried out and the process came to be known as *Telegnosis.* This was done by scanning the radiograph with light, then transmitting analog signals, which were received by a photographic plate in the form of light. This plate was then processed.

Applications

- Dental insurance authorization
- Consultation and referrals
- Continuing education
- Forensic identifications
- Compatibility with electronic record retrieval systems

A basic teleradiology system consists of three major components which are interconnected. They are:

a. An image sending station
  i. Image digitizer
  ii. Network interface device
b. A transmission network
c. An image receiving/review station
  i. Network interface device (modem)
  ii. Personal computer with storage medium
  iii. One or two TV monitors
  iv. Optional hard copy printer device

a. Image sending station

i. Image Digitizer

Transmission of dental radiographic images requires the image files to be in a digital format. Conventional dental radiographic films can be scanned to convert them from analog to digital formats and this process is known as digitization. To avoid scanning of conventional radiographs, two basic types of digital dental systems can be used to acquire images. They are:

- **Direct digital system:** Direct digital system with the electronic sensor having CCD or CMOS. These systems allow a range of image processing procedures. In addition, these systems offer a reduced radiation dose and a wide range of contrast.
- **Indirect digital system:** Early projects used video cameras to analog radio-

13

13

graphic images by photographing them. This resulted in a reduction in quality. Two new technologies have been developed recently for the digitization of conventional radiographs. They are laser digitizers and CCD digitizers.

The image can also be acquired by indirect computed radiography systems using storage phosphor image receptors. These systems have the advantage of reducing radiation dose to the patient and post-processing image manipulation over digitization of conventional film-based radiography.

ii. Network Interface Device (modem)

To transmit digital information using voice lines it is necessary to convert the data into voice or modulated analog signal through a modem at the transmitting end. It has to be reconverted to digital form by demodulation through a modem at the receiving end.

b. Transmission network

Approaches to Telecomputing

- Dedicated lines or private leased lines
- Shared telephone lines
- Wide band electronic mail

A line is a configured physical equipment for telecommunications and a channel is a path along which information flows. These channels are of three types:

- *Simplex:* This allows transmission in one direction only. To get feedback it requires loop configuration.

- *Half duplex:* This is a two-way channel but allows unidirectional transmission at each time.

- *Full duplex:* This is also a two-way channel which allows simultaneous transmission of information to both the ends.

Image Communication Protocol

The transfer of any information between two computer systems requires a communication protocol that is understood by both systems. A communication protocol is simply a set of rules governing how two systems communicate.

Some types of naming and addressing protocols allow computers to identify themselves and the systems they want to communicate with. For radiology the standard is DICOM -3.0 which was jointly published by the American College of Radiology and the National Electrical Manufacturers Association in 1996. Maxillofacial radiology also uses the DICOM standard, which specifies the roles played by systems that participate in image exchange. It also specifies the protocol to be used by computer systems when they communicate with each other to exchange images. The DICOM standard is complete and consists of several parts. It includes message exchange protocols and specifications for image formats for various types of medical images.

Connections

Point-to-point connection: This consists of the basic sending and review station directly connected by a dedicated transmission network (single wire or fiber-optic cable). This is commonly used in a single building to accommodate image transmission from one location to another.

Local area network (LAN) connection: A LAN consists of a dedicated transmission network like in point-to-point connection but is attached to multiple sending stations.

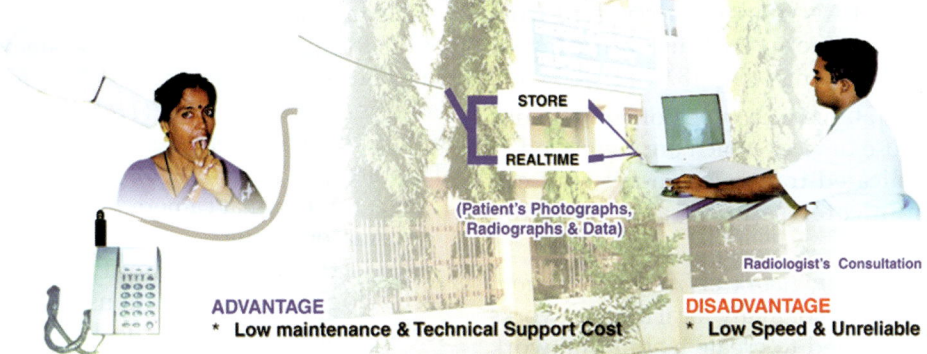

STORE

REALTIME

(Patient's Photographs, Radiographs & Data)

Radiologist's Consultation

ADVANTAGE
* **Low maintenance & Technical Support Cost**

DISADVANTAGE
* **Low Speed & Unreliable**

Fig. 13.9: Type 1 – Plain old telephone line system

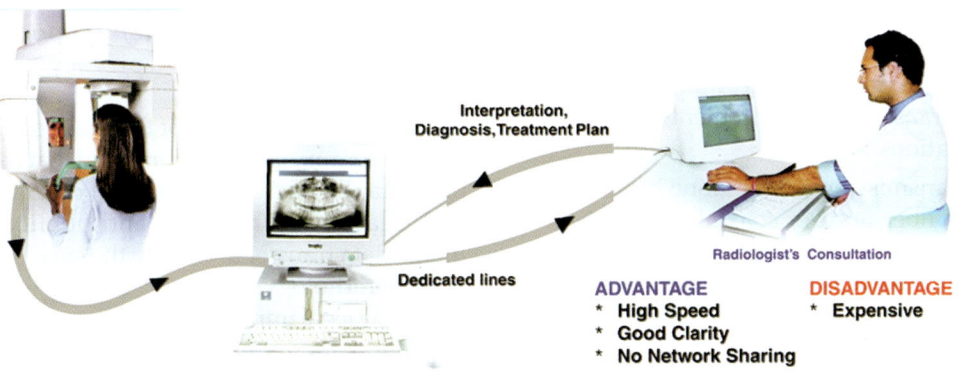

Interpretation, Diagnosis, Treatment Plan

Radiologist's Consultation

Dedicated lines

ADVANTAGE
* **High Speed**
* **Good Clarity**
* **No Network Sharing**

DISADVANTAGE
* **Expensive**

13

Fig. 13.10: Type 2 – Integrated services digital network

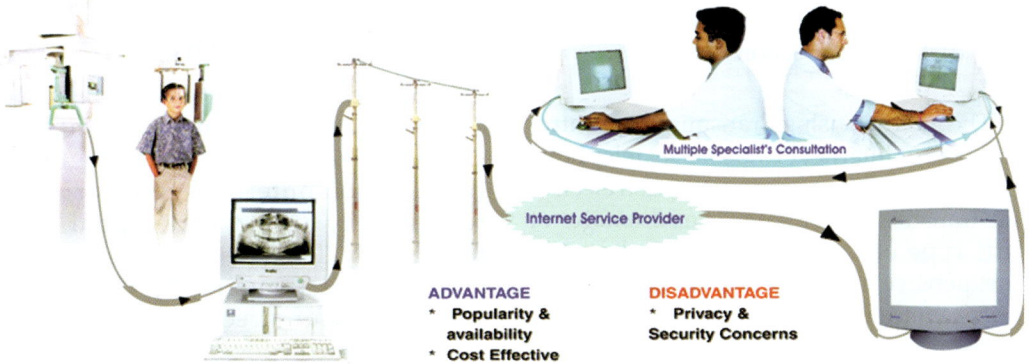

Multiple Specialist's Consultation

Internet Service Provider

ADVANTAGE
* **Popularity & availability**
* **Cost Effective**

DISADVANTAGE
* **Privacy & Security Concerns**

Fig. 13.11: Type 3 – Web based technology.
[Figs 13.9 to 13.11—*Courtesy:* JSS Dental College and Hospital, Mysore]

13

Thus in a LAN, images can be sent from several locations within a building or multiple buildings (Fig. 13.9).

In the above two types of connections only those devices which are connected to the dedicated transmission network can communicate (sending and receiving images).

Wide area network (WAN) connection: WAN consists of many local area networks interconnected to create a super network (Fig. 13.10 and 13.11).

Image transmission: Digital image files may be transmitted over short or long distances using a WAN. The choice of WAN depends upon the type of image, number of images, data transfer rate requirements and financial limitations.

Transmission can be done by telephone lines, fiber-optic or coaxial cables, lasers or microwave transmission links, to communication towers or satellites.

The telephone network can be considered a WAN. It has **advantages** like:

- It is already widely existent
- Transparency of inner working and complexity of networking
- Readily available long and short distance connections
- Low cost

The internet, using Transmission Control Protocol or Internet Protocol over telephone lines can also be used to accomplish electronic transmission of data. The *advantages* of this type of transmission are that it is inexpensive and widely available and the *disadvantage* is the unpredictable speed of transmission.

The speed of transmission can be increased by data compression using compression algorithms.

Digital images may be saved in a variety of file formats in data retrieval systems for future use. The commonly used file format is *Tagged Image Format File (TIFF)*. Two types of hard copy imagers are used commonly. They are:

- A multiformat camera
- A laser printer

As is the case commonly with new technologies and applications of existing technologies, unique medical and ethical implications have arisen with the maturation of teleradiology. These issues include professional licensure, credentials and clinical privileges, liability, doctor-patient relationships, privacy and confidentiality.

The existence and use of teleradiology in the 21st century is given in any field that uses radiographic images for medical diagnosis and treatment. The speed and fidelity of image data transfer are key to the success of any teleradiology program.

All the legal implications of teleradiology in general and in the area of oral radiology may not be addressed; however, teleradiology will soon be the standard method of diagnosis in many practices.

COMPUTED TOMOGRAPHY

Other names for computed tomography are computerized axial tomography (CAT), computerized transaxial tomography (CTAT), computerized reconstruction tomography (CRT) and digital axial tomography (DAT).

Computed tomography (CT) is the combination of direct digital electronic imaging and tomography. In this technique, an X-ray source and electronic detectors positioned opposite to each other move synchronously around the long axis of the patient over a span of 360 degrees to produce images.

Advantages

- *Imaging of hard and soft tissues:* This feature makes CT especially useful when the pathologic process extends beyond the limits of bone into the surrounding soft tissues; soft tissue imaging is not possible in conventional radiography.

- *Differentiates between normal and diseased tissue:* CT can demonstrate minute differences in tissue densities more effectively than conventional radiography.

- *Tomographic sections in axial plane can be made*: CT has the advantage of producing axial cross sectional images routinely over conventional tomography in which only frontal (coronal) and lateral (sagittal) images are possible. Each slice can be viewed individually without superimposition of adjacent structures.

- *Image manipulation and reconstruction is possible:* This can be accomplished in the absence of the patient since all the data are stored in the computer. CT has the ability to reconstruct a sequence of axial images into images of other planes or into 3-D images. The 3-D images can be rotated on the computer screen, color can be added to selected structures and unwanted images can be removed.

- *Contrast CT* can also be made.

Disadvantages

- High cost of the equipment
- Not easily accessible to the patient
- Very thin contiguous or overlapping slices may result in repetition and high radiation dose to the patient

- Metallic objects produce artefacts (restorations)

Head and Neck Applications

- Examination of benign and malignant tumors.
- Tumors and swellings of extra-organ or intra-organ origin of parotid gland.
- Staging of tumors of the maxillary sinus, base of skull, pterygoid region, pharynx, and larynx.
- Evaluation of bony changes affecting the condyle and articular eminence. Images of the articular disc are only moderately well defined but not to the anticipated level.
- Preoperative assessment of the alveolar bone of maxilla and mandible for dental implants.
- Assessment of fractures of facial bones, cranial base and cervical vertebrae.
- Assessment of intracranial diseases, intracranial and spinal cord injury.
- Head and neck infections.

Components

There are three major components which include:
  i. Gantry
 ii. Computer
iii. Operating console

i. Gantry

This comprises of subparts such as:
- X- ray source
- Detector assembly
- High voltage generator
- Patient positioning and supporting unit

X-ray Source

The X-ray source of CT scanners consists of an X-ray generator and an X-ray tube. The

13

X-ray tube has a rotatory anode which has a large focal spot with heating capacity between 1 and 4 MHU (Mega Heat Units). The X-ray generator produces a 400 mA beam at a continuous rate. The X-ray beam is collimated twice, once before it passes through the patient (pre-patient), which reduces the radiation dose to the patient and again at the detector array (post-patient), which reduces the amount of scattered radiation and improves the quality of the image. Co-ordination of pre-patient and post-patient collimators determines the thickness of the image slice.

Detector Assembly

Tremendous advances have been made in the technology of CT. One of the significant advancements is the detector assembly.

Detectors are classified into:
- Scintillation detectors
- Gas detectors

Both the detector systems are 45% efficient in detection with 55% of the remnant X-rays exiting the patient. This contributes to patient dose.

Scintillation Detectors

Previously used detector arrays contained crystal photo-multiplier tube assemblies. These required a power supply for each tube and it was not possible to pack them very tightly together. Recently, they were replaced by crystal-photodiode assemblies. These assemblies are smaller, cheaper, do not require a power supply and are efficient. Early scanners used sodium iodide as the detector. In recent days, bismuth germanate, cesium iodide and cadmium tungstate have been used. Generally, one to eight detectors per centimeter or one to five detectors per degree are used.

Gas Detectors

These are made of a large metallic chamber divided into many small chambers of 1 mm dimension. Each small chamber acts as a separate detector. These chambers are sealed and contain a high atomic number inert gas such as xenon or a xenon-krypton mixture under pressure. Ionization of these gases occurs when they are exposed to X-rays which is proportional to the incident radiation.

ii. Computer

CT requires high-speed computers since each scan requires solving 30,000 equations simultaneously. These computers use an array processor to permit the simultaneous solution of all the equations generated during the scan. The time taken for the production of a visible image of a slice after receiving the data (known as reconstruction time) is about one second. The cost of the computer is approximately one third the cost of a CT scanner.

iii. Operating Console

Most consoles have at least two monitors to allow the radiographer and the radiologist to manipulate the image. Image data are stored in the computer so that images can be reformatted. Data can be stored in magnetic tapes or on discs. CT images are commonly viewed on a film by transferring the electronic data in it using a laser camera. Film size to be used is 14 × 17 inches which accommodates 4 to 15 images.

Procedure/Technique

CT utilizes X-rays to produce slice images as in conventional tomography, but uses very sensitive crystals or gas detectors

13

instead of the radiographic film. The detectors measure the intensity of X-rays exiting from the patient and convert them into digital data, which are stored and can be manipulated by a computer. The digitized information is displayed in gray-scale representing densities of various tissues as a visual image. The usual range of CT image slice thickness varies between 1.5 mm to 6.0 mm.

CT images are made with the patient in a lying down posture, by positioning the part to be examined within the circular gantry which contains the X-ray source and detectors. Depending on the level, thickness and plane, usually axial, the X-ray source rotates around the patient and scans the area of interest. The X-rays generated penetrate the patient and reach a set of detectors depending on the attenuation and penetration profile of the part being examined. Once this is completed the computer calculates the absorption at each point on a matrix formed by the intersection of the generation profiles. A matrix is formed typically by 512 × 512 or 1024 × 1024 pixels. As the size of the pixels decreases, the resolution of the image increases. Each pixel has a volume known as *voxel*, which depends on the selection of thickness of the tomographic slice. Depending on the amount of absorption within that area of tissue, each voxel is given a number between +1000 and −1000 known as CT number. Some scanners can differentiate sign between CT numbers that range from 2000 to + 6000. Each CT number produces a different scale of gray and produces a visual image. Selected images are photographed to produce a copy of pictures. The presence of metallic restorations can produce significant artefacts in a scan of the head and neck region.

The information gained from the original axial scan can be manipulated to reconstruct images in the coronal, sagittal or any other plane as necessary or to construct 3-D images.

Image Characteristics

The image characteristics of CT images are different from other plain film images because the image receptor is not a film but a direct digital sensor. The image characteristics for film based images are based on H and D curve. The H and D curve indicates that a loss of contrast occurs at extremes of density. The image receptors used in CT have a linear response to exposure. Thus images at the extremes of density can be visualized with CT when they would not be visible in a film based image.

The parameters used to evaluate the quality of any digital image are spatial and contrast resolution, linearity and noise.

Spatial Resolution

It describes the ability to discriminate between two objects that are close together. For CT images spatial resolution could be defined by pixel size whereas for conventional films spatial resolution is described in terms of line pairs per millimeter.

The modulation transfer function (MTF) defines spatial resolution for CT and is used to determine the limit of a system's ability to provide an accurate representation of the image.

Contrast Resolution

What CT lacks in terms of spatial resolution, it more than makes up for with contrast resolution. Contrast resolution is the ability to discriminate between small differences in density. Modern CT units can image up to

13

8000 different densities (Hounsfield units) in a single view. The process called *windowing* allows these subtle differences to be amplified.

Linearity

It refers to the ability of the CT system to assign CT numbers accurately to known structures in an image. Linearity is determined by plotting the linear attenuation coefficients of known structures against their known CT numbers. The line generated should be straight and intersect '0' (Water) for the CT unit to be functioning properly.

Noise

Noise degrades the quality of an image. It is defined as a fluctuation in the optical density of the image. Many factors such as pixel size, detector efficiency, slice thickness and radiation dose to the patient affect the amount of noise in an image. Noise also affects contrast and spatial resolution.

Patient Exposure to Radiation

CT is considered a high radiation dose technique. Several parameters affect the patient dose. These include the region being imaged, number of slices, slice thickness, pitch and kVp. The effective dose has been calculated as 2 to 4 mSv for a head scan and 5 to 15 mSv for a body scan.

Image Reconstruction

This is a complex procedure that is performed by the computer system of the CT scanner. Several different algorithms are used to reconstruct CT images: back projection, iterative reconstruction and analytical reconstruction.

Back projection reconstruction also known as summation reconstruction is no longer used. Iterative reconstruction came into being when CT scans became faster and not every area of interest was imaged. The iterative methods can be used to calculate values mathematically for missing data. The analytical methods were developed as a result of mathematical shortcomings of the iterative methods. These methods use complex mathematical equations to address minute variations in tissue density when data is missing.

Image Enhancement Tools

CT images can be viewed in different orientations and with different density parameters with the use of the same data set. All images are acquired from an axial orientation. Three dimensional reconstructions can be used to show only the surface of the object-surface rendering or the relationship of the object to the surrounding structures. Volumetric reconstructions or 3-D reconstructions require thin slices and are sensitive to patient movement. A different form of reconstruction is used for implant site assessment.

Windows and Levels

The ability to view a CT image using different ranges of density can be achieved through the process of *windowing* of an image. It allows the operator to select the range of densities to be viewed (window level) and the number of gray levels to be viewed (window width). Soft tissue and bone windows are frequently used in CT images. The components of the regions being imaged are used to determine window width. For example, a narrow width is used to image the brain whereas a wide window width is indicated for evaluation of bony pathology. Contrast media can be used to enhance subtle differences in density in some situations. A contrast medium is commonly used to enhance the vasculature of a structure. In these instances, an iodine-based contrast medium or the compound meglumine glycate is used. A typical head scan with contrast uses approximately 120 ml of contrast medium. Less contrast medium is needed with spiral CT.

Artefacts

Some artefacts are specific to the type of CT system, for example, ring artefact with third generation scanners, whereas others are products of the objects being imaged. Common artefacts are motion, partial volume, beam hardening, metallic objects and stair step.

Motion: Patient movement and faster patient couch movement can cause distortion of images of the structure of interest. Some electron beam CT scans (EBCT) are so fast that the pulsation of blood vessel can be captured, which may sometimes be misinterpreted as stenosis.

Partial volume: They have the greatest impact at the interface between two high contrast objects. Objects smaller than the size of a pixel (or voxel) cannot be imaged accurately. The effects of partial volume averaging can be minimized by using thin slices and then combining those slices or by changing the plane of reconstruction. However, it is important to remember that the use of thinner slices increases radiation dose to the patient.

Beam hardening: The thick bone in the cranium acts as a filter that removes lower energy. The resultant beam is actually more energetic and generates a false lower attenuation coefficient for the tissue traversed by it. Beam hardening can produce streaking, a dark ring adjacent to the center of the image.

Metallic objects: These are commonly encountered when imaging the head and neck with CT. These artefacts appear as a streak or a star and result from scattered radiation.

Stair step: This artefact is specific for spiral CT. It is more apparent when linear structures such as blood vessels are imaged.

GENERATIONS OF CT

The operation mode of CT has developed through four generations. The first and second generations are no longer produced.

First Generation

This utilized a finely collimated pencil shaped X-ray beam and a single detector. This assembly translates across the patient and rotates between successive translations. The scan requires 180° translations each separated by one degree rotation. The major drawback of this generation was that it required five minutes to produce one scan.

Second Generation

This is also a translating rotate type. This utilizes a fan shaped X-ray beam instead of a pencil beam and multiple (5 to 30) detectors. A single translation results in the same number of data points due to multiple detector arrays. So each translation is separated by five degrees or more as compared to the 1st generation where each translation is separated by one degree. This results in a reduced number of translations required to produce a scan and thus saves time. The use of multiple detectors increases the quality of image. This generation required 20 seconds or more to produce one scan. The image quality is not significantly improved compared to the 1st generation due to increased scattered radiation by the fan beam.

Third Generation

The X-ray tube and detector array rotate concentrically around the patient but there is no translational movement. This employs a curvilinear detector array which contains at least 30 detectors and a fan beam. The number of detectors and width of the fan beam are larger than in the second generation and encompass the whole body of the patient at all times. The time required for each scan is as low as one second. The disadvantage of this generation is the occasional appearance of the ring artefact.

Fourth Generation

In this generation, as in the third generation, the only motion is rotation. The X-ray source rotates but the detector assembly does not. A fixed circular array of detectors containing as many as 1000 individual elements detects the radiation. The fan-shaped X-ray beam remains similar to the one in the 3rd generation. These units are capable of producing one scan per second and do not have the drawback of the ring artefact. The disadvantages of these units are higher radiation dose to the patient as compared to previous three generations and a higher cost of equipment.

SPECT or Single Photon Emission Computed Tomography

SPECT or single photon emission computed tomography is a recently developed technique that involves a gamma camera that rotates around a patient, generating circumferential projections. SPECT is used to assess condylar activity, carcinomas and in facial imaging protocols.

Helical or spiral CT is a variation of the fourth generation scanners. The principal difference is that the patient couch moves continuously during image acquisition.

Multislice spiral CT overcomes the limitations of spiral CT but complicates fan beam reconstruction techniques by adding a divergence of the fan beam along the longitudinal axis (Z-axis).

Electron Beam CT (EBCT) can produce a scan in as little as 50 milliseconds. The principal applications of EBCT are cardiac studies. EBCT differs from other CT techniques in that it contains no moving parts. The limiting factor in EBCT is the speed of data processing rather than the heating capacity of the X-ray source.

Localized CT or micro CT is based on the same principles as CT; however sampling volume and reconstruction of cross-sections are more relevant to dental applications.

PET-CT is a unique combination of cross-sectional details provided by CT and metabolic inflammation provided by PET. It has revolutionized detection work-up further. PET-CT has a single tube with a combined gantry of CT and PET.

The development of stereolithography (rapid prototyping or RP) to make plastic models of the skull has made it possible to reproduce more complex structures. Plastic models may make 3-D analysis of facial bones easier than it is from CT reconstructions (Fig. 13.12).

Optical Coherence Tomography (OCT)

Here, cross-sectional images of tissues are generated using a near infrared light source. This light is able to penetrate tissue without biologically harmful effects. Differences in the reflection of light are used to generate a signal that corresponds to the morphology and composition of the underlying tissues.

Tuned Aperture Computed Tomography (TACT)

This is a three-dimensional radiographic data acquisition technique based on the optical aperture theory, which extends and completely generalizes the better known laminographic process termed tomosynthesis. This technology can accommodate patient movement between exposures with no appreciable effect on image quality or projection accuracy underlying the resulting 3-D display.

Fifth Generation

It is under development with innovative modifications.

CONE BEAM COMPUTED TOMOGRAPHY (CBCT)

Cone beam computed tomography is a fast emerging imaging modality, which shows much promise in the field of oral diagnostics. It uses a cone-shaped beam of X-rays, as opposed to the fan-shaped beam used in conventional computed tomography (CT). CBCT utilizes an X-ray tube and a flat detector placed opposing each other. The conical beam rotates 360° around the patient, generating an image for each degree of rotation (i.e. a series of 360 images). The X-rays are detected by the detector, transmitted by a high-resolution charge-coupled device camera, and reconstituted with a digital processor. A three-dimensional view of the part being examined is thus obtained. Depending on the

13

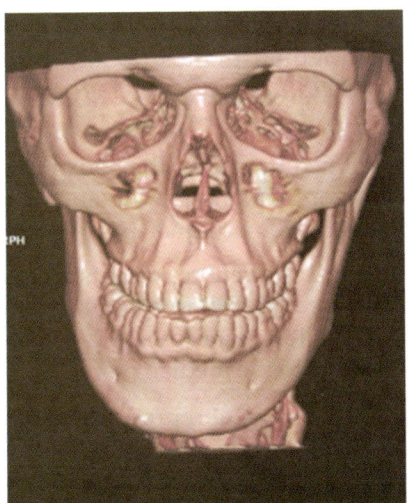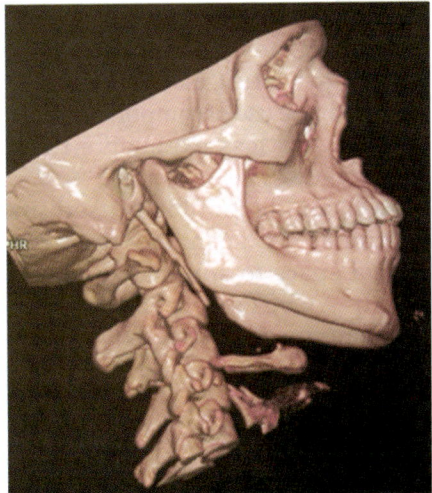

Fig. 13.12: 3D CT of skull. [*Courtesy:* JSS Dental College and Hospital, Mysore]

equipment, scan times range from 17 seconds to a little over one minute. Final images may be printed on a 1:1 scale. CBCT images have been shown to be fairly accurate when compared with anatomical structures.

Advantages

- A major advantage of cone beam CT over conventional CT is its higher spatial resolution.
- Mean skin dose with CBCT has been found to be comparable with intraoral or panoramic examination, which is a fraction of the exposure received during a CT scan.
- A CBCT scanner requires far less electrical energy for its operation. It utilizes a two-dimensional, or panel, detector, which allows for a single rotation of the gantry to generate a scan of the entire head. Reduction in the number of rotations makes CBCT much more cost-effective than conventional CT.
- The use of a cone beam instead of a fan beam significantly increases X-ray utilization. Cone beam technology employs X-rays much more efficiently, and allows for the use of components that are smaller and less expensive than conventional CT.
- The fan-beam technology used in conventional CT scanners requires significant space to spiral around the entire body. A CBCT scanner on the other hand requires much less space.

Applications

The combination of plain X-ray transmission projections and panoramic radiography is adequate in many uncomplicated clinical situations; however, CBCT adds the third dimension for better exploration. This imaging system can evaluate various radiolucent, radiopaque and mixed density lesions at various locations in the maxillofacial complex. A complete view of all oral and maxillofacial structures is possible, providing the clinician with thorough diagnostic information. A series of cases is presented to illustrate the benefits of this imaging system.

Before exploring various CBCT clinical applications, it is important to understand various preset formats that can be applied through CBCT software. Once a scan is complete, the data can be reconstructed to produce two-dimensional views of three-dimensional images using programmed presets. A variety of renderings can be viewed including: Soft tissue, hard tissue, maximum intensity projection (MIP) and Ray Sum. Programmed presets range from full cranial views to temporomandibular joint (TMJ) views.

The volumetric data set is presented to the clinician on the computer screen as secondary reconstructed images in three orthogonal planes (axial, sagittal, and coronal).

An **axial view** represents a cross-section obtained by slicing the body structure in a horizontal plane, i.e. a plane, which intersects the longitudinal axis at a right angle.

A **sagittal view** represents a cross-section obtained by slicing anatomic structures in the sagittal plane, which is a vertical plane parallel to the median plane.

A **coronal view** represents a cross-section attained by slicing any anatomic structure in the coronal or frontal plane, which is a vertical plane perpendicular to the median or sagittal plane.

13

Most CBCT software provides for various non-axial two-dimensional images, referred to as multiplanar reformation (MPR). Such MPR modes include oblique (used for two-dimensional reformatted panoramic images), and curved planar reformation and serial transplanar reformation. Cross-sections can be viewed along the maxillary or mandibular arch. Section thickness can be varied from 0.1 mm to 40 mm. All images are scaled at a 1:1 ratio with 0.1 mm of precision for measurement and analysis purposes. Images are reconstructed directly into a standard digitally compatible (DICOM) format for easy transfer to other practitioners and software programs. Three-dimensional virtual models can be created by volume rendering for thorough image analysis and surgical planning. Indirect volume rendering, called segmentation, is technically demanding and compu-tationally difficult but provides volumetric surface reconstruction with depth. Direct volume rendering, also called maximum intensity projection, is simpler but does not give detailed information.

The cases presented here were scanned with I-Cat CBCT machine at higher resolution, 0.20 mm voxel sizes and 120 kVp. The I-Cat software was used to create orthogonal views consisting of axial, coronal and sagittal views, multiplanar views like reformatted panoramic view, and the corresponding cross-sectional views. A three-dimensional virtual model was created using 3D volume surface rendering with Dolphin imaging 3D software. This software provides tools for onscreen manipulation, segmentation and analysis of volumetric datasets.

In a clinical setup, CBCT can be used frequently for localization of impacted teeth,

placement of dental implants, assessment of various pathological lesions and TMJ evaluation.

Localization of Impacted Teeth

Impacted teeth generally present a challenge to the clinician. They vary greatly in their inclination and approximation to various anatomical features such as the inferior alveolar canal, the lower border of the mandible (mandibular teeth) and the maxillary sinus (maxillary teeth). They may also cause resorption of adjacent teeth and may undergo cystic changes. Maxillary cuspids are the most frequently impacted teeth after the third molars, with a prevalence ranging from approximately 1% to 3%. Orthodontic-surgical management of impacted maxillary or mandibular cuspids requires an accurate diagnosis and localization.

Case 1: *Localization of impacted mandibular cuspids*

A 12-year old female was evaluated for impacted mandibular cuspids. A review of the CBCT scan provided information about cystic degeneration of the enlarged follicle of a left horizontally impacted mandibular cuspid and resorption and thinning of the facial cortex (Figs 13.13, 13.14A, B, C, 13.15, 13.16).

Case 2: *Localization of impacted maxillary and mandibular third molars and inferior alveolar canal*

The relationship of right maxillary third molar roots with the floor of the maxillary sinus and relationship of mandibular molars with the inferior alveolar canal and lower border of mandible is being assessed. The radiopaque lesion posterior to the left

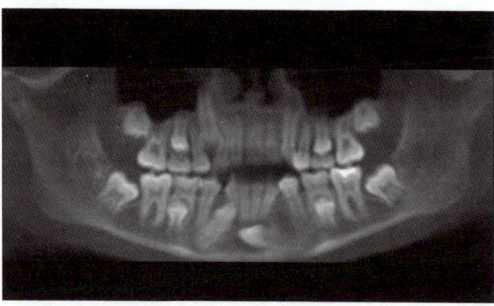

Fig. 13.13: Reformatted panoramic view (10.8 mm thick layer) showing impacted mandibular right and left cuspids

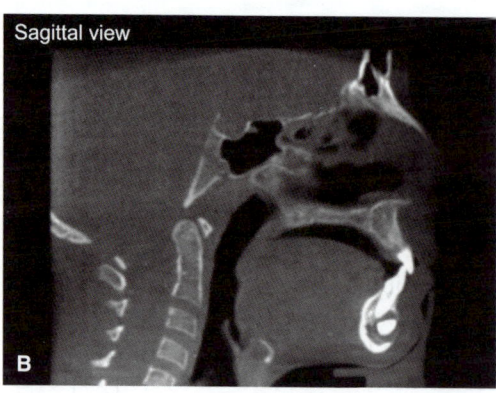

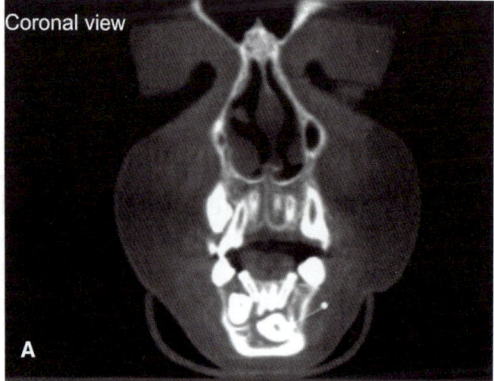

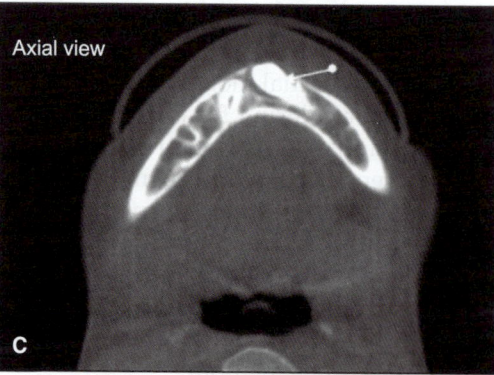

Figs 13.14A to C: Multiplanar reformatted view showing mandibular left canine with enlarged follicle (C, arrow) causing resorption of facial cortex (B), mandibular right cuspid causing tilting and resorption of mandibular right lateral incisor (A)

mandibular third molar is also evaluated (Figs 13.17, 13.18A, B, C, 13.19 to 13.21).

Placement of Dental Implants

The dental implant is a successful treatment modality. A conventional panoramic radiograph can be considered as the basic image in this context. However, the ortho-gonal views, and reformatted panoramic and cross-sectional views of alveolar bone height, width, and angulation generated by CBCT are useful.

Case 3: *Implant site assessment*

A 31-year old female complained of a persistent, annoying, dull ache in the area of the right mandibular first molar since the time the implants were placed two months earlier. Her postoperative conventional radiographic survey had shown the implants and the adjacent teeth to be within normal limits (Figs 13.22, 13.23A, B, C, 13.24 to 13.27).

The initial utilization of this tool in the preoperative planning stage increases the

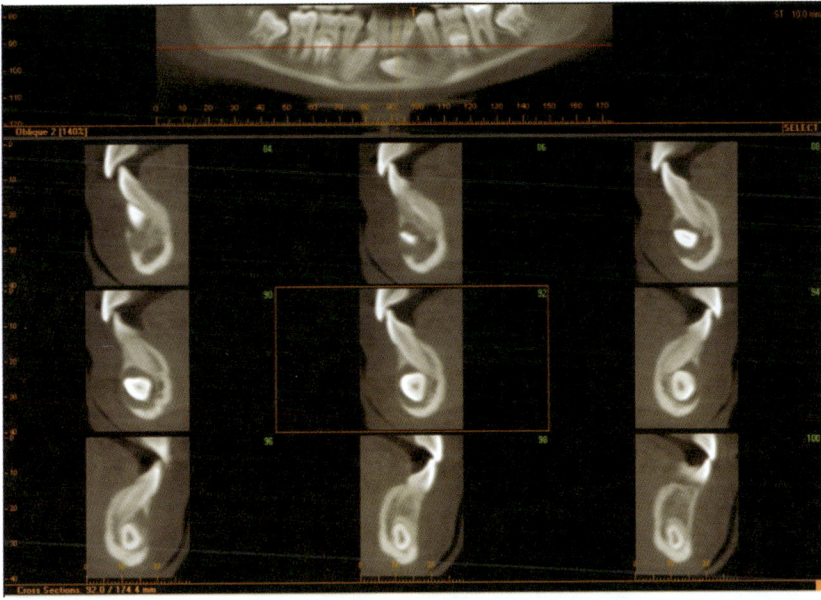

Fig. 13.15: Reformatted panoramic view with dotted red line corresponding with cross-sections of crown of mandibular left cuspid. Note the enlarged follicle and resorption of facial cortex

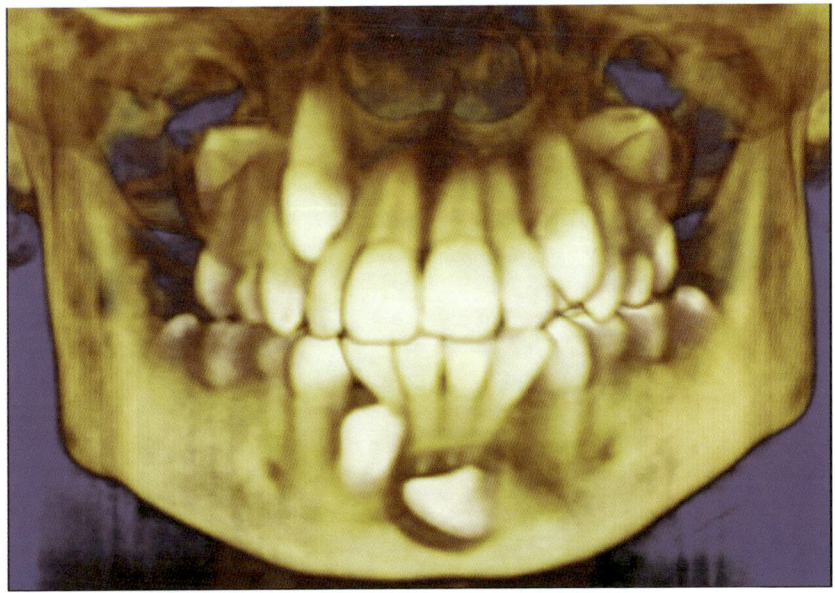

Fig. 13.16: Volume rendered 3D virtual model; frontal view showing impacted mandibular cuspids. Enlarged follicle associated with left mandibular cuspid gives impression of cystic degeneration. Right mandibular cuspid causing tilting and resorption of root of left mandibular right lateral incisor

13

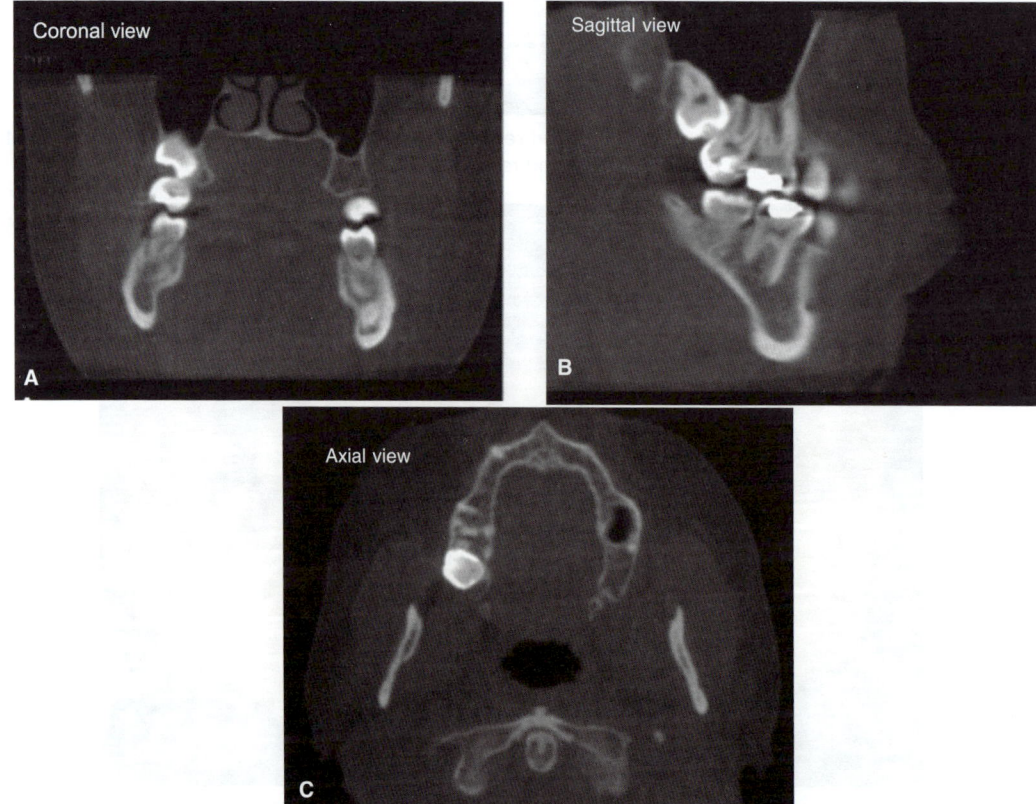

Fig. 13.17: Reformatted panoramic view (10.8 mm thick layer) showing impacted maxillary right and mandibular right and left third molars. Note a radiopaque lesion posterior to left mandibular third molar

Figs 13.18A to C: Multiplanar reformatted view: coronal and sagittal view showing the maxillary right third molar in close approximation to the floor of maxillary sinus

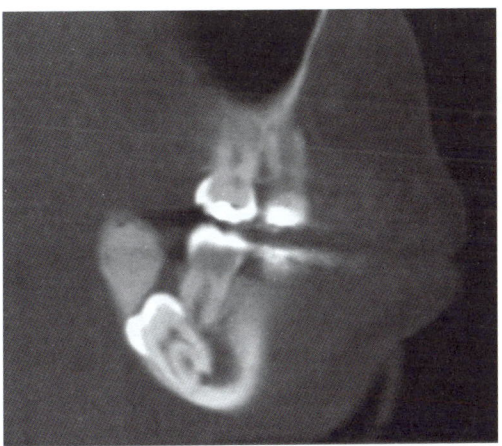

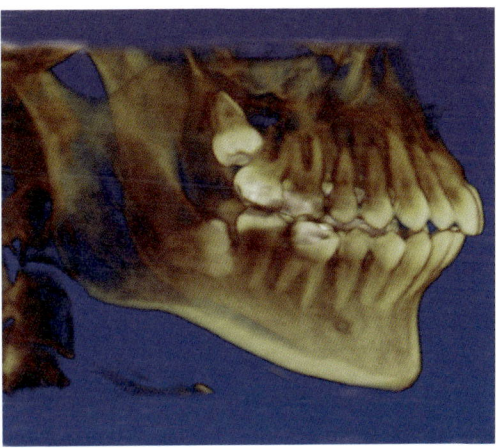

Fig. 13.19: Left sagittal view showing distoangular impacted mandibular left molar near to the lower border of mandible. Note a dense radiopaque lesion occluding the path of eruption of third molar, lying coronal to the impacted tooth and approximating the alveolar crest

Fig. 13.20: Volume rendered 3D virtual model; right sagittal view showing impacted maxillary and mandibular right third molars

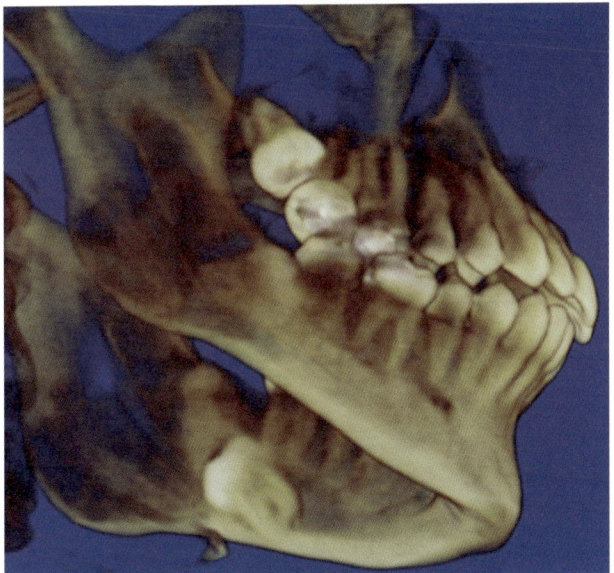

Fig. 13.21: Volume rendered 3D virtual model; left lateral oblique view showing impacted mandibular left molar and radiopaque lesion occluding its path of eruption, displacing it to the lower border of the mandible

13

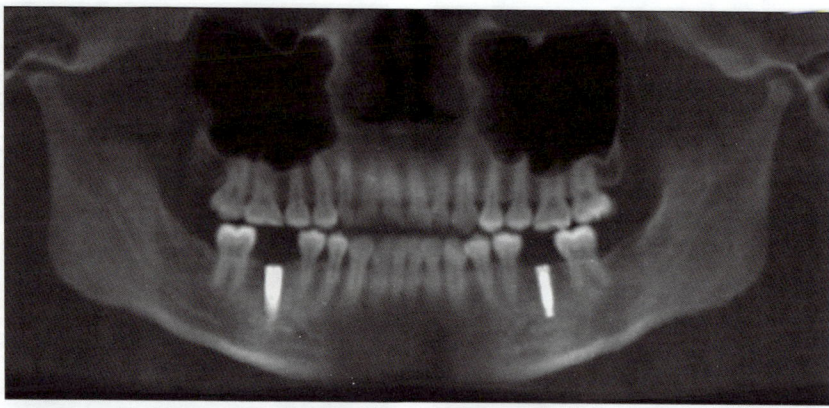

Fig. 13.22: Reformatted panoramic view (10.8 mm thick layer) showing right and left implants in place of extraction spaces of mandibular first molars. The implants seem to be placed appropriately and doing well

13

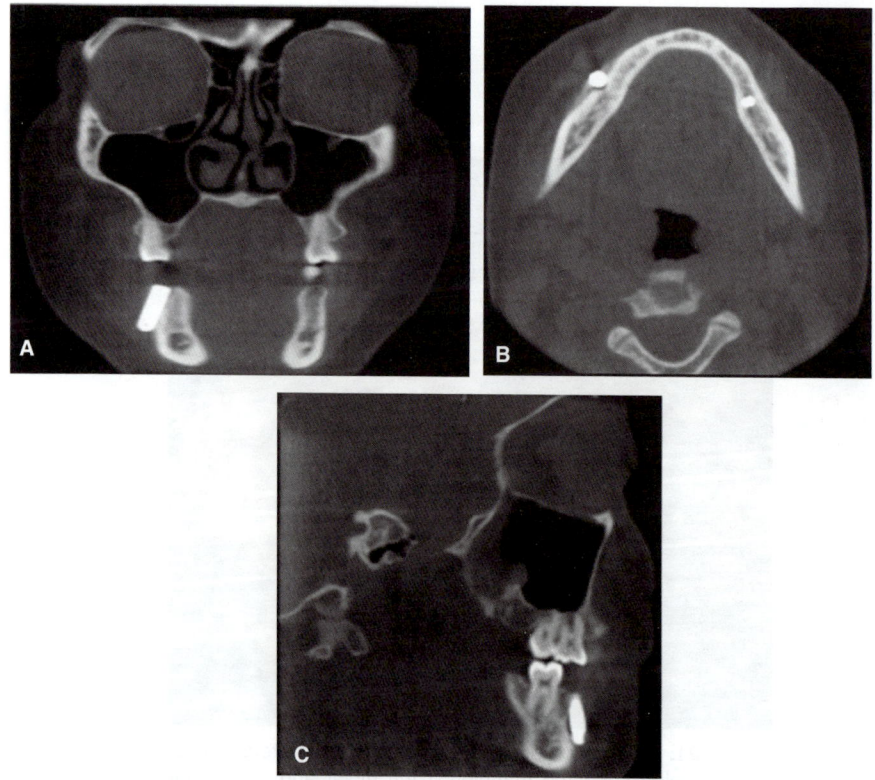

Figs 13.23A to C: Multiplanar reformatted view showing the right implant perforating the facial cortex and lying in soft tissue

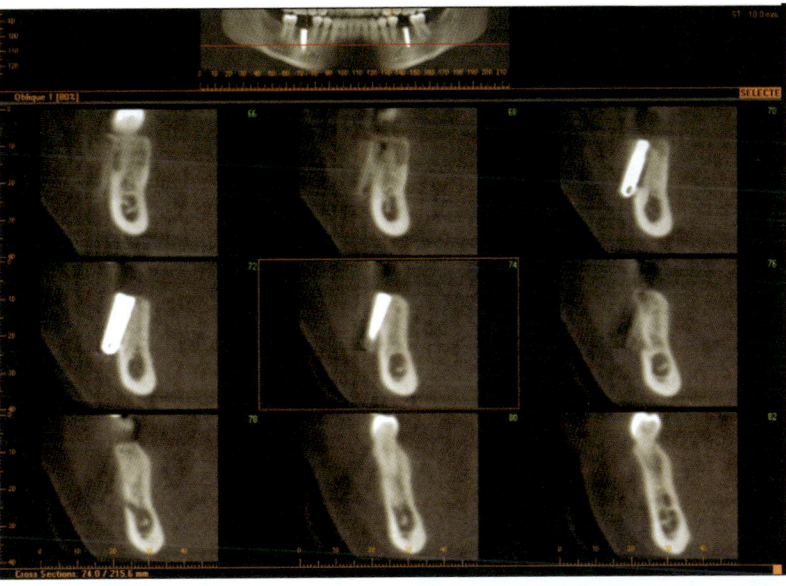

Fig. 13.24: Reformatted panoramic view with dotted red line corresponding with cross-sections of right mandibular implant showing perforation of facial cortex

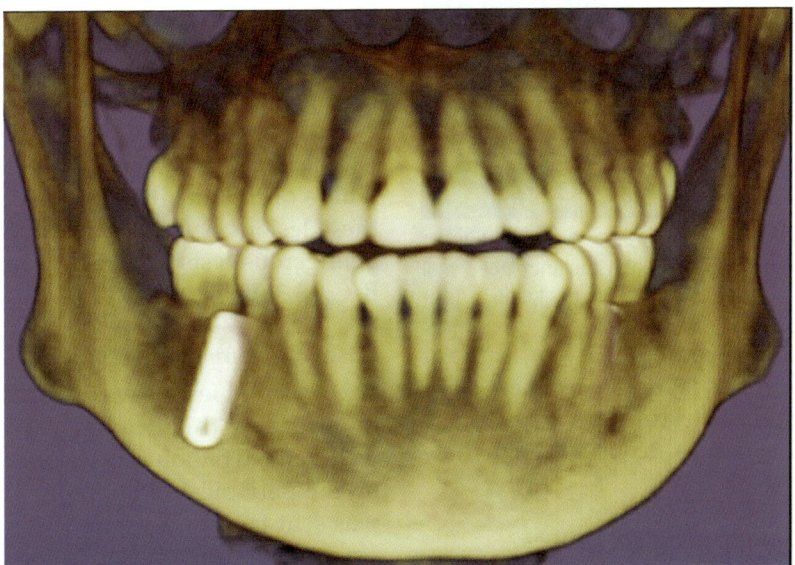

Fig. 13.25: Volume rendered 3D virtual model; frontal view showing right dental implant lying on the surface of mandibular bone

13

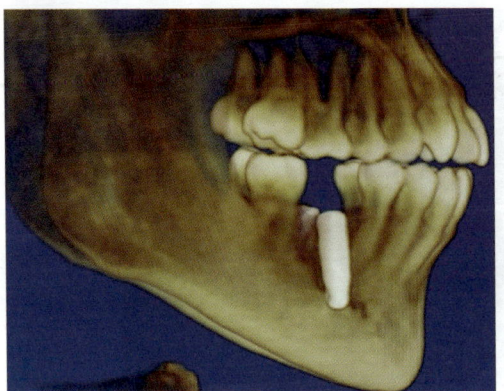

Fig. 13.26: Volume rendered 3D virtual model; right sagittal view showing perforation of facial cortex

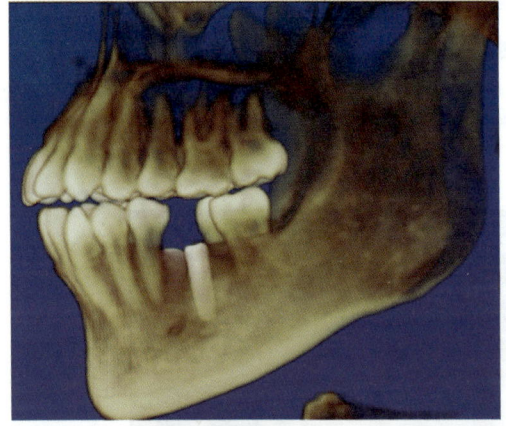

Fig. 13.27: Volume rendered 3D virtual model; left sagittal view showing left dental implant placed well within the bone. Compare it to the right side

accuracy and predictability of implant orientation at less favorable recipient sites. A more favorable implant position is assured if the tissues are visualized in three dimensions.

Evaluation of Pathological Lesions

Two-dimensional radiographs are of limited value in the detection of the borders of osseous lesions. The radiographic depiction of lesions of the alveolar bone depends on adjacent teeth complexity, superimposition of bilateral structures and projection geometry. Benign and malignant lesions, various diseases of bone and metabolic conditions manifesting in the jaws could be evaluated using CBCT. Cross-sectional imaging provides insight into the lesion and helps the clinician determine its accurate definition and the effect it may have on the surrounding structures.

Cysts of the Jaws

Case 4: *Multiple radiolucent lesions*
A 57-year old male patient with a chronic dull ache of both the jaws was evaluated. A conventional panoramic radiograph showed two large mandibular posterior lesions but did not reveal much information about the soft tissue density in the left maxillary sinus. A CBCT scan on this patient revealed the borders of the mandibular lesions more clearly and a third maxillary cystic lesion surrounding the crown of the left maxillary third molar and filling up the whole of the maxillary sinus. On biopsy these lesions were diagnosed as multiple dentigerous cysts (Figs 13.28, 13.29, 13.30A, B, C, 13.31).

Case 5: *Solitary radiolucent lesion*
A 21-year old female was evaluated for left mandibular third molar extraction. A well-defined radiolucent lesion was sighted on the periapical radiograph. The patient was sent for CBCT examination. The cyst was curetted and on biopsy, the lesion was diagnosed as an odontogenic keratocyst (Figs 13.32, 13.33A, B, C, 13.34 and 13.35).

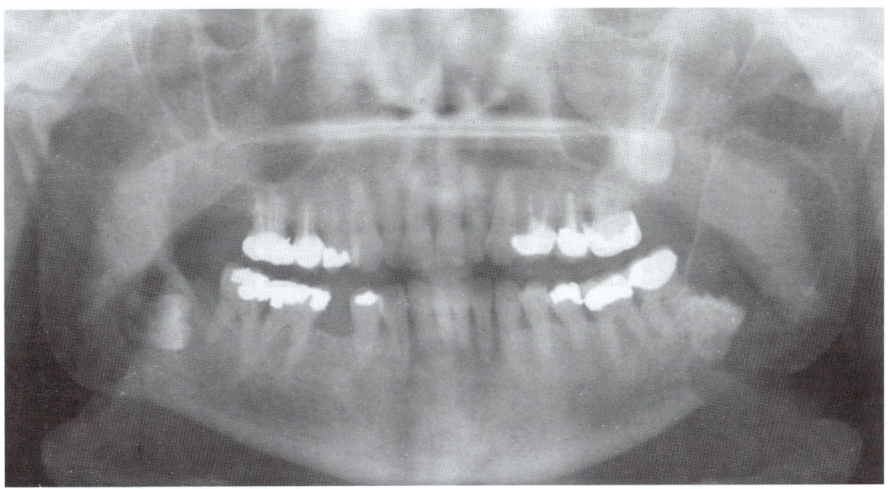

Fig. 13.28

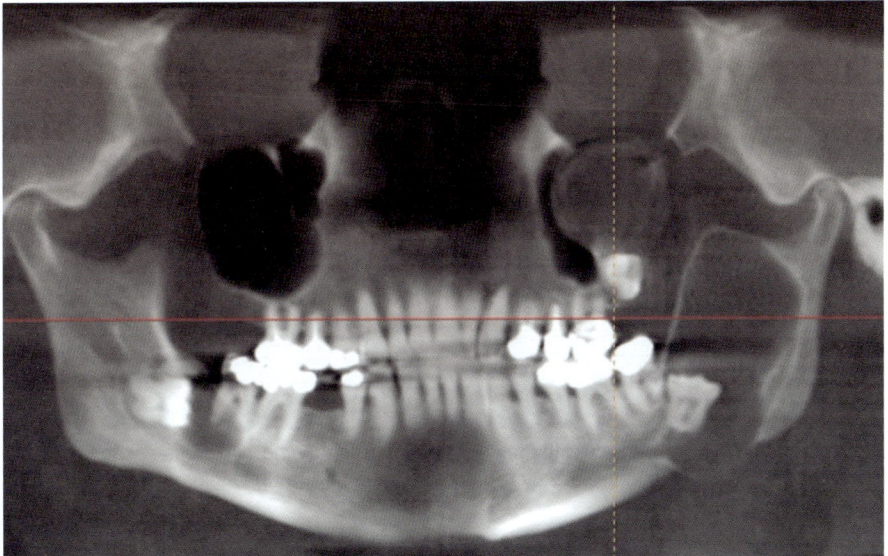

13

Fig. 13.29

Figs 13.28 and 13.29: Conventional panoramic radiograph showing large radiolucent lesions associated with impacted mandibular right and left third molars. Also note radiopacity associated with impacted maxillary left third molar; compare it to reformatted panoramic view in Figure 13.29 where left relative radiopaque lesion is defined more clearly associated with impacted maxillary third molar, filling up whole of maxillary sinus

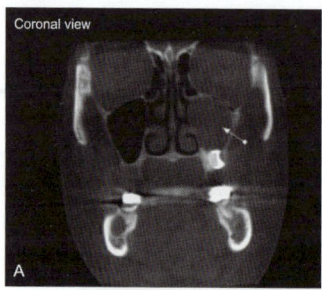 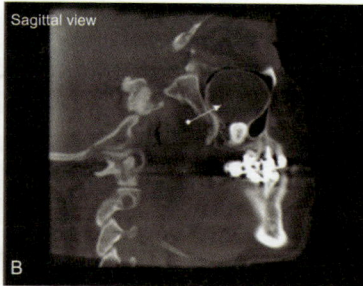 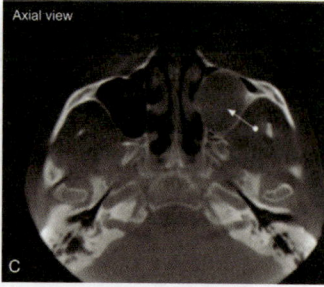

Figs 13.30A to C: Multiplanar reformatted view showing the left maxillary lesion surrounding the crown of impacted molar and filling up whole of the maxillary sinus

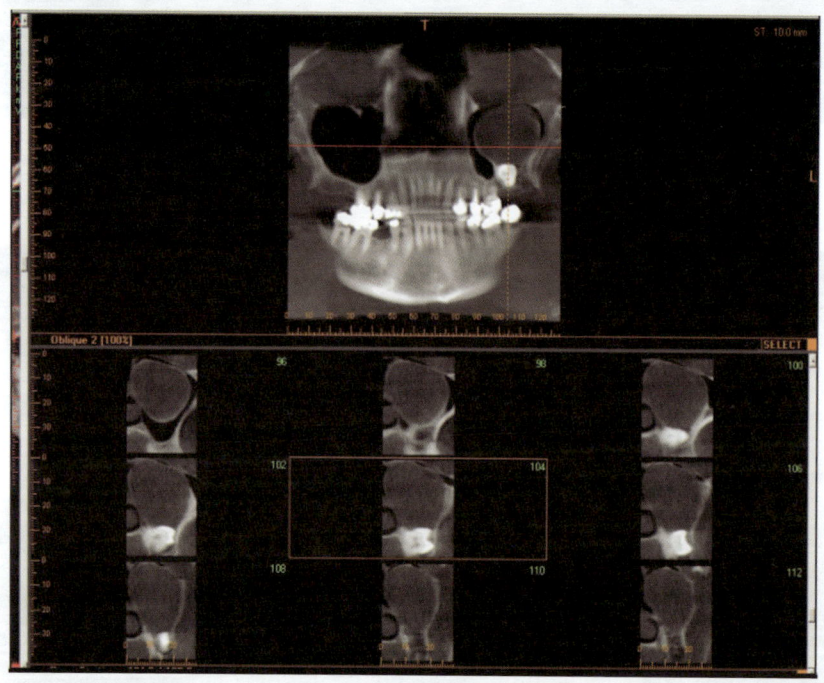

Fig. 13.31: Reformatted panoramic view with dotted red line corresponding with cross-sections of left maxillary lesion showing rounded well defined relatively radiopaque lesion filling up whole of maxillary sinus

Benign Tumors of Jaws

Case 6: *Expansile radiolucent lesion*

A 58-year old African-American female was evaluated for a continuously enlarging right mandible. The case was diagnosed as unicystic ameloblastoma after biopsy (Figs 13.36, 13.37A, B, C, 13.38).

Case 7: *Mixed density lesion*

A 53-year old Hispanic man presented with a mixed, well-defined, corticated lesion in

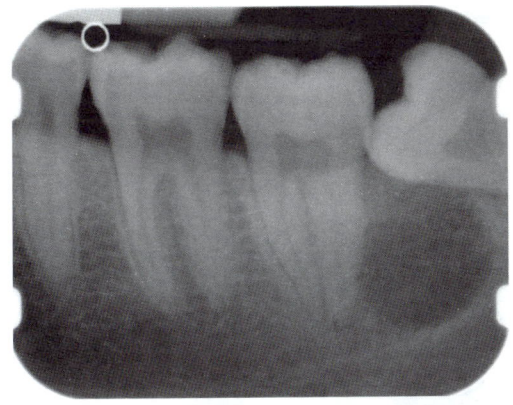

Fig. 13.32: Conventional periapical view showing a well-defined rounded radiolucent lesion between left mandibular second and mesially inclined impacted third molar

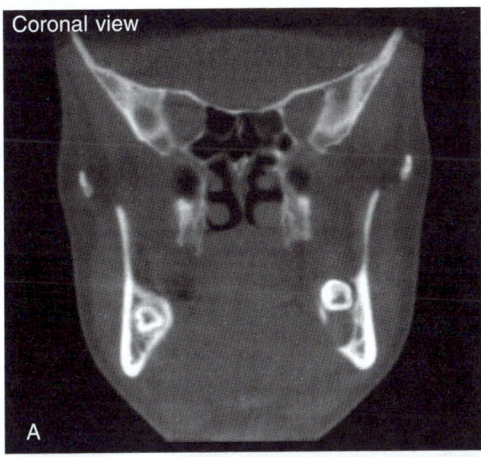

Coronal view

A

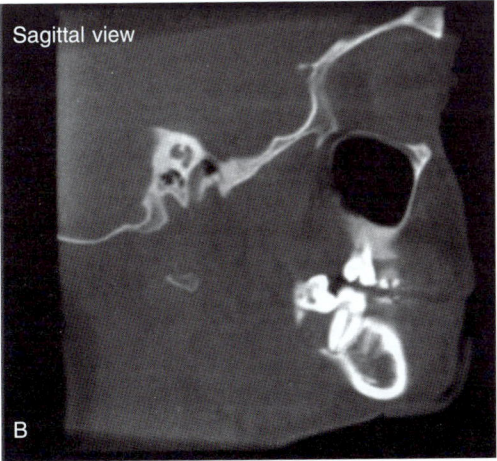

Sagittal view

B

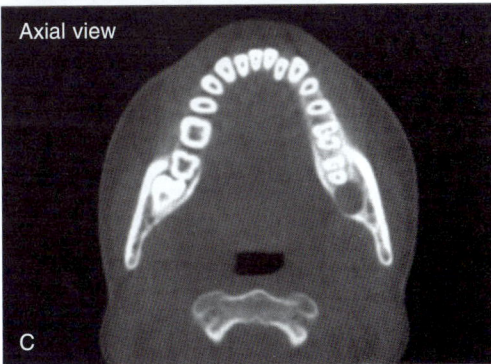

Axial view

C

Figs 13.33A to C: Multiplanar reformatted view showing well-defined radiolucent lesion causing resorption and thinning of lingual cortex

13

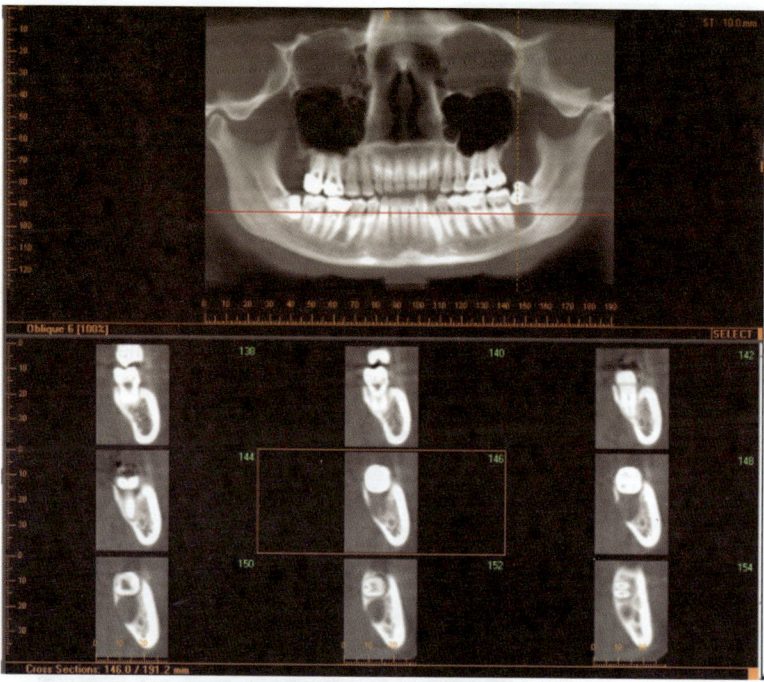

Fig. 13.34: Reformatted panoramic view (10 mm thick section) with dotted red line corresponding with cross-sections of radiolucent lesion showing perforation of lingual cortex

13

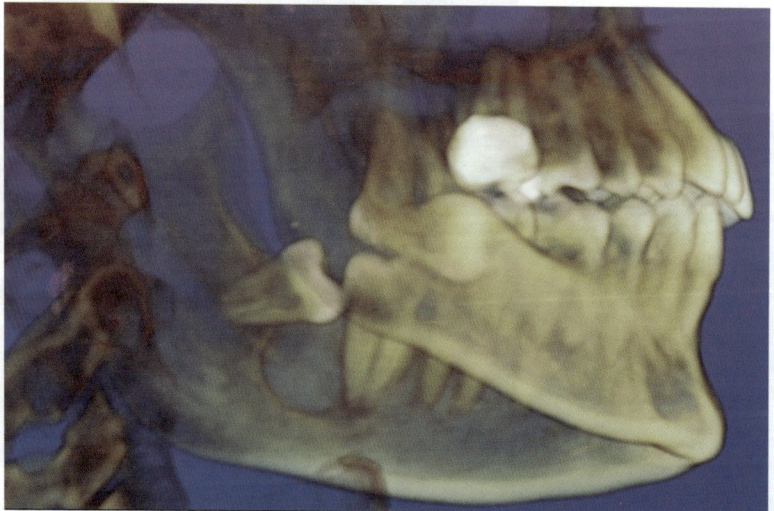

Fig. 13.35: Volume rendered 3D virtual model; left lateral oblique view showing well-defined borders and its relation to the associated teeth

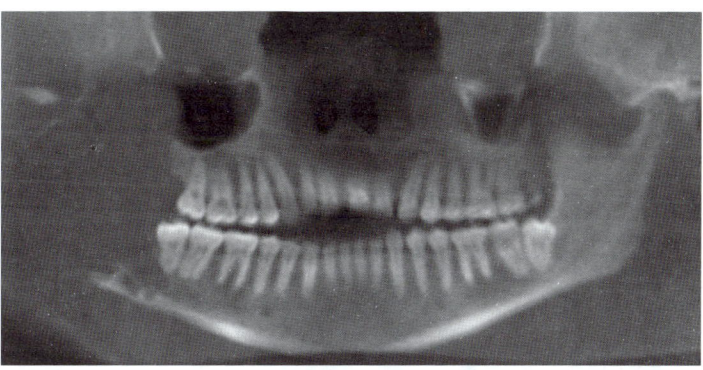

Fig. 13.36: Reformatted panoramic view showing expansile large radiolucent lesion of posterior right mandible. The posterior and anterior walls of the right ramus along with the right condyle and coronoid processes cannot be seen. The borders of the lesion cannot be delineated

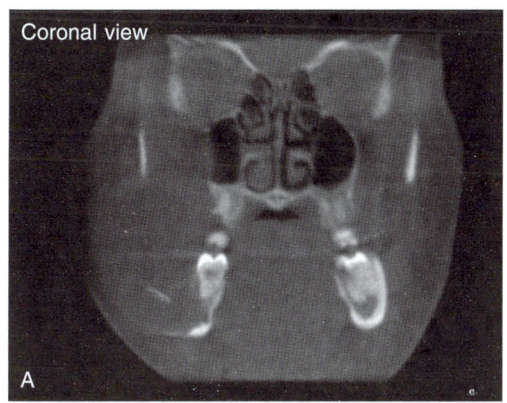

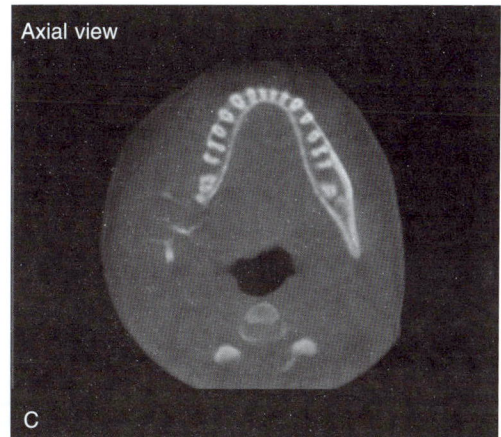

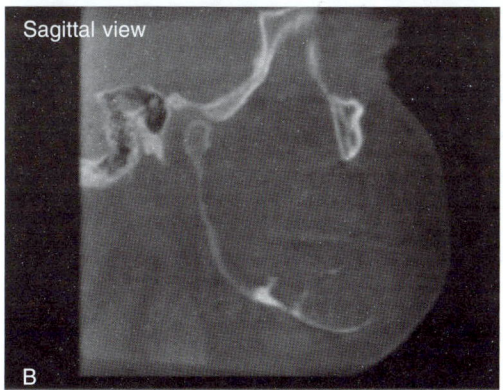

Figs 13.37A to C: Multiplanar reformatted view; axial and coronal views showing expansile large radiolucent lesion extending posteriorly from mesial of mandibular right first molar to right condyle and coronoid process involving the whole of ramus. The posterior wall of ramus which was not visible in other views can be delineated in sagittal view. It is thinned and resorbed by the expanding lesion and there is some evidence of coarse and curved septa formation in the anterior part of lesion creating internal compartments

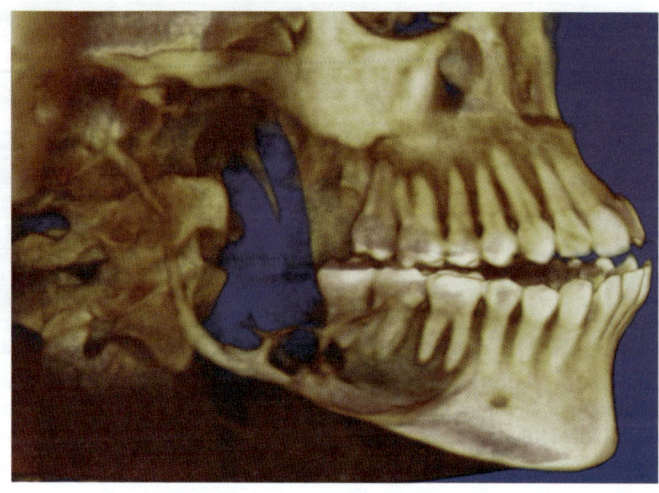

Fig. 13.38: Volume rendered 3D virtual model; right sagittal view. Showing complete destruction of right mandibular posterior body and ramus of mandible with condyle and coronoid processes. Also note the bony septa creating internal compartments. Posterior border of the ramus is thinned and resorbed and show evidence of pathological fracture. Tumor seems to have infiltrated in the zygomatic process and glenoid fossa too

the right maxilla. Mucous retention phenomenon was noted as an incidental finding. Pathological diagnosis of this lesion was established as Pindborg tumor or calcifying epithelial odontogenic tumor (Figs 13.39A, B, C, 13.40, 13.41).

Case 8: *Radiopaque lesion*
A relatively radiopaque lesion may be a complex odontoma, impeding the eruption of the mandibular right second molar and pushing it to the lower border of the mandible (Figs 13.42, 13.43A, B, C).

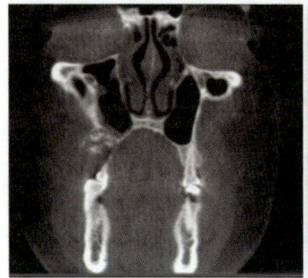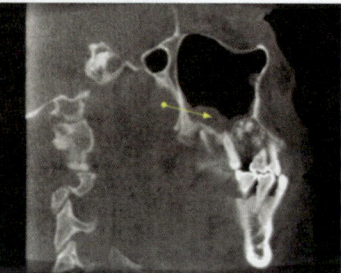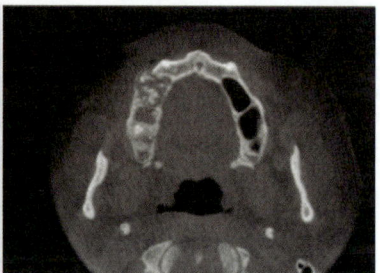

A. Coronal view   B. Sagittal view   C. Axial view

Fig. 13.39: Multiplanar reformatted view showing mixed density expansile maxillary lesion causing thinning and resorption of buccal cortex and extending superiorly in the sinus. Floor of sinus is intact. Also note mucous retention phenomenon in right maxillary sinus, an incidental finding (arrow) in sagittal section

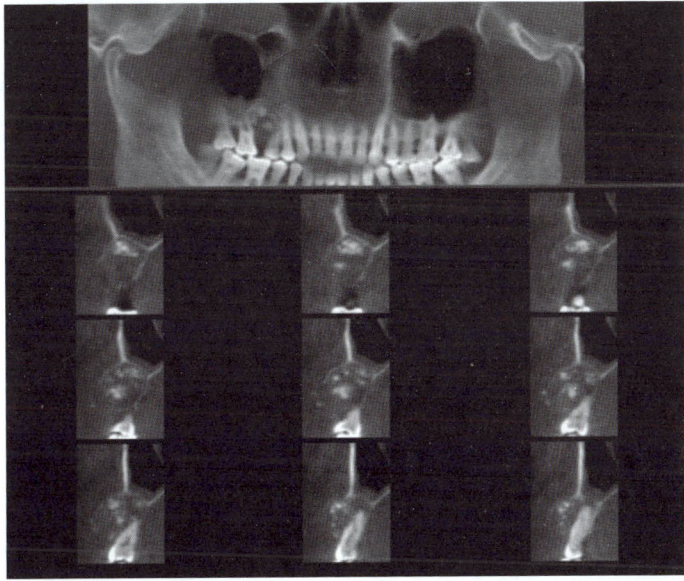

Fig. 13.40: Reformatted panoramic view (10 mm thick section) corresponding with cross-sections of well-defined mixed density lesion with various amounts of internal calcifications

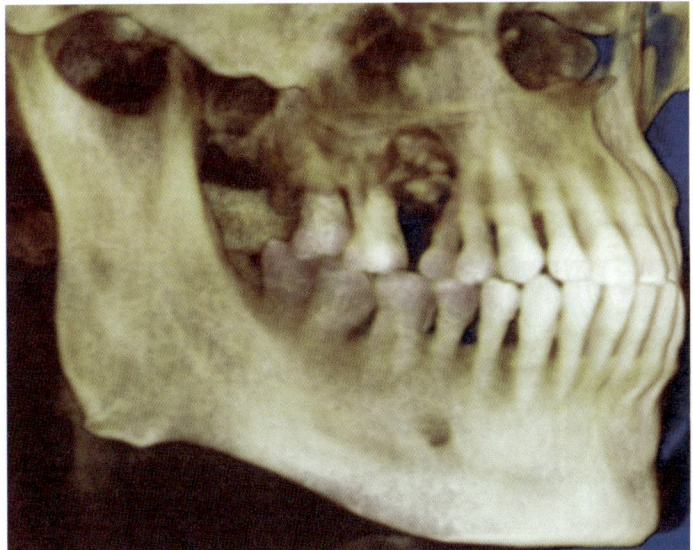

Fig. 13.41: Volume rendered 3D virtual model; right oblique view; showing well-defined maxillary mixed density lesion displacing maxillary right second premolar and first molar. Internal calcifications are also visible

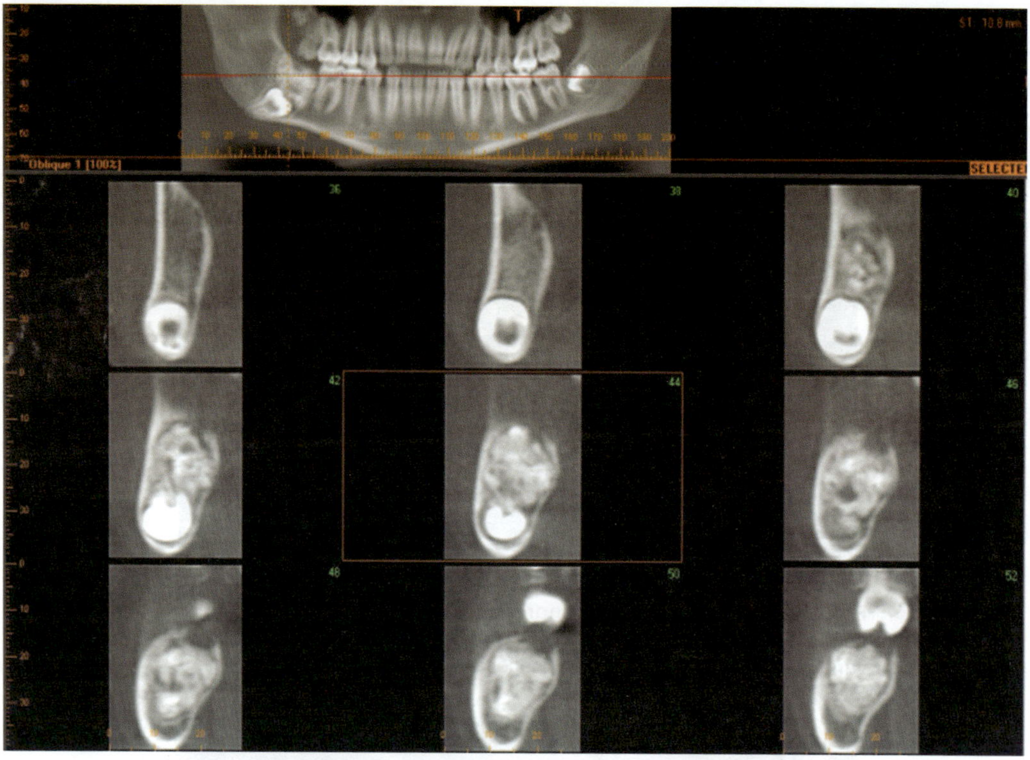

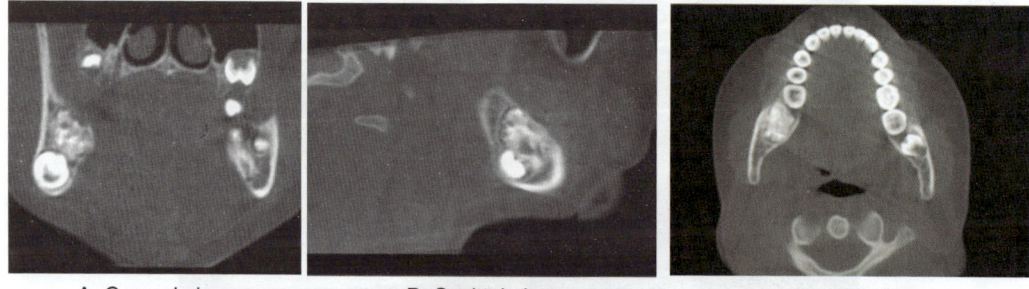

Fig. 13.42: Reformatted panoramic view (10 mm thick section) with dotted red line corresponding with cross-sections of radiopaque lesion in right posterior body of mandible impeding eruption of right second molar, displacing the tooth to the inferior border of mandible

A. Coronal view B. Sagittal view C. Axial view

Figs 13.43A to C: Multiplanar reformatted view showing tooth-like density of the internal structure, a radiolucent capsule interfering with eruption of second molar, displacing it to inferior border of mandible

13

Malignant Lesions of Jaws

Case 9: *Ill defined multiple radiolucent lesions*

A 39-year old female patient was evaluated for a persistent, dull ache in the whole of the lower jaw (Figs 13.44A, B, C, 13.45, 13.46). This case was identified as metastasis of *adenocarcinoma of breast* to jaw.

Case 10: *Punched out multiple radiolucencies*

In these CBCT generated images, classical

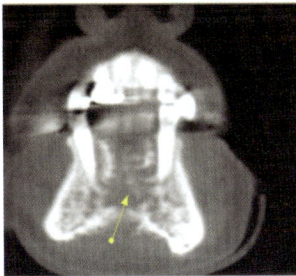 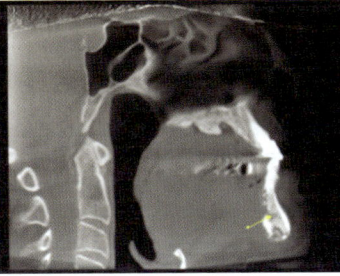 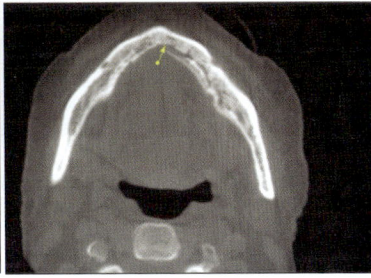

| A. Coronal view | B. Sagittal view | C. Axial view |

Figs 13.44A to C: Multiplanar reformatted view showing ill-defined radiolucent lesion in anterior mandible (A); lamina dura and periodontal ligament space are irregular in mandibular anterior teeth (B); Inferior border of mandible is also eroded by invasive margins of the lesion in this region (C)

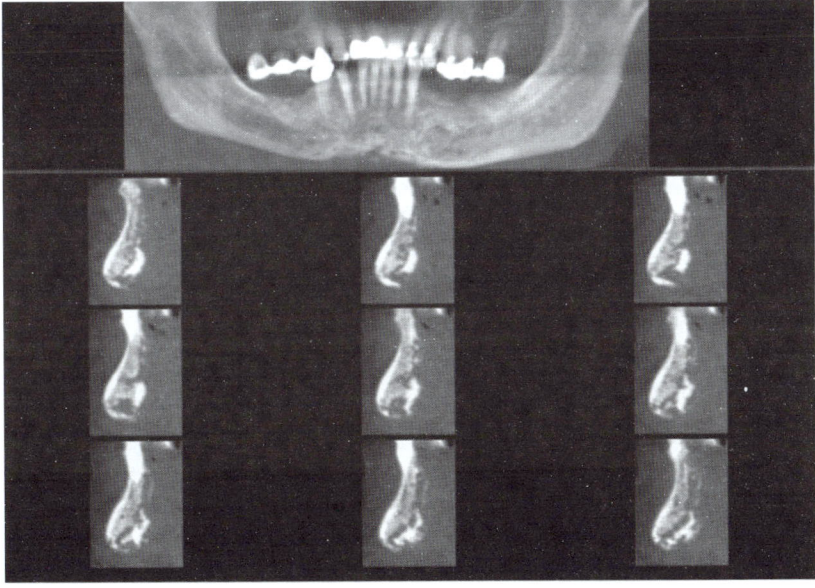

Fig. 13.45: Reformatted panoramic view (10 mm thick section) with corresponding cross-sections of lesion area shows destruction of body and inferior border of anterior mandible

13

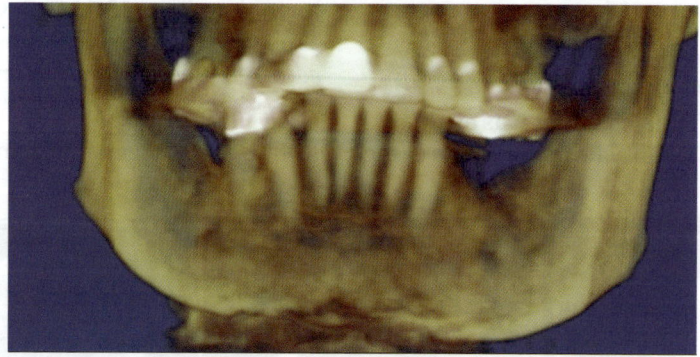

Fig. 13.46: Volume rendered 3D virtual model; frontal view showing destruction of anterior mandible and teeth seem to be standing out without much bone support

punched out lesions of multiple myeloma can be appreciated throughout the maxilla and mandible representing lost bone mineral, teeth too opaque and standing out conspicuously from their osseous background. The head and necks of both right and left condyles and the temporal bone are also affected. Thinning of the lower

border of mandible is visible and both the sinuses are pneumatized (Figs 13.47, 13.48A, B, C, 13.49, 13.50).

Bone Dysplasia

Cemento-osseous dysplasias are a group of disorders known to originate from periodontal ligament tissues and involve

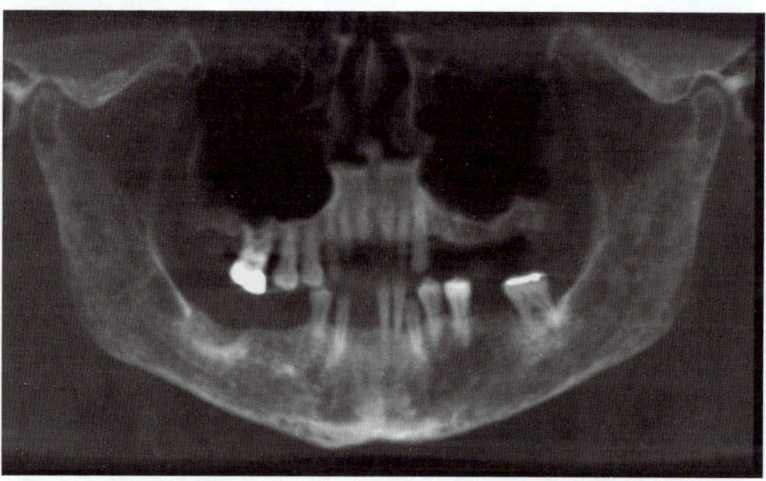

Fig. 13.47: Reformatted panoramic view (10 mm thick section) shows multiple punched out radiolucent lesions intersperse throughout maxilla and body of mandible involving both the ramii, condyle and coronoid processes

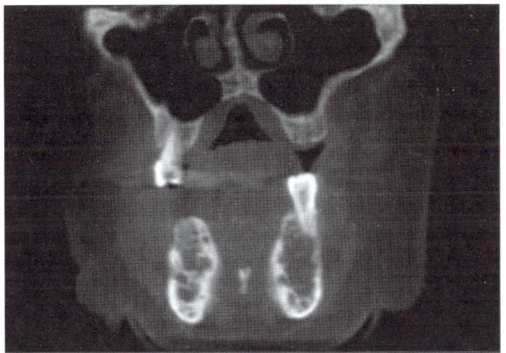

A. Coronal view

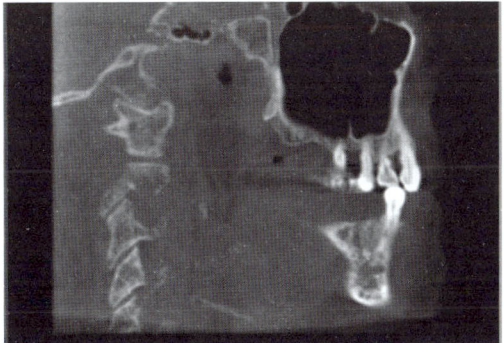

B. Sagittal view

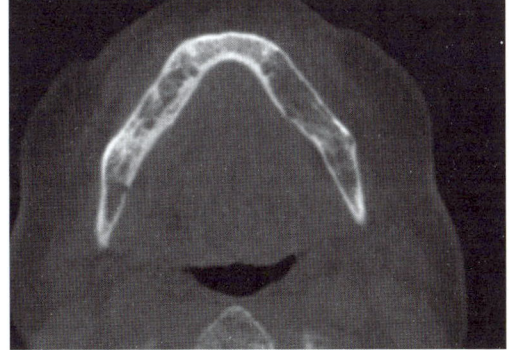

C. Axial view

Figs 13.48A to C: Multiplanar reformatted view showing multiple ragged and infiltrative lesions, general destruction of bone, inferior border of mandible is thinned and teeth show areas of profound bone destruction

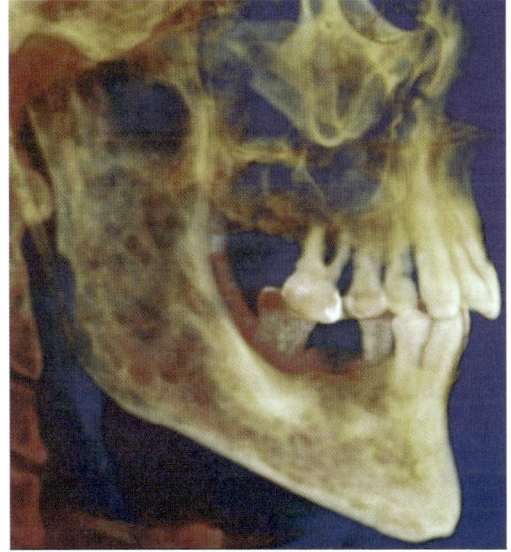

Fig. 13.49

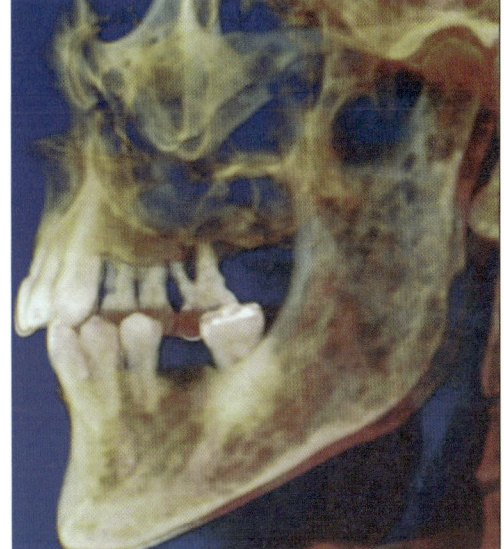

Fig. 13.50

Figs 13.49 and 13.50: Volume rendered 3D virtual model; right sagittal view and left sagittal view showing general bone destruction, multiple punched out lesions and teeth standing out without much bone support

13

13

essentially the same pathological process. A benign fibro-osseous lesion in which mature bone is replaced with woven bone in a matrix of fibrous connective tissue may be totally asymptomatic, and in such cases, the lesion is detected when radiographs are taken for some other purpose. The radiographic appearance can vary from areas of lucency to mixed lesions and to rather opaque masses. Over time, the lesions tend to become increasingly radiopaque. They can be found in multiple quadrants in both the maxilla and the mandible and are mostly confined to the tooth bearing regions. The lesions are usually benign and require no treatment. A review of the literature shows that the classification of fibro-osseous lesions of the jaw has been an area of concern for pathologists and clinicians alike. To complicate the diagnosis further, many other pathological lesions mimic fibro-osseous lesions. There is also considerable overlap in the histological features.

Therefore, in most cases histological features alone are inadequate to make a definite diagnosis, and in contrast to other pathologic lesions, rely on radiology and clinical findings.

Case 11: *Mixed density fibro-osseous lesions*
A 51-year old African-American male patient was evaluated for a left maxillary posterior swelling. The unilateral occurrence with the characteristic cotton wool appearance involving the maxillary posterior region gave the impression of monostotic fibrous dysplasia (Figs 13.51A, B, C, 13.52, 13.53).

Case 12: *Relatively radiolucent*
fibro-osseous lesion
A 55-year old African-American female patient was evaluated for a mandibular swelling. Compare the conventional panoramic radiograph to the reformatted panoramic image generated from a CBCT scan. A mixed density lesion without

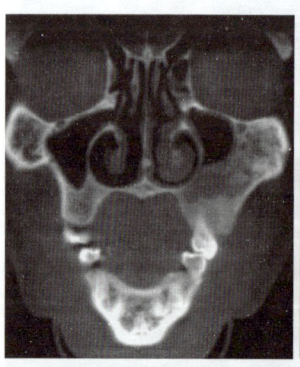 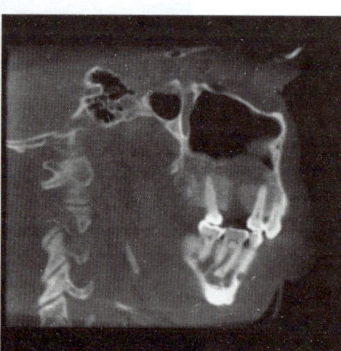 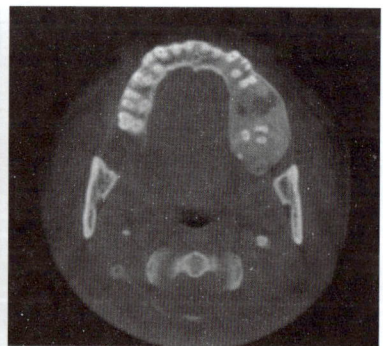

A. Coronal view   B. Sagittal view   C. Axial view

Figs 13.51A to C: Multiplanar reformatted view showing predominately radiopaque expansile lesion in the left posterior maxillary region extending from left maxillary canine posteriorly involving lamina dura and periodontal ligament spaces of premolars and molars and left tuberosity and the zygomatic process of the maxilla. The lesion extends into the left maxillary sinus displacing its inferior cortical boundary and occupying half of the sinus supero-inferiorly. The internal pattern gives cotton wool appearance

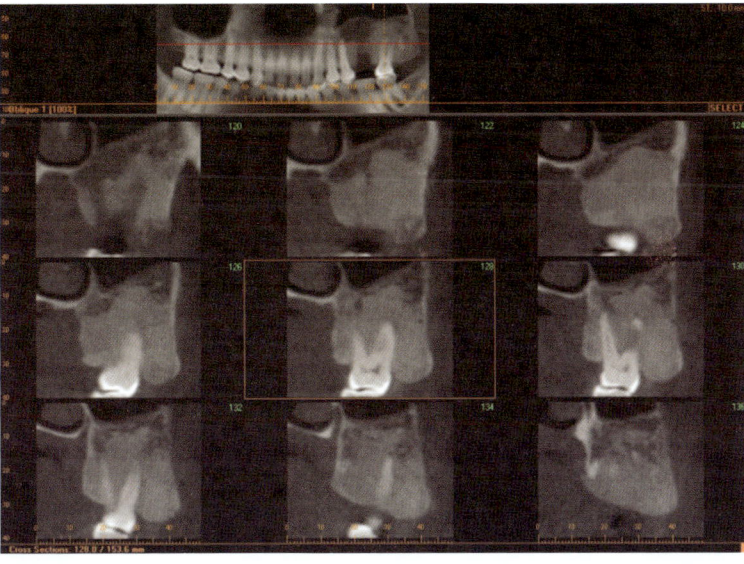

Fig. 13.52: Reformatted panoramic view with dotted red line corresponding with cross-sections of left maxillary lesion showing predominately radiopaque expansile lesion in the left posterior maxillary region. Lamina dura and periodontal ligament space of involved molar is not visible

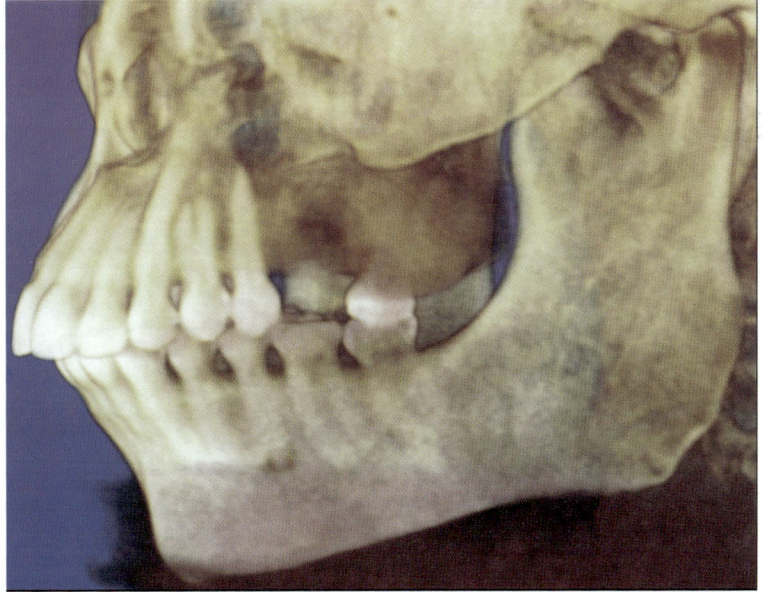

Fig. 13.53: Volume rendered 3D virtual model; right sagittal view showing unilateral expansile lesion with altered bone around involved teeth

13

13

expansion was observed extending from the distal of the extraction space of the mandibular left first molar, causing notable expansion of the buccal and lingual cortices of the mandible. The lesion was (predominantly radiopaque and showed chunks of calcifications) with bone-like density in the anterior region (Figs 13.54A, B, 13.55A, B, C, 13.56). It was excised and biopsied, and the pathological diagnosis was established as ossifying fibroma associated with florid osseous dysplasia.

Evaluation of Temporomandibular Joint

The temporomandibular joint is another area where pain and dysfunction provide a diagnostic challenge. Temporomandibular disorders (TMD) are usually diagnosed by means of a thorough patient history and comprehensive clinical examination.

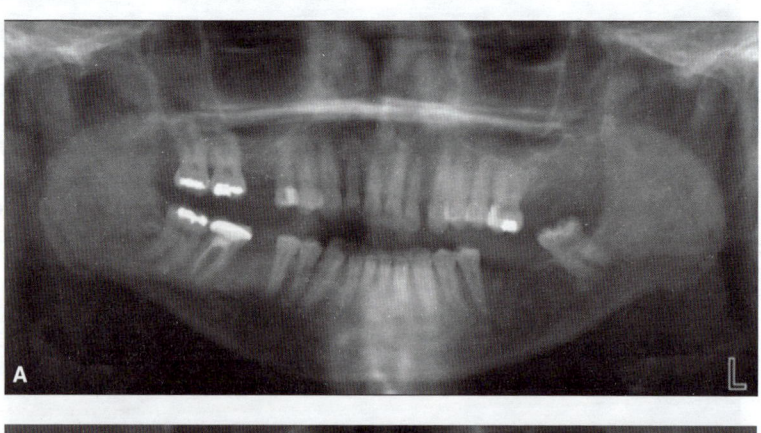

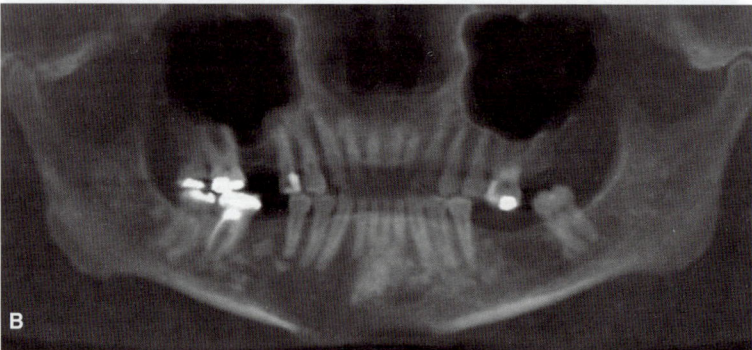

Figs 13.54A and B: Conventional and CBCT generated panoramic views. (A) Conventional panoramic radiograph with various superimposing structures and ghost images. Lesion borders and its internal structure cannot be appreciated adequately. Compare it to reformatted panoramic view (B) with no superimposition of spine shadow in the center, note the mixed density pattern of internal structure of the lesion and expansion of body of mandible in supero-inferior directions

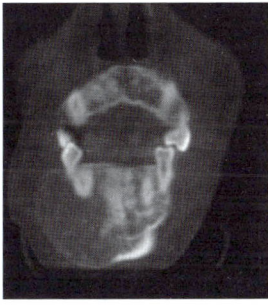
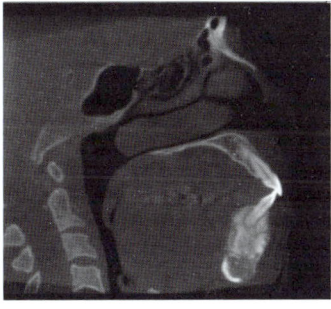
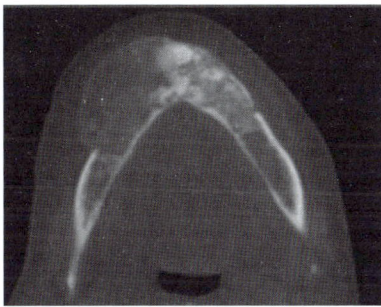

| A. Coronal view | B. Sagittal view | C. Axial view |

Figs 13.55A, B, C: Multiplanar reformatted view. Note the expansion of right side of body of mandible. The outer cortical plates have been displaced and thinned but are still intact

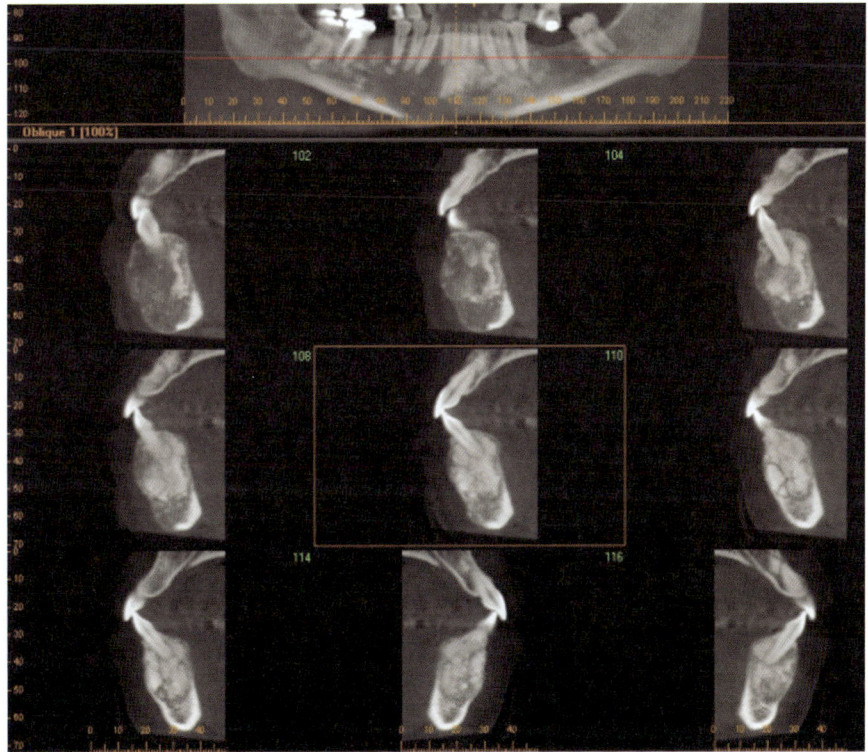

Fig. 13.56: Reformatted panoramic view (10 mm thick section) with dotted red line corresponding with cross-sections of middle of lesion shows flocculent pattern of bone with large tufts of bone formation in the anterior mandible

13

However, additional diagnostic tests, such as imaging of the TMJ area, are necessary in cases where the signs do not explain the symptoms. CBCT imaging is a cost and radiation dose effective alternative to computed tomography.

Case 13: *Temporomandibular Joint Study*
A 65-year old female patient was evaluated for chronic pain in the left joint. Evaluation of frontal and the corresponding lateral

cross-sections of the right and left condyles indicated arthritic changes in the left joint (Fig. 13.57).

Case 14: *Temporomandibular Joint Study*
The patient was evaluated for continuously increasing mandibular asymmetry and minimal jaw opening. CBCT scan generated data revealed enlargement and deformity of the condylar head and corresponding glenoid fossa (Figs 13.58, 13.59, 13.60). This

13

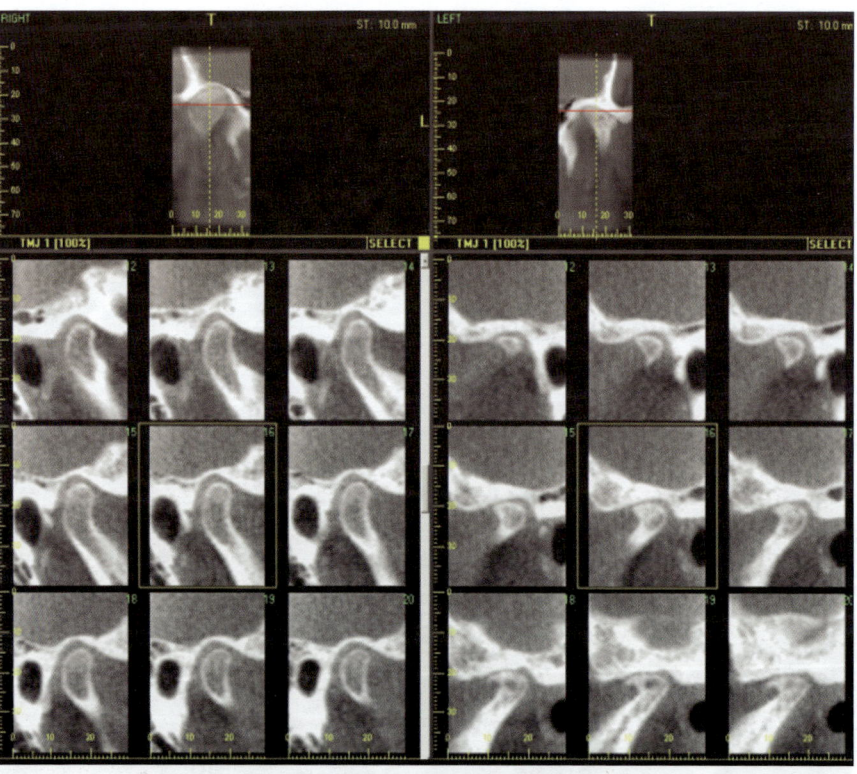

Fig. 13.57: Frontal and the corresponding lateral cross-sections of the right and left condyle. Note flattening and erosions of the articulating surfaces of the left condyle and the temporal component. Osteophyte formation is evident on the anterior surface of the condyle. The joint space is narrow. Round radiolucent areas with irregular margins consistent with Ely cysts are visible deep to the articulating surfaces. Compare it to right condyle. All these observations indicate arthritic changes in the left joint

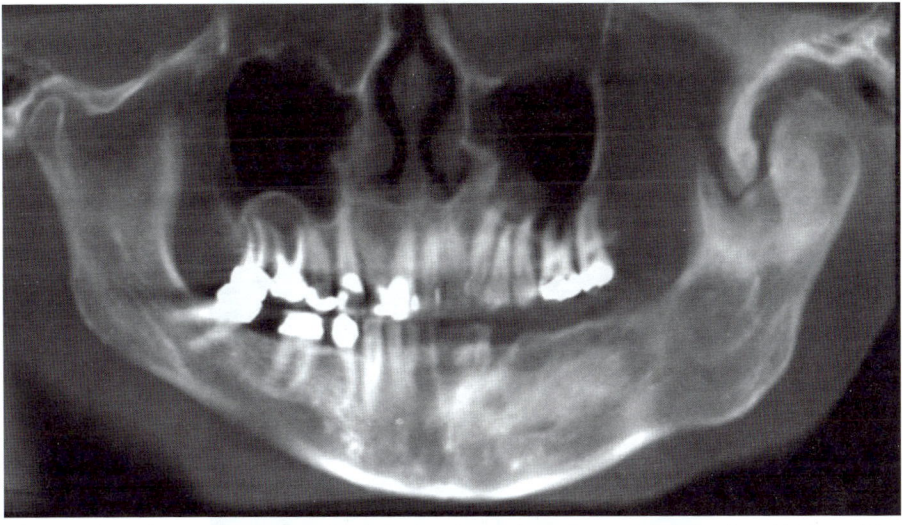

Fig. 13.58: Reformatted panoramic view showing enlargement and deformity of left condylar head and mandibular asymmetry

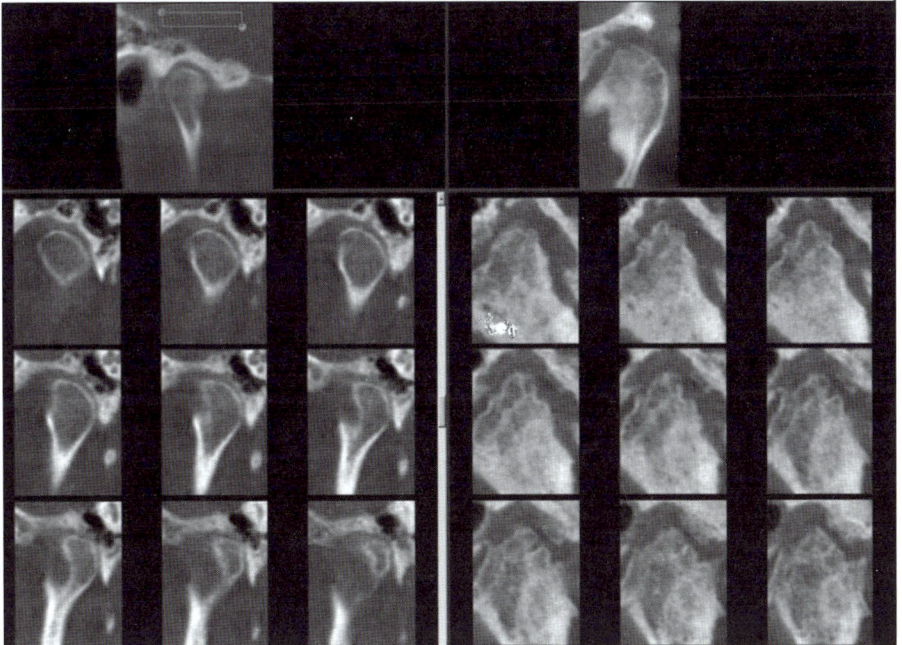

Fig. 13.59: Frontal and the corresponding lateral cross-sections of the right and left condyle. Note irregular altered shape of condyle. Head of condyle and corresponding glenoid fossa seem to be enlarged and radiopaque

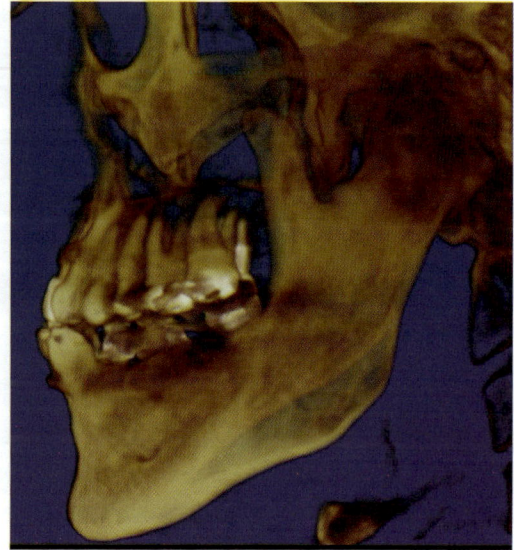

Fig. 13.60: Volume rendered 3D virtual model; left sagittal view showing enlarged head of left condyle and glenoid fossa

13

example demonstrates that CBCT scan is a valuable tool in establishing developmental abnormalities.

Magnetic Resonance Imaging (MRI)

MRI is a recently developed imaging technique that offers the best visualization of soft tissues. This imaging modality uses hydrogen atoms which are abundant in the human body to form the image. The technique depends upon the hydrogen atoms in the body reacting in a particular way in a magnetic field since nuclei of hydrogen atoms are especially susceptible to the force of an external magnetic field (Figs 13.61A and B).

Hydrogen nuclei have one proton and one neutron each and possess their own motion called *spin*. These spinning nuclei are randomly oriented in the human body. Since the hydrogen nuclei are also electrically charged, they generate a magnetic field about themselves that has a north pole and a south pole.

Indications

- Evaluation of the size, site, and extent of all soft tissue tumors and tumor-like lesions involving the salivary glands, pharynx, larynx, paranasal sinuses, and orbits.
- Imaging of the TMJ to demonstrate bony and soft tissue components including position of the disc to diagnose suspected internal derangement and as a preoperative analysis before disc surgery. The major advantage of MR imaging of the temporomandibular joint is the exquisite definition of the internal joint anatomy, especially the joint disc. The associated bony abnormalities of the articular eminence and the mandibular

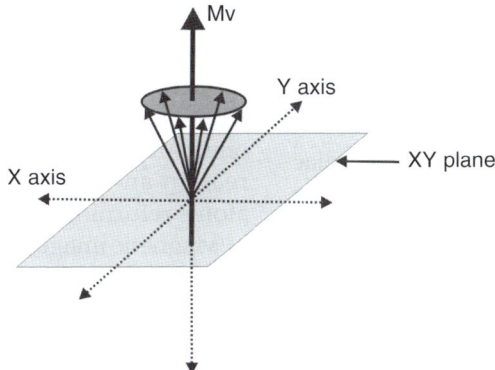

Fig. 13.61A: When hydrogen nuclei are subjected to an external magnetic field, two energy fields result, one is the spin up, which is in the direction of the field, and the other is the spin down, which is in the direction opposite to the field. The combined effect of these two energy states is a weak net magnetic moment, or the magnetization vector (Mv), parallel to the applied magnetic field

13

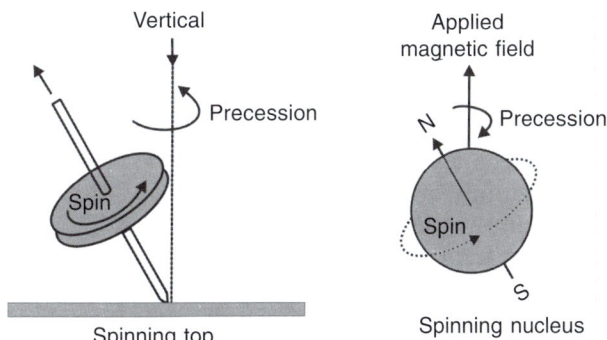

Fig. 13.61B: The tilting or wobbling of the spinning hydrogen nuclei around the direction of the external magnetic field is called precession. The rate or frequency of precession is called the resonant or Larmer frequency. The Larmer frequency is specific for the nuclear species and depends on the strength of the external magnetic field

condyle are also well visualized by MR imaging.

- Evaluation of developmental anomalies, inflammatory lesions and cysts of the head and neck.

Advantages

- Non-invasive procedure
- No ionizing radiation is used
- No reported adverse effects
- Image manipulation and reconstruction in all the planes possible
- High resolution and excellent capability to differentiate between different soft tissues and between normal and abnormal/pathologic tissues which is better than CT
- Direct flow measurements
- No bone or air artefacts

Disadvantages

- Bone does not produce MR signal, only bone marrow gives MR signal
- Lengthy scanning
- Contraindicated in patients with cardiac pacemakers, surgical clips and cochlear implants and those in the 1st trimester of pregnancy
- Equipment is noisy and claustrophobic
- Metallic objects to be removed or replaced by non-ferromagnetic alternatives
- Very expensive equipment
- Positioning of equipment is difficult due to powerful magnets
- Facilities are not widely available

Procedure/Technique

MR scanners are cylindrical devices within which a patient is made to lie on a specially designed table, so that his/her body is surrounded with electromagnets of known strength. Because of the extremely strong external magnetic field randomly oriented nuclei of hydrogen atoms in the patient's body are aligned with the long axis of magnetic field, the degree of which is proportionate to the strength of the magnetic field. The spinning hydrogen nuclei wobble as they struggle against the external magnetic field to return to their randomly oriented state. This state is disrupted by a radio frequency (RF) energy pulse emitted by a body coil transmitter at 90 degrees to the magnetic field. This energy is absorbed by protons which are knocked out of alignment. The disrupted nuclei begin to realign within a fraction of a second. First they begin to precess and their long axes move away from the long axis of the magnetic field. So the longitudinal movements diminish and the transverse magnetic movements grow. Secondly, their spins synchronize in phase with each other. This realignment process emits distinctive RF signals which are stored in the computer. Different tissues can be differentiated based on the rate at which their hydrogen nuclei realign and on the number of hydrogen atoms returning signals.

Magnetic images are made by applying a series of RF pulses to tissues located in a strong magnetic field so that they interact with hydrogen nuclei and produce weak but detectable radio signals. These signals are influenced by the T1 and T2 relaxation times and the number of hydrogen nuclei in tissues.

T1 relaxation

When the RF pulse is shut off, the protons begin to relax or return to their baseline state. The time period for this relaxation is called T1 relaxation or spin lattice relaxation or longitudinal relaxation.

T2 relaxation

RF causes all the protons to precess in the same direction or to be 'in phase'. However, in a little while they are out of phase due to magnetic movements of hydrogen nuclei interfering with those of nearby nuclei and causing the precession to get out of phase. This is T2 relaxation or spin-spin relaxation.

T1 and T2 relaxations occur concurrently but T2 times are always less than or equal to T1 times.

The most helpful scan technique for most lesions is a combination of T1 weighted sequences (short repetition time or TR, short echo time or TE) for definition of anatomy and T2 weighted sequences (long TR, long TE) for assessment of lesions infiltrating through tissue planes and in lymph nodes.

MR Images

T1 weighted Images

T1 relaxation time is the major determinant of tissue contrast. It is commonly used to produce images of normal anatomy.

T2 weighted Images

This technique uses suppression of signals in order to obtain additional information of tissues. It is used to produce images of disease.

The weighting of an image is controlled by the parameters set by the operator before the MR scan. The most important parameters responsible for image contrast are TR (repetition time) and TE (echo time).

In T1 weighted images, both the TR and TE are short. In T2 weighted images, both the TR and TE are long. If the TR is long and TE is short, then the image is proton density weighted.

In a T1 weighted image, tissues with short T1 times appear bright and tissues with long T1 times appear dark, whereas in a T2 weighted image, tissues with short T2 times appear dark and tissues with long T2 times appear bright.

Fast MR Imaging Techniques

Since MR scan time is too long and it can be uncomfortable for the patients to lie motionless in a small space, and some body parts such as the abdomen have respiratory motion, two methods of reducing scan times have been developed.

i. Speeding of the spin-echo sequence by fractional acquisition or multiple echo trains.

ii. Using different methods of producing a signal for readout known as gradient-echo imaging instead of spin-echo sequence.

Echo sequence is the manner in which RF is pulsed for transmission into the patient. It refers to the timing pattern in which the pulse is transmitted.

The different echo sequences available are:

- Static spin-echo and fat suppression sequences
- Time-lapse subtraction used for vascular imaging
- Cineloop or pseudodynamic used mainly for TMJ
- Echo planar or dynamic used mainly as a research tool

Imaging Planes for Head and Neck Lesions

For midline lesions sagittal images are most useful. If the lesion is congenital, a T1 weighted sequence is usually the best for assessment of anatomic interrelationships.

An axial scan is a part of almost all head and neck studies. It is usually T1 weighted, with and without contrast for tumors and infections, and without contrast for congenital lesions. Most tumors are also studied with T2 weighed sequences in axial projections.

Coronal scans are especially useful in assessing lesions at the base of the skull, perineural extension of tumors and lesions of the oral and nasal cavities.

Contrast Enhancement

Image contrast can be enhanced by paramagnetic contrast agents such as gadolinium diethylene triaminepenta acetic acid which is well tolerated by the body. These agents shorten the T1 and T2 times of water, which results in significant brightening of highly vascular tissues.

When an extension of a tumor or infection is present in muscle, brain or blood vessels,

13

13

contrast enhancement is helpful in defining the lesion extent. Bright enhancement may be difficult to differentiate from bright fat. Therefore, fat suppression techniques are generally used when available, alongwith contrast enhancement in the head and neck.

The problems of magnetic susceptibility artefacts are aggravated by the use of fat suppression techniques, and metallic restorations in the mouth may render the fat suppression images useless. Enhancement is seen with processes that cause hyperemia, including tumors, abscesses, cellulitis, and even trauma.

The margins of surgical resection commonly get enhanced, with the degree of enhancement decreasing to a variable extent with time. Enhancement has been seen following surgery for more than a year in some cases.

Normally, enhancement is seen in structures with a large blood supply and should not be confused with a pathologic process. The normally enhanced structures include the mucosa, nasal turbinates, tonsils and salivary glands. Significant for the lack of normal enhancement are muscle, fat, bone, vocal cords and epiglottis.

Perineural spread, seen commonly along the third division of the trigeminal nerve and facial nerves from lesions in the masticator and parotid spaces is difficult to diagnose clinically and is almost invisible to all imaging modalities. Contrast enhanced MR imaging is of definite use in diagnosing this historically difficult clinical problem.

Contrast should be used in evaluating lymph nodes for possible tumor invasion. Most lymph nodes larger than 1.0 cm in size or with central inhomogeneity are considered malignant. The digastric nodes are normally somewhat larger (1.0–1.5 cm)

than the submandibular nodes (1.0 cm). The presence of central cavitation greater than 1.0 mm, surrounded by contrast enhancement is highly specific for tumor necrosis. Contrast enhancement is the only way to assess the inhomogeneity of the internal architecture of the lymph node. MR imaging with contrast enhancement has improved the ability to detect metastatic lymph node involvement with a reported sensitivity and specificity of 80 percent.

Bibliography

1. Aarthus Wenzel Ann: Direct digital radiography in the dental office. *IDJ* 1995;45:27.
2. Ahlqvist J, Eliasson S, Welander U: The effect of projection errors on cephalometric length measurements. *European Journal of Orthodontics*. 1986;8:141.
3. Bender IB: Factors influencing the radiographic appearance of bony lesions. *J. Endod.* 1997; 23:5.
4. Bolin A, Eliasson S, von Beetzen M, et al.: Radiographic evaluation of mandibular posterior implant sites: correlation between panoramic and tomographic determinations. *Clinical Oral Implants Research*. 1996;7:354.
5. BouSerhal C, Jacobs R, Quirynen M, et al.: Imaging technique selection for the preoperative planning of oral implants: a review of the literature. *Clinical Implant Dentistry and Related Research*. 2002;4:156.
6. Brooks SL, Miles DA: Advances in diagnostic imaging in dentistry. *Dent Clin North Am*: 1993;37:91.
7. Conley RS, Boyd SB, Legan HL, et al.: Treatment of a patient with multiple impacted teeth. *Angle Orthod.* 2007;77:5.
8. Dooms GC, Fisher MR, Hricak H, Richardson M, Crooks LE, Genant HK. Bone marrow imaging : Magnetic resonance imaging studies related to age and sex. *Radiology* 1985;155:429.
9. Dula K, Mini R, van der Stelt PF, et al.: The radiographic assessment of implant patients: decision-making criteria. *The International journal of Oral & Maxillofacial Implants*. 2001;16: 80.

10. Estrela C, Bueno MR, Leles CR, et al.: Accuracy of cone beam computed tomography and panoramic and periapical radiography for detection of apical periodontitis. *J. Endod.* 2008; 34:273.

11. Farahani RM, Zonuz AT: Triad of bilateral duplicated permanent teeth, persistent open apex, and tooth malformation: a case report. *The journal of Contemporary Dental Practice.* 2007; 8:94.

12. Garg AK: Dental implant imaging: TeraRecon's Dental 3D Cone Beam Computed Tomography System. *Dental Implantology Update.* 2007;18: 41.

13. Grassl U, Schulze W: In vitro perception of low contrast features in digital, film and digitized dental radiographs: A receiver operating characteristic analysis. *O Surg, O Med, O Path*: 2007;103:694.

14. Grondahl K, Grondahl HG, Webber RL. Digital subtraction radiography for diagnosis of periodontal bone lesions with simulated high-speed systems. *O Surg, O Med, O Path* 1983;55: 313.

15. Guerrero ME, Jacobs R, Loubele M, Schufyser F, Suetens P State of the art on cone-beam CT imaging for pre-operative planning of implant placement. *Clin Oral Invest* 2006;10:1.

16. Halse A, Stuart C. White: Detection of mineral loss in approximal enamel by subtraction radiography. *O Surg, O Med, O Path.* 1994;77: 177.

17. Hashimoto K, Arai Y, Iwai K, Araki M, Kawashimo S, Terakodo M: A comparison of a new limited cone beam computed tomography machine for dental use with a multidetector row helical CT machine. *O Surg, O Med, O Path* 2005;95:371.

18. Hilgers ML, Scarfe WC, Scheetz JP, et al.: Accuracy of linear temporomandibular joint measurements with cone beam computed tomography and digital cephalometric radiography. *Am J Orthod Dentofacial Orthop.* 2005;128:803.

19. Hussain AM, Packota G, Major PW, et al.: Role of different imaging modalities in assessment of temporomandibular joint erosions and osteophytes: a systematic review. *Dento maxillofac Radiol* 2008;37:63.

20. Johnson DH: CT of maxillofacial trauma. *Rad Cl North Am* 1984;22:131.

21. Kalathingal SM, Tyndall DA, Caplan DJ: *In vitro* assessment of cone beam local computed tomography for proximal caries detection. *O Surg, O Med, O Path* 2007;104:699.

22. Kaneda T, Minami M, Ozawa K, Akimoto Y, Utsunomiya T. Yamamoto H. *et al.*: Magnetic resonance imaging of osteomyelitis in the mandible: Comparative study with other radiologic modalities. *O Surg, O Med, O Path* 1996;82:229.

23. Katsmata A, Hirukawa A, Okumura S, Naitoh M, Fujishita M, Ariji E, Langlan R: Effect of image artefacts on grey nature dentistry in limited volume cone beam computerized tomography. *O Surg, O Med, O Path* 2007;104: 829.

24. Katsumata A, Hirukawa A, Fujishita M, Noujein M, Okumura S, Naitoh M. Image artefacts in dental cone beam CT. *O Surg, O Med, O Path* 2006;101:652.

25. Kau CH, Richmond S, Palomo JM, Hans MG: Three dimensional cone beam computed tomography in orthodontics. *J Ortho* 2005;32:282.

26. Kawamata A, Ariji Y, Langelis RP: Three dimensional computed tomography imaging in dentistry. *Dental Clin North America* 2000;44:395.

27. Kumar V, Ludlow J, Soares Cevidanes LH, et al.: In vivo comparison of Conventional and Cone Beam CT Synthesized Cephalograms. *Angle Orthodontist.* 2008;78:873.

28. Kumar V, Kumar A, Ferguson, B, Katz J: The influence of adding third dimension in diagnosis and treatment planning. *Missouri Dental Journal Focus* 2009;89:1.

29. Lim KF, Loh EEM, Hong YH: Intraoral computed radiography – an in vitro evaluation. *J Dent* 1996;24:359.

30. Lou L, Langravere MO, Compton S, Major PW: Accuracy of measurements and reliability of landmark identification with computed tomography (CT) techniques in the maxillofacial area: a systematic review. *O Surg, O Med, O Path.* 2007;104:402.

31. Ludlow JB, Davies-Ludlow LE, Brooks SL, et al.: Dosimetry of 3 CBCT devices for oral and maxillofacial radiology, CB Mercuray, NewTom 3G and i-CAT. *Dento-maxillofac Radiol.* 2006;35:219.

13

13

32. Ludlow JB, Laster WS, Bailey LT, Hershey GH : Accuracy of measurements of mandibular anatomy in cone beam computed tomography images. *O Surg, O Med, O Path*. 2007;103:534.

33. Maverna R, Gracco A: Different diagnostic tools for the localization of impacted maxillary canines: Clinical considerations. *Progress in Orthodontics*. 2007;8:28.

34. Misch KA, Yi ES, Sarment DP: Accuracy of cone beam computed tomography for periodontal defect measurements. *J Periodontol* 2006;77:1261.

35. Mischkowski RA, Pulsfort R, Ritter L, Zoller JE, Keeve E, Brochhagen GH, Neugebauer J: Geometric accuracy of a newly developed cone-beam device for maxillofacial imaging. *O Surg, O Med, O Path*. 2006;101:652.

36. Molteni R: Direct digital dental X-ray imaging with Visalix/VIXA. *O Surg, O Med, O Path* 1993;76:235.

37. Molteni R: Visualix, a new system for direct dental X-ray imaging: A preliminary report. *Dentomaxillofacial Radiol* 1992;21:222.

38. Mozzo P, Procacci C, Taccom A, Martini PY, Andreis IA: A new volumetric CT machine for dental imaging based on the cone beam technique: Preliminary result. *Eur Radiology* 1998;8:1558.

39. Nair MK, Tyndall DA, Ludlow JB, May K: Timed aperture computed tomography and detection of recurrent caries. *Caries Res*: 1998;32:23.

40. Parissis N, Kondylidou SA, Tsirlis A, Patias P: Conventional radiographs vs digitized radiographs: Image quality assessment. *Dentomaxillofacial Radiol*: 2005;34:353.

41. Preda L, La Fianza A, Di Maggio EM, et al.: The use of spiral computed tomography in the localization of impacted maxillary canines. *Dentomaxillofacial Radiol*. 1997;26:236.

42. Queguinner L: Computer tomography and complete dentures. Morphometric analysis. *O Surg, O Med, O Path* 1994;77:90.

43. Ricalde P, Horswell BB: Craniofacial fibrous dysplasia of the fronto-orbital region: a case series and literature review. *J Oral Maxillofac Surg*. 2001;59:157.

44. Rudolf DJ, White SC: Film holding instrument for intraoral subtraction radiography. *O Surg, O Med, O Path* 1988;65:767.

45. Rurkart AJ, Dove SB, McDavid WD. Direct digital radiography for the detection of periodontal bone lesions. *O Surg, O Med, O Path* 1992;74:652.

46. Sanderimk GCH: Imaging: New versus traditional technological aids. *Int Dent J* 1993;43:335.

47. Scarfe WC, Farman AG, Sukovic P. Clinical applications of cone-beam computer tomography in dental practice. *J Can Dent Assoc* 2006;72:75.

48. Schropp L, Wenzel A, Kostopoulos L: Impact of conventional tomography on prediction of the appropriate implant size. *O Surg, O Med, O Path* 2001;92:458.

49. Shrout MK, Russel CM, Potter BJ, Powell BJ and Hildebolt CF. Digital enhancement of radiography: Can it improve caries diagnosis ? *JADA* 1996;127:469.

50. Syriopoulos K, Sanderink GC, Velders XL, Vanderstelt PF: Radiographic detection of approximal caries: A comparison of dental films and digital imaging systems. *Dentomaxillofacial Radiol* 2000;29:312.

51. Terakado M, Hashimoto K, Arai Y, Honda K, Sekiwa T, Sato H: Diagnostic imaging with newly developed ortho super high resolution computed tomography (ortho CT) *O Surg, O Med, O Path* 2000;89:509.

52. Tsiklakis K, Syriopoulos K, Stamatakis HC: Radiogrpahic examination of the temporo-mandibular joint using cone-beam computed tomography. *Dentomaxillofacial Radiol* 2004;33:196.

53. Tyndall DA, Brooks SL: Selection criteria for dental implant site imaging: a position paper of the American Academy of Oral and Maxillofacial radiology. *O Surg, O. Med, O Path* 2000, 89, 30.

54. Tyndall DA, Kapa SF, Bagnell CP: Digital subtraction radiography for detecting cortical and cancellous bone changes in the periapical region. *J Endo* 1990;16:173.

55. Van Daatselaar AN, Tyndall DA, Vandor Stelt PF: Detection of caries with local CT. *Dentomaxillofacial Radiol* 2003;32:235.

56. Vandenberghe B, Jacob R, Yang J: Diagnostic validity (acuity) of 2D CCD versus 3D CBCT images for assessing periodontal breakdown. *O Surg, O Med, O Path* 2007;104:395.

57. Vander Stelt PF: Principles of digital imaging. *Dent Clinic North Am* 2000;44:237.

58. Vander Stelt PR: Improved diagnosis with digital radiography. Editorial review: *Orthodontitis and Pedodontics* 1992;2:1.

59. Vogler JB, Murphy WA: Bone marrow imaging. *Radiology* 1988;168:679.

60. Walker A, Horner K, Czajka J: Quantitative assessment of a new dental imaging system. *Br J Radiol* 1991;64,:529.

61. Walker L, Enciso R, Mah J: Three-dimensional localization of maxillary canines with cone-beam computed tomography. *Am J Orthod Dentofacial Orthop.* 2005;128:418.

62. Welander U, Nelvig P, Tronje G: Basic technical properties of a system for direct acquisition of digital intraoral radiographs. *O Surg, O Med, O Path* 1993;75:506.

63. Wenzel A, Haiter N: Influence of spatial resolution and bit depth on detection of small caries lesions with digital receptors. *O Surg, O Med, O Path* 2007;103:418.

64. Wenzel A, Hintze H, Mikkelsen L, Mouyen F: Radiographic detection of occlusal caries in non-cavitated teeth. A comparison of conventional film radiographs digitized film radiographs and radiovisiography. *O Surg, O Med, O Path* 1991;72:621.

65. Wenzel A, Larsen MJ, Fejerskov O: Detection of occlusal caries without cavitation by visual inspection, film radiographs, xeroradiographs and digitized radiographs. *Caries Res* 1991;25:365.

66. Wenzel A, Sewerin I. Sources of noise in digital subtraction radiography. *O Surg, O Med, O Path* 1991;71:503.

67. Wenzel A. Effect of image enhancement for detectability of bone lesions in digitized intra oral radiographs. *Scand J Dent Res* 1988;96:149.

68. White SC, Yoon DC: Comparative performance of digital and conventional images for detecting proximal surface caries. *Dentomaxillofacial Radiol* 1997;26:32.

69. White SC: Computer aided differential diagnosis of oral radiographic lesions. *Dentomaxillofacial Radiol.* 1989;18:53.

70. Zeigler CM, Woertche R, Brief J, Hassfeld S: Clinical indications for digital volume tomography in oral and maxillofacial surgery. *Dentomaxillofac Radiol* 1999;28:245.

71. Zubery Y: Computerised image analysis in dentistry : Patient status and future application. *Compend Cont Educ Dent* 1992;13:964.

13

Infection Control in Dental Radiology

Human beings are prone to various types of infections. Medical and dental health care workers in general are more exposed to potentially infectious organisms. These organisms can be airborne, waterborne, or saliva/blood borne. Dental surgeons, students and patients in particular are more prone to saliva and blood-borne infections. Many apparently healthy looking patients suffer from various infectious diseases. It is mandatory to use strict infection control regimes and universal precautions to protect both the patient and the operator. The infection can spread from patient to operator, from operator to patient or from patient to patient.

Apart from general precautions in the dental operatory, certain guidelines should be followed in the radiology department during exposure, processing and other handling procedures. Disease transmission can occur either through direct contact or cross contamination. It has been established that bacteria can survive in used dental radiographic developer and fixer solutions for up to two weeks. The radiographic films can be contaminated in the developer and fixer and vice-versa. The risk of transmission of infectious diseases is more during intraoral radiography than with extraoral, panoramic and other radiographic techniques.

The *Environment Protection Agency (EPA)* sets regulations for disinfection procedures in the environment. The chemicals used to disinfect and sterilize objects in the radiography area must have EPA registration. Certain other agencies regulate the guidelines for infection control regimes such as *The Centers for Disease Control (CDC)* and the *Office of Sterilization and Asepsis Procedures (OSAP)*. These agencies are responsible for developing overall guidelines for medical and dental practitioners. The term *universal precautions* was devised, which refers to a set of precautions designed to prevent transmission of HIV, Hepatitis B and Hepatitis C, and other saliva/blood borne infections. The universal precautions consider all body fluids, secretion and excretion (except sweat) as potentially infectious. Infection control procedures should be followed for everyone who comes in contact with saliva and/or blood.

The infection control programme for dental radiology is discussed under the following heads:

i. Personal protection
ii. Surface disinfection
iii. Disinfection during exposure
iv. Disinfection during film processing
v. Panoramic radiograph
vi. Digital imaging

i. Personal Protection

It is necessary to wear gowns, long sleeves, masks and protective eyewear during routine radiological procedures. Gloves should be worn when taking intraoral radiographs and handling contaminated film packets, equipments and instruments. Powder-free gloves are recommended because powder can affect the film's emulsion layer, causing artefacts. It is advisable to change the gloves after single use. Washing and/or disinfection of the gloves will not be effective.

ii. Surface Disinfection

The items/objects in any clinic are divided into three subgroups:

• Critical items – are those items that penetrate the oral mucosa or contact bone. These items are to be sterilized.
• Semi-critical items – are those items that touch but do not penetrate the mucosa. Semi-critical items should also be sterilized; however proper disinfection will suffice.
• Least critical items – are those items that do not touch the oral mucosa but may come in contact with saliva or blood-contaminated hands. These items should be disinfected.

Most of the items in dental radiology are of a semi-critical nature. These items should be sterilized; however, high level disinfection should be sufficient. The categorization of items in the dental radiology department vis-à-vis their disinfection regime is given in Table 14.1.

High touch surfaces require sanitation and disinfection frequently. It should be carried out at least three times a day; one at the start of working, one at the finish and the other during routine procedures. This includes removing or cleaning of potentially infectious material followed by spraying a disinfectant agent for five to ten minutes. Usual spray disinfectants contain phenols or alcohol-phenol combinations.

Non-disposable film holding devices should be properly decontaminated. These are preferably sterilized by autoclaving and/or dry heat. Disposable items such as film holders (Fig. 14.1) and bitewing tabs (Fig. 14.2) can be disinfected. Sterilized plastic covers are available to cover the surfaces prone to routine touch by the operator and the patients (Figs 14.3 to 14.5). If uncovered surfaces are contaminated they should be disinfected after the patient leaves. Surface barriers should be changed between patients.

iii. Disinfection During Exposure

During routine intraoral radiography, certain disinfection regimes should be followed. The patient is given 0.1–0.2% chlorhexidine for rinsing for 30 seconds before the exposure. The patient is also instructed to remove dentures, eye-glasses etc. to avoid cross-contamination. The surface cover should be properly applied to the head rest, arm rest, control unit and other related surfaces. To further avoid cross-contamination, a foot switch can be used.

14

Table 14.1: Items in dental radiology and disinfection protocol

Categories	Contaminated Items	Level of Decontamination
Critical	Items that penetrate tissues and/or contact blood. Usually not used in routine radiographic procedures	Sterilization required OR Disposable instruments
Semi-critical	No tissue penetration, but contacts mucous membrane. Most intraoral devices and materials used in radiological procedures, e.g. Intraoral films, film holders, position-indicating devices, panoramic guides, digital image receptors	Sterilization or high-level disinfection
Least-critical	No tissue penetration, no contact with mucous membrane or saliva by equipment/devices, touches intact skin only. Most extraoral and panoramic radiographic devices, e.g. Lead aprons, collars, cones, handles and knobs, tubeheads, control units, chair seats, handles and head and arm rests	Disinfection and use of barriers
Environmental surfaces	No direct patient contact-Environmental surfaces that do not normally touch the patient but may be contaminated by the care provider, e.g. High-touch surfaces on which exposed films/instruments are placed, table tops and working surfaces in the operatory.	Sanitization and use of barriers

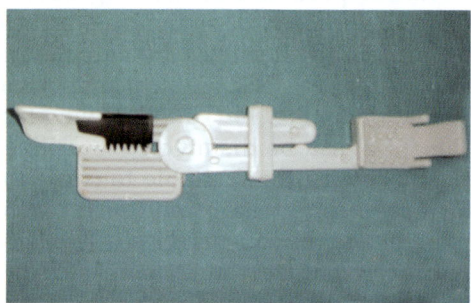

Fig. 14.1: Film holder

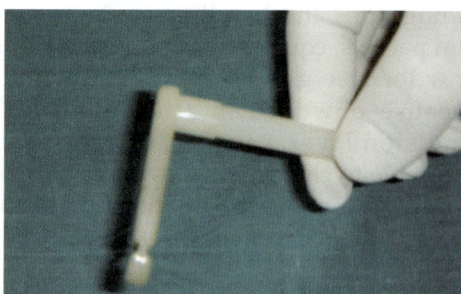

Fig. 14.2: Bitewing tab

14

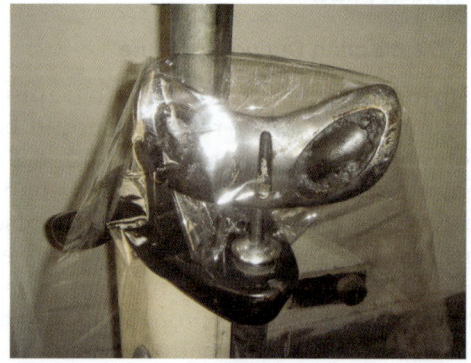

Fig. 14.3: Head rest covered by sterilized plastic cover

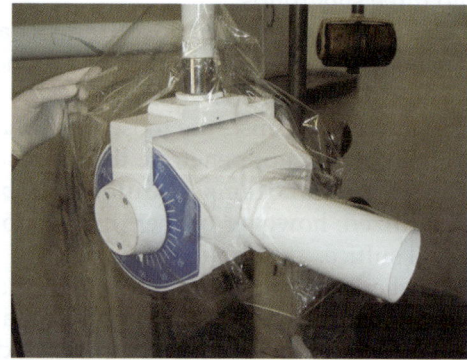

Fig. 14.4: X-ray tube covered by sterilized plastic cover

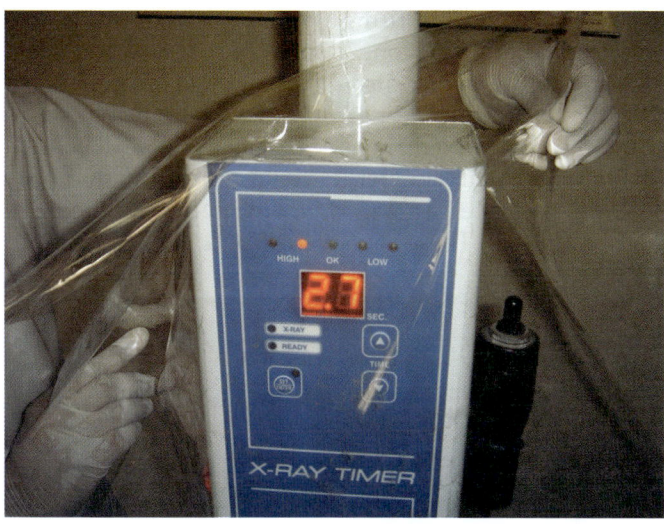

Fig. 14.5: The timer covered by sterilized plastic cover

The operator should wear a sanitized apron (Fig. 14.6) and put a collar over the patient. Vinyl unpowdered gloves should also be worn. Before wearing gloves, the hands should be washed thoroughly using soap and water or preferably with an appropriate antimicrobial soap containing chlorhexidine or parachlorometaxylenol. The X-ray machine switches, light, etc. should be adjusted prior to wearing the

14

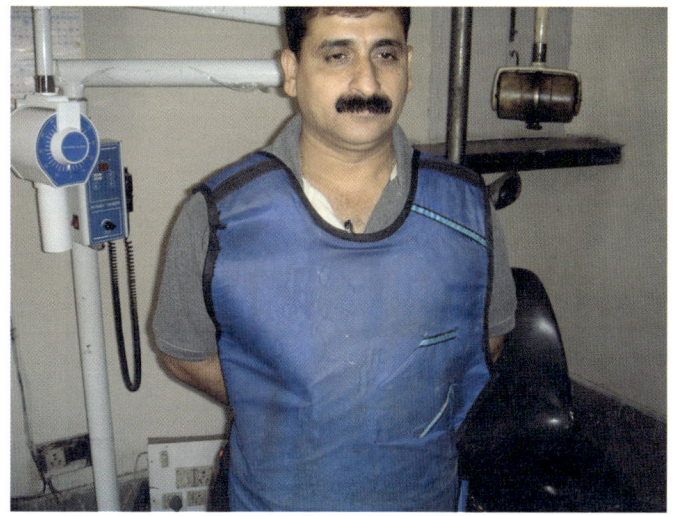

Fig. 14.6: Operator wearing sanitized apron

gloves. The polycoat radiographic film packets can be disinfected after a 30 second immersion in 5.25% sodium hypochlorite. The pack containing the sterile film holding devices is opened and the film is fixed onto the disposable film holder. This film holder along with the film is adjusted in the patient's mouth (Figs 14.7 to 14.9). These film packets can be further enveloped in plastic envelopes, which protects the film from contact with blood and saliva (Fig. 14.10). These envelopes are opened during processing. In case the films are contaminated with blood and saliva, they are wiped with sterilized napkins and dropped into a paper cup. Sensors and

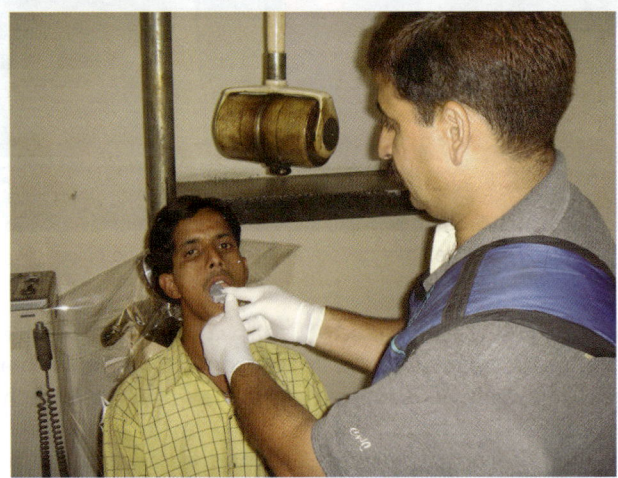

Fig. 14.7: Film packet adjusted in patient's mouth

14

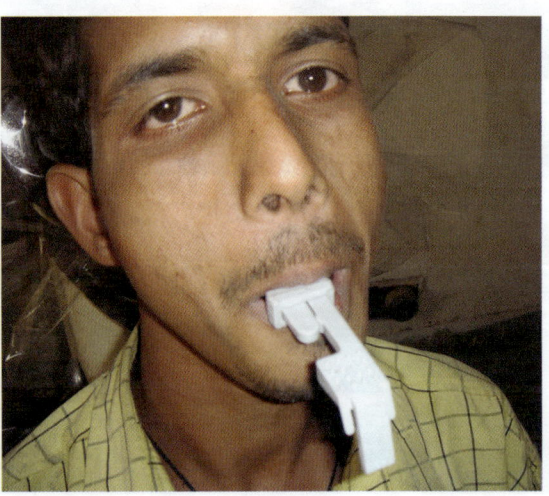

Fig. 14.8: Film packet adjusted with disposable carrier

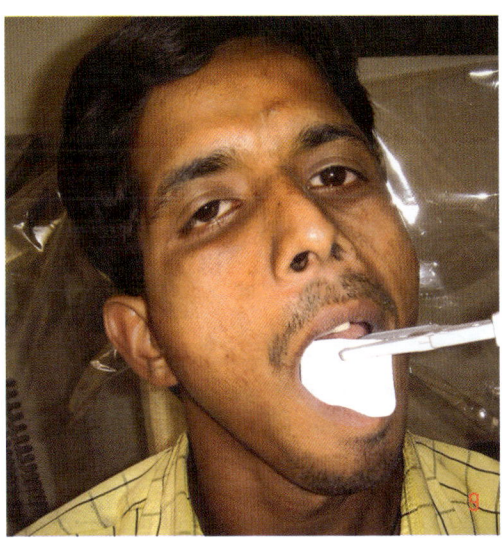

Fig. 14.9: Film packet held with artery forceps

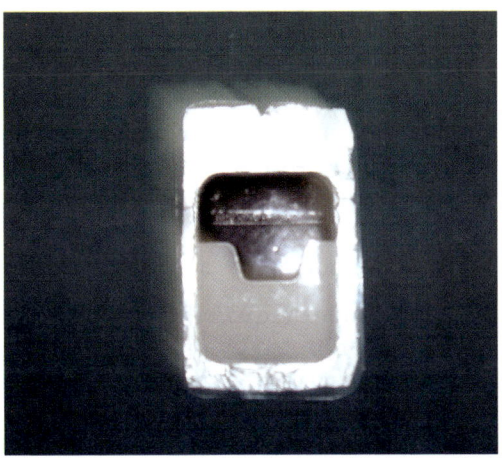

Fig. 14.10: Enveloped film packet

digital imaging tools are usually not sterilizable, thus it is important to use barriers to protect them from contamination when placed in the patient's mouth.

iv. Disinfection during Film Processing

The exposed films are immediately dropped into a paper cup without touching the outer surface of the cup. The films in the cups are carried to the processing areas.

An overglove can be worn over the contaminated gloves before transporting the exposed films to the darkroom. The operator can pick up the cup containing exposed films with overgloved hands. Alternatively, the contaminated gloves can be removed, hands cleaned and another pair of sterilized gloves can be worn after taking the paper cup to the dark room. Unpowdered gloves are recommended because the powder might result in artefacts in the X-ray images.

a. Film Processing in Daylight Loader

The lid of the daylight loader is opened, preferably wearing overgloves. The paper cup is placed on the base of the loader.

The lid is then closed. The overgloved hands are inserted into the sleeves provided on both sides of the loader. Inside the loader, the overgloves are removed. The film packet is carefully opened with the contaminated gloves on. As the films are opened, the lead foil and other accessories are kept on one side of the loader. The gloves are then removed and the films are processed using clean hands. After all the films have been put to the processing cycle, the operator takes his/her hands out of the sleeves of the loader gloves. The overgloves are worn, once again the sleeves are entered and the waste is removed from the loader. Alternatively, instead of using overgloves, two separate pairs of gloves can be used. The second pair is donned after removing the first one and thoroughly cleaning the hands (Figs 14.11A and B).

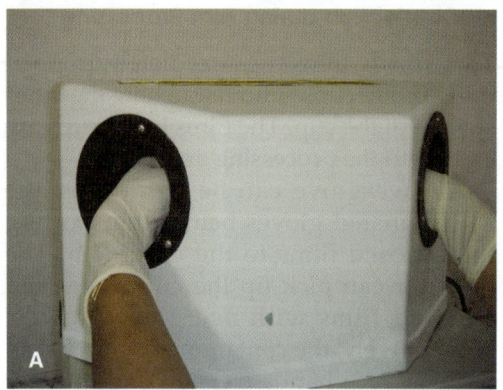 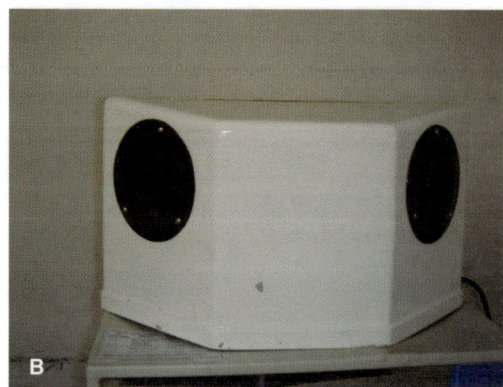

Figs 14.11A and B: Daylight film processor

b. Film Processing in Dark Room

The film packets in the paper cup are transported to the dark room area. The film is taken out from the packet without touching the film (Figs 14.12A to E). When all the film packets have been removed, the operator is to discard the waste at one corner. The contaminated gloves can be carefully removed and discarded. Immediately after removing the gloves, the hands are thoroughly washed with an antimicrobial soap. After placing the films in the processing unit, the hands should be washed again. The films are removed from the processor and dried. They are then mounted in presterilized plastic containers. The contaminated film holders should be placed in solution before further sterilization. The operator should wear new gloves, etc. to remove waste material from the dark room. This material is discarded into the regular waste bin. The apron/collar is also disinfected.

v. Panoramic Radiographs

During panoramic radiography, the operator should wear no gloves. However, the hands are washed. The patient is asked to rinse with a mouth wash. Bite blocks if required, should be used in covers and the patient is instructed to replace the same without touching the operator's hands. The bite blocks are discarded into a waste bin. The patient's chin rest, head rest and other parts of the panoramic machine should be thoroughly cleaned after the exposure. Routine procedures are followed for processing.

vi. Digital Imaging

The equipment required during digital imaging is protected by properly covering with barrier wrappers. The central processing unit is covered except for the air vent to prevent overheating. The keyboard is covered with a plastic wrapper, which is also cleaned regularly with disinfectants. The monitor is wrapped in high touch areas only (Fig. 14.13). A screen shade is used to prevent aerosols from contaminating the monitor screen. The screen and the cover are disinfected in routine. The printer is also covered with wrappers.

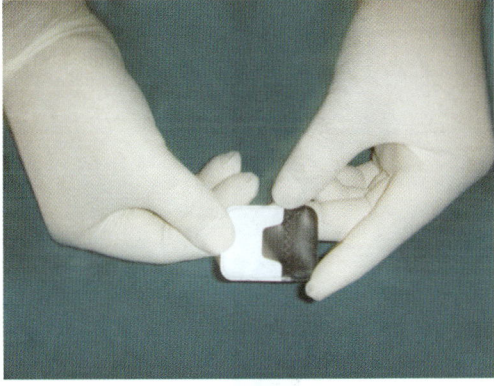

A. Holding the film

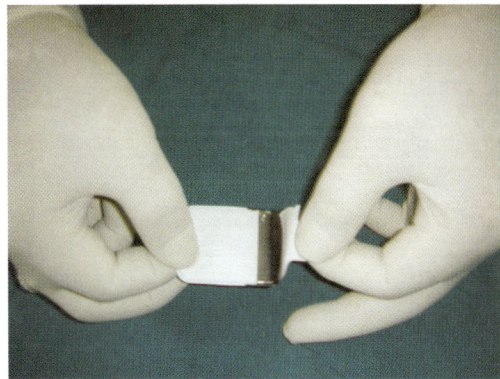

B. Opening the film

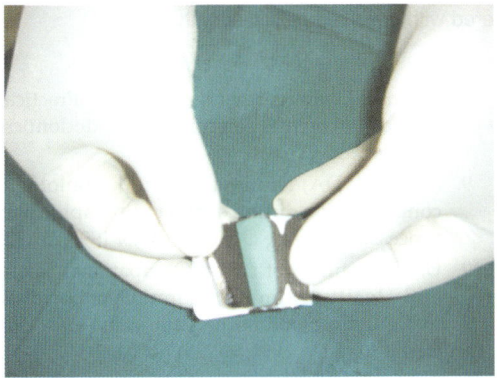

C. Opening the film

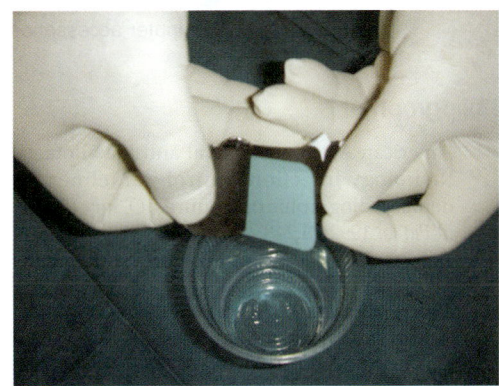

D. Shifting the film to cup

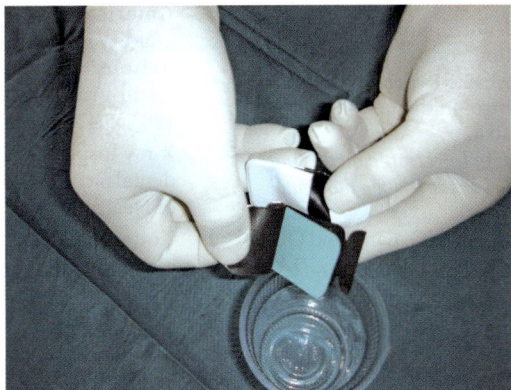

E. The film being shifted to cup

Figs 14.12A to E: Transportation of film to the dark room

14

14

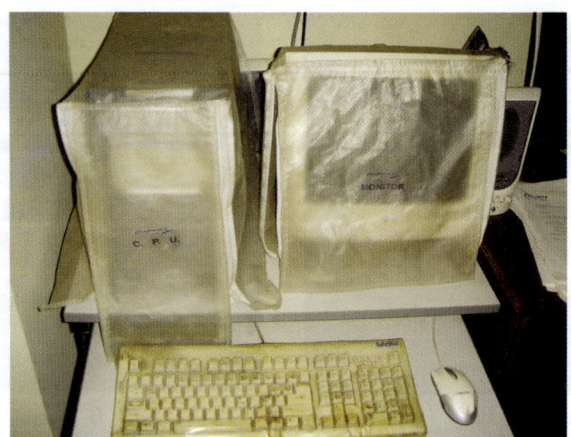

Fig. 14.13: Computer accessories covered with sterilized plastic sheaths

Bibliography

1. American Academy of Oral and Maxillofacial Radiology infection control guidelines for dental radiographic procedures, *O Surg O Med, O Pathol* 1992;73:248.
2. American Dental Association: Infection control recommendations for the dental office and dental laboratory. *JADA* 1996;127:672.
3. American Dental Association Council on Scientific Affairs and American Dental Association Council on Dental Practice: Infection Control recommendations for the dental office and the dental laboratory, *JADA* 1996;127:672.
4. Centers for Disease Control and Prevention: Recommended infection control practices for dentistry, *MMWR* 1993;42(RR-8):1.
5. Glass BJ: Infection control in dental radiology, *NY State Dent J*. 1994;60:42.
6. Miller CH, Palenik CJ: *Infection control and management of hazardous materials for the dental team*, St. Louis, Mosby, 1998.
7. Puttaiah R, Langlais RP, Katz JO, Langland OE: Infection control in dental radiology, *CDAJ* 1995;23:21.
8. Reams GJ,Baumgartner JC, Kulild JC: Practical application of infection control in endodontics, *J Endod* 1995;21:281.
9. Stanczyk DA, Paunovich ED: Microbiologic contamination during dental radiographic film processing. *O Surg O Med O Pathol* 1993;76:112.
10. US Department of Labor, Occupational Safety and Health, Administration: Occupational exposure to blood borne pathogens. *Final rule federal Register*. 1991;56(235):64004.
11. ADA council on Scientific Affairs: An update on radiographic practices: Information and recommendations, *J Am Dent Assoc* 2001; 132:234
12. American Academy of Dental Radiology Quality Assurance Committee: Recommendations for Quality Assurance in dental Radiography, *O Surg O Med O Pathol*. 1983;55:421.
13. X-ray Inspection Service: Quality assurance for dental facilities, Ontario, Canada, 1990 Ministry of Health.
14. Kodak Dental Radiography Series: *Quality assurance in dental radiography*, N-416, Rochester, NY, Eastman Kodak, 1995.

Interpretation of Radiographs

15

Radiographic interpretation is a science in itself. Correct interpretation of radiographs requires thorough knowledge of basic anatomical landmarks, both radiolucent and radiopaque. All the relevant and normal anatomical landmarks may not be seen on a single radiograph. This does not imply that the landmarks do not exist; but the angulation of X-radiations and other factors change their presentation over the radiograph.

Detailed knowledge of the normal landmarks helps in differentiating them from various pathological lesions. Normal landmark, either radiopaque or radiolucent, embraces both hard and soft tissues. The landmarks related to head and neck region are studied in dental and oral radiology.

Before proceeding to study the anatomical landmarks, the following terms used in routine, must be understood.

- *Anterior and Posterior:* The terms 'Anterior' and 'Posterior' describe the front-to-back relationship of one part of the body to another. For example, the ear is posterior to (in back of) the eye; the

nose is anterior to (in front of) the ear, etc.

- *Internal (medial) and external (lateral):* These two terms describe the sideway relationship of one part of the body to another following the mid-sagittal plane as a reference. For example, the ear is external (or lateral) to the eye because the ear is farther from the mid-sagittal plane; the eye is internal (or medial) to the ear because it is closer to the mid-sagittal plane.

- *Long axis:* It is an imaginary central line passing longitudinally through the body or any of its parts.

- *Body planes:* In radiology, a plane is a real or an imaginary slice made through a body. The slices are made to study the details of the cut surfaces. These cut surfaces are called sections or views. Planes can pass through a body in an infinite number of ways.

The common and standard planes are:

- *Sagittal plane:* A plane that is parallel to the long axis of a body and divides it into right and left parts. Mid-sagittal plane divides the body equally into right and left parts.

- *Frontal plane:* A plane that is parallel to the long axis of a body and divides it into anterior and posterior parts.
- *Transverse (Horizontal) plane:* This plane divides a body into upper and lower parts. More specifically, it is a one that passes through a body at right angle (90 degrees) to the sagittal and frontal planes.

The anatomical structures can be broadly divided into two types:

A. *Hard tissues:* The mineralized tissues having firm intercellular substance are called hard tissues. For example: Skull, Mandible, Teeth, Vertebrae, Hyoid bone, Clavicle etc.

B. *Soft tissues:* These are non-mineralized tissues that connect, envelope, support and/or move the structures around. For example: Scalp, Eyes, Ears, Tongue, Nose, Lips, Cheeks, Pharynx, Larynx, Muscles etc.

A. HARD TISSUES

Skull/Cranium

The skeleton of head, called skull, is formed by a number of separate bones, which are joined together with each other with linear sutures. Earlier these sutures are narrow gaps that are filled with dense fibrous tissue that ossifies after the age of 30 years. The skull at birth consists of 45 separate bones while an adult skull consists of 22 bones. The skull bones are classified as:

- Bones of Calvaria (Brain Box)
- Facial bones

Calvaria/Brain case/Brain Box: It encloses the brain with the meninges surrounding it. This part of skull is made up of eight bones that are classified as:

Paired bones
- Parietal
- Temporal

Unpaired bones
- Frontal
- Sphenoid
- Occipital
- Ethmoid

Facial Bones

The bones in the region of face collectively constitute the facial skeleton. 'Face' is defined as 'the surface in front of head extending from the top of the forehead to the base of the chin vertically and from right auricle to left auricle horizontally'.

Osteologically, it extends superiorly from frontal bone and inferiorly to base of mandible. On each side, it extends to external acoustic meatus of temporal bone.

The facial part is made up of the bones that are classified as:

Paired bones
- Maxilla
- Palatine
- Zygomatic
- Nasal
- Lacrimal
- Inferior Nasal concha

Unpaired Bones
- Mandible
- Vomer

Cavities of Skull

These are the hollow spaces surrounded by calvarial or facial bones. These cavities harbour some soft tissues. The cavities are as follows:

I. *Cranial cavity:* This is the superior most cavity of the skull that harbours brain along with its meninges, venous sinuses, all cranial nerves, four petrosal nerves, parts of internal carotid artery and 4th part of vertebral artery.

II. *Orbital cavities/orbit:* These are pyramidal bony cavities, situated one on each side of the root of the nose. Each orbit is occupied by eye and the related structures (muscles, nerves, blood vessels etc.). Each orbit resembles an irregular pyramid. The anatomical configuration of the orbit is constituted as follows:

1. *Apex:* An apex is situated at the posterior end of orbit, at the opening of optic canal.
2. *Base:* The base is the opening of orbit on the face.
3. *Medial wall:* The medial walls of two orbits are parallel to each other and are formed from front to backwards by the following bones:
   - Maxilla
   - Lacrimal
   - Ethmoid
   - Sphenoid.
4. *Lateral wall:* The lateral walls of two orbits are at right angle to each other and each is formed by greater wing of sphenoid and frontal process of zygomatic bone.
5. *Roof:* The major part of roof of the orbit is formed by orbital plate of frontal bone and a small triangular area near the apex is formed by the lesser wing of sphenoid.
6. *Floor of orbit:* It is formed by zygomatic, palatine and maxillary bones.

III. *Nasal cavity:* These are paired cavities that are present inferior to the cranium, superior to oral cavity and medial to the maxillary sinus and orbit.

Anatomically, the nasal cavity is constituted as follows:

1. *Nasal septum:* It separates two nasal cavities and is formed by:
   - Perpendicular plate of ethmoid
   - Vomer bone
2. *Floor:* It is smooth, concave in shape and communicates with oral cavity through incisive foramen. The *'Greater Anterior Part'* is formed by palatine processes of maxillae and the *'Smaller Posterior Part'* is formed by horizontal plates of palatine bones
3. *Roof:* The roof is formed anteriorly by nasal part of frontal bone, the middle part by ethmoid bone and the posterior part by body of the sphenoid bone.
4. *Lateral wall of nose:* It is occupied by nasal conchae—Superior and Middle nasal conchae are a part of ethmoid bone while inferior nasal concha is an independent bone.

IV. *Oral cavity:* The oral cavity is bounded anteriorly by lips and laterally by cheeks. The roof is formed by hard palate anteriorly and soft palate posteriorly while floor is formed by tongue and sublingual tissues. It communicates with the exterior through oral commissure present between upper and lower lips anteriorly and with the pharynx posteriorly. Also, it communicates with the nasal cavity through the incisive foramen via naso-palatine canal. It is divided into two parts by teeth and their alveolar processes:

- *Vestibule:* It is the space that is bounded by lips anteriorly; cheeks laterally; and by teeth and their alveolar process posteriorly. It

15

communicates with oral cavity through small interdental spaces present between the teeth.

- *Oral cavity proper:* It is the space that is bounded anterolaterally by teeth and their alveolar processes and posteriorly opens into pharynx through oropharyngeal isthmus. The roof is formed by the hard and soft palate while floor is formed by tongue and sublingual tissues.

V. *Para nasal sinuses:* These are air filled spaces that are present in certain bones of skull and face. These are:
  - Maxillary sinus
  - Frontal sinus
  - Ethmoid sinus
  - Sphenoidal sinus

Different views for Studying the Skull

The skull can be studied from different views according to the line of vision. Their clinical importance lies in the fact that the different extra-oral radiographs are taken, studied and diagnosis is given on the basis of these lines of vision e.g. in PA/AP projections structures in frontal or coronal plane are studied and diagnosed. The different views for studying the skull are discussed below:

1. **Norma Verticalis:** If the skull is viewed and studied from above, the view is called Norma Verticalis.

The following bones can be viewed (Fig. 15.1) in it:
- Frontal
- Parietal
- Part of occipital

Other features identified are:
- Coronal suture
- Sagittal suture
- Lambdoid suture
- Bregma
- Lambda
- Parietal foramen

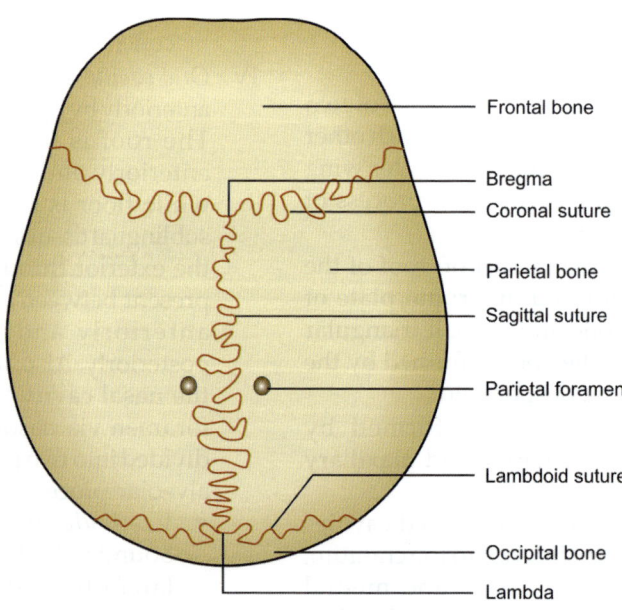

Frontal bone

Bregma
Coronal suture

Parietal bone

Sagittal suture

Parietal foramen

Lambdoid suture

Occipital bone

Lambda

Fig. 15.1: Norma Verticalis

15

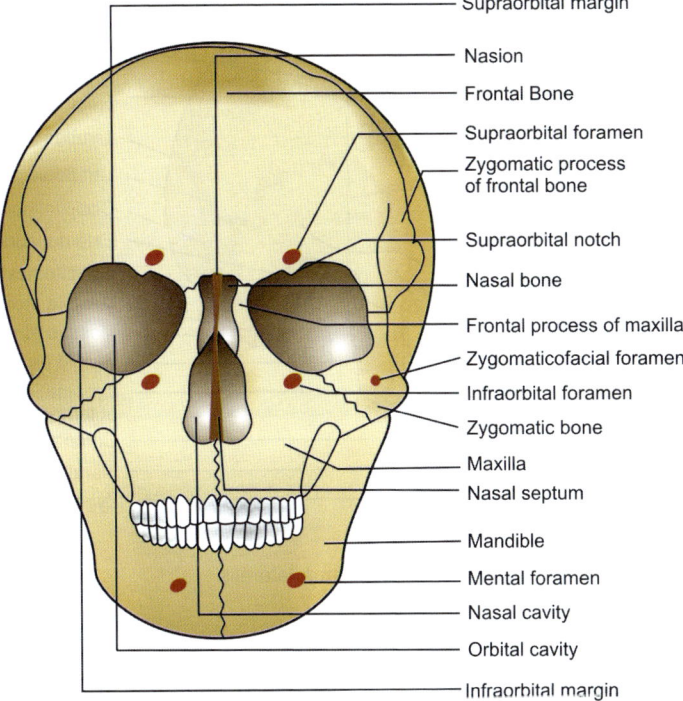

Supraorbital margin

Nasion

Frontal Bone

Supraorbital foramen

Zygomatic process of frontal bone

Supraorbital notch

Nasal bone

Frontal process of maxilla

Zygomaticofacial foramen

Infraorbital foramen

Zygomatic bone

Maxilla

Nasal septum

Mandible

Mental foramen

Nasal cavity

Orbital cavity

Infraorbital margin

Fig. 15.2: Norma Frontalis

2. **Norma Frontalis:** If the skull is viewed and studied from front, the view is called Norma Frontalis.
   The following bones can be viewed (Fig. 15.2) in it:
   • Frontal bone
   • Nasal bones
   • Maxillae
   • Zygomatic bones
   • Two orbital cavities
   • Two nasal cavities.
   Other features identified are:
   • Nasion
   • Supra-orbital margins
   • Supra-orbital notches
   • Supra-orbital foramina
   • Infra-orbital margins

   • Infra-orbital foramina
   • Zygomatic-facial foramina
   • Frontal processes of maxilla
   • Nasal septum
   • Zygomatic process of frontal bone
   The features/structures of mandible visible in Fig. 15.2 are elaborated separately.

3. **Norma Lateralis:** If the skull is viewed and studied from the sides, the view is called Norma Lateralis. Most of the features mentioned in other views are also seen in this view. It is demarcated from other views by the salient temporal lines.
   The bones viewed (Fig.15.3) are:
   • Frontal
   • Parietal bone

15

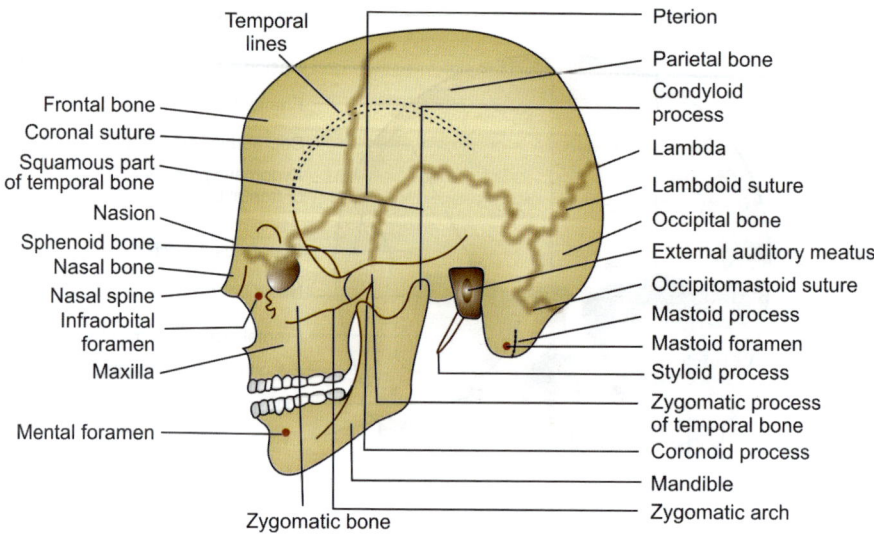

Fig. 15.3: Norma lateralis

- Sphenoid
- Temporal
- Zygomatic
- Maxilla
- Occipital

Other features identified are:
- Temporal lines
- Zygomatic arch
- External auditory meatus
- Occipito-mastoid suture
- Lambdoid suture
- Mastoid process
- Mastoid foramen
- Styloid process
- Pterion
- Nasal bone
- Nasal spine
- Lambda
- Zygomatic process of temporal bone

The features/structures of mandible visible in Fig.15.3 are elaborated separately.

4. **Norma Basalis and Base of Skull:** If the skull is viewed and studied from an inferior aspect, the view is called Norma Basalis. It has the most irregular appearance.

Norma Basalis is divided into three parts (Figs 15.4 and 15.5):

a. *Anterior part* is formed by hard (bony) palate and alveolar arches.

b. *Middle part* is the part of skull, which is between anterior part and a transverse line drawn across anterior margin of foramen magnum.

c. The part behind the transverse line drawn across anterior margin of foramen magnum is the *posterior part* of base of skull.

a. *Anterior part of Norma Basalis*

The bony palate lies within the arch formed by teeth of maxillae and alveolar processes. The bony palate is made up of (i) palatine processes of maxillae and (ii)

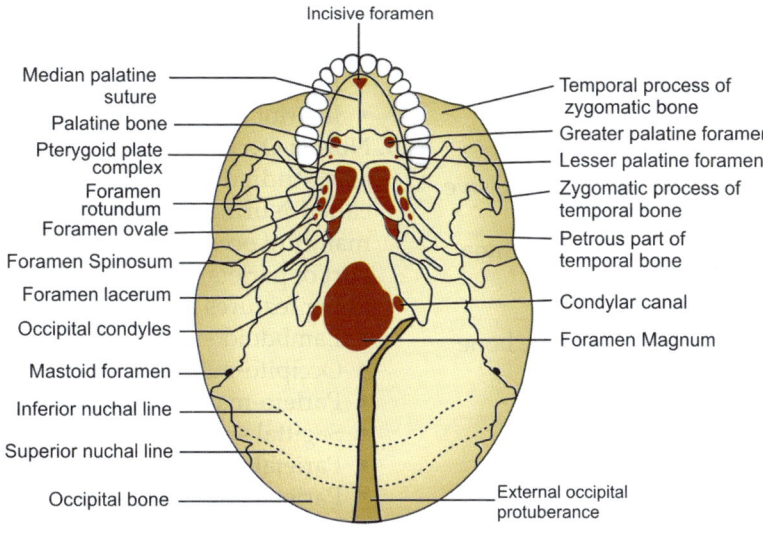

Fig. 15.4: Norma basalis

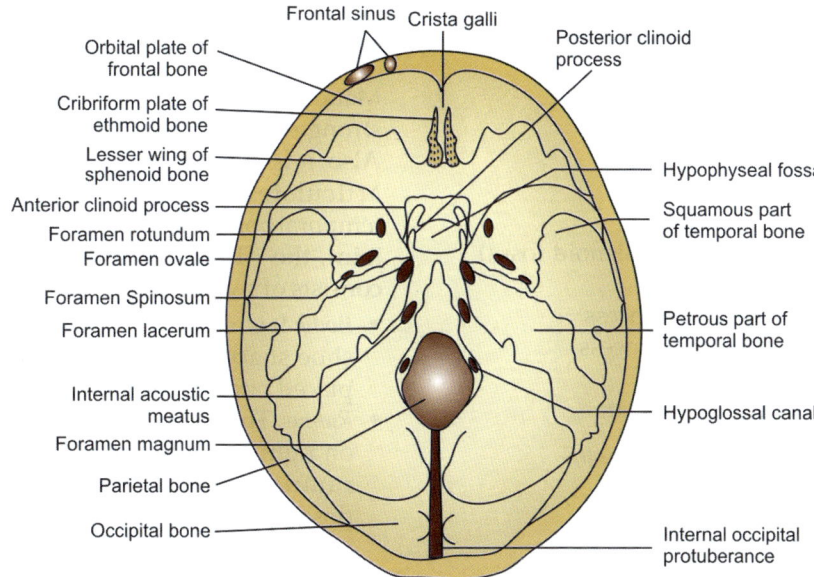

Fig. 15.5: Base of skull

15

horizontal plates of palatine bones and has inter-maxillary, inter-palatine and palato-maxillary sutures.
Other features identified are:

- Incisive canal
- Incisive foramen opening into incisive canal
- Greater and lesser palatine foramina
- Alveolar arch
- Palatine bone
- Temporal process of zygomatic bone
- Median palatine suture
- Ethmoid bone
- Frontal bone
- Frontal sinus
- Crista galli

b. *Middle part of Norma Basalis*
The bones viewed are:
- Sphenoid
- Pterygoid plates
- Occipital
- Temporal
Other features identified are:
- Occipital bone
- Pterygoid plates
- Pterygoid hamulus
- Foramen ovale
- Foramen spinosum
- Foramen lacerum
- Mandibular fossa (Glenoid fossa)
- Articular tubercle
- Anterior clinoid process
- Posterior clinoid process
- Hypophyseal fossa
- Internal acoustic meatus.

c. *Posterior part of Norma Basalis*
The bones viewed are:
- Occipital
- Temporal
Other features identified are:
- Foramen Magnum
- Occipital condyles

- Hypoglossal canal (Condylar canal)
- Mastoid foramen
- External occipital protuberance
- Inferior and superior nuchal lines.

5. **Norma Occipitalis:** If the skull is viewed and studied from behind, the view is called Norma Occipitalis. It comprises mainly of occipital bone along with some part of parietal bone (Fig.15.6).
Other features identified are:
- Lambdoid suture
- Occipito-mastoid sutures
- Parieto-mastoid sutures
- Sagittal suture
- Parietal foramen
- Parietal bone
- Mastoid foramen
- Mastoid process
- External occipital protuberance
- Highest nuchal lines
- Superior-nuchal lines
- Inferior-nuchal lines

Mandible

Mandible or the 'lower jaw' is the largest and strongest bone of face (Figs 15.7 and 15.8). Also, it is the only movable bone of face. It articulates with the glenoid fossa of temporal bone of the skull to form a movable joint, the 'Temporomandibular joint'. It consists of two major parts:

- *Body:* It is an unpaired, u-shaped or horse shoe shaped, convex and horizontally placed part of mandible.
- *Ramus:* These are paired parts present each on right and left side of mandible. Each ramus projects upwards from the posterior end of the body and ultimately joins the glenoid fossa of temporal bone of skull through its *condylar process* to form Temporomandibular joint. It has another flattened process known as *coronoid*

15

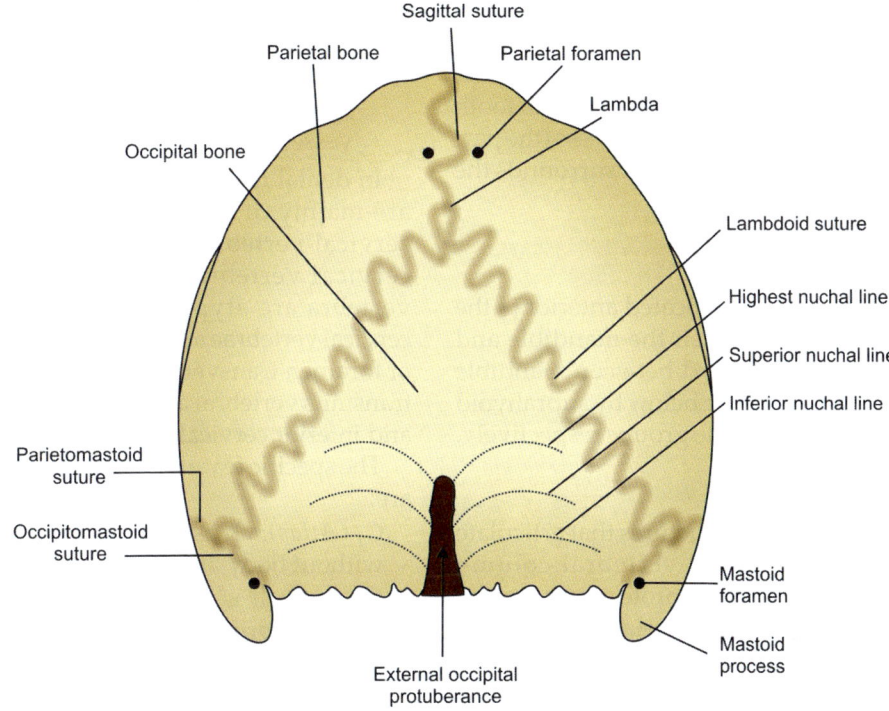

Sagittal suture

Parietal bone

Parietal foramen

Lambda

Occipital bone

Lambdoid suture

Highest nuchal line

Superior nuchal line

Inferior nuchal line

Parietomastoid suture

Occipitomastoid suture

Mastoid foramen

Mastoid process

External occipital protuberance

Fig. 15.6: Norma Occipitalis

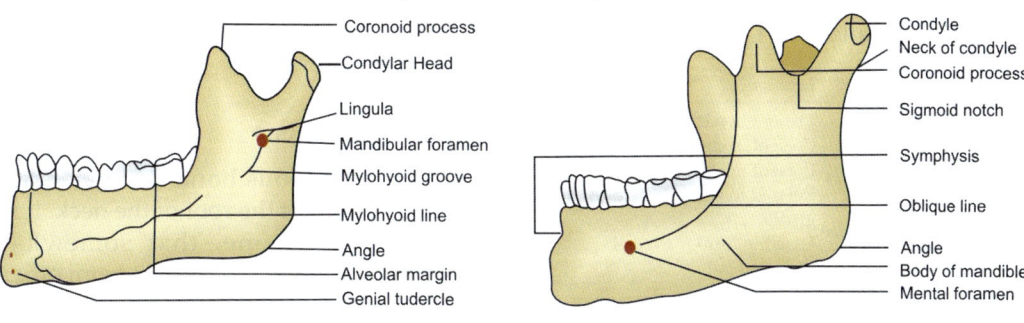

Coronoid process

Condylar Head

Lingula

Mandibular foramen

Mylohyoid groove

Mylohyoid line

Angle

Alveolar margin

Genial tudercle

Condyle
Neck of condyle
Coronoid process

Sigmoid notch

Symphysis

Oblique line

Angle
Body of mandible
Mental foramen

Fig. 15.7: Medial surface of the mandible

Fig. 15.8: Lateral surface of the mandible

15

process, which is placed anterior to condylar process with a concavity in between two that is known as sigmoid notch.

Teeth and their Alveolar Processes

Teeth are defined as hard bone like structures rooted in sockets in jaws of vertebrates, typically composed of a core of soft pulp surrounded by a layer of hard dentin that is coated with cementum at root or enamel at crown and is used for biting/chewing food or as a mean of attack or defense. Each tooth is supported by its alveolar process (the part of mandible and maxilla that surrounds the tooth root).

Hyoid Bone

It is a u-shaped bone located anterior to the spinal column between the mandible and larynx. It is suspended between mandible above and the clavicle below by suprahyoid and infrahyoid muscle groups respectively.

Vertebrae

These are the bony structures that articulate together to form the vertebral column (backbone). It acts as a protective covering for the spinal cord and related structures lying in the mid dorsal line of neck and trunk. It is made up of 33 vertebrae but consists of 26 bones because of fusion of five sacral and four coccygeal vertebrae. The vertebral formula is $C_7T_{12}L_5S_{(5)}C_{(4)}$.

Notation	Vertebrae	Location	Number
C	Cervical	Present in neck	7
T	Thoracic	Present in chest	12
L	Lumbar	Present in abdomen	5
S	Sacral	Related to pelvic girdle	5
C	Coccygeal	Fused to form vestigeal tail	4

A typical vertebra has following parts:
- *Vertebral body:* The anterior or ventral part of the vertebra is called its body.
- *Vertebral arch/neural arch:* The posterior or dorsal part of the vertebra is called its arch.
- *Vertebral foramen:* This foramen lies between the body and arch of each vertebra. These foramina are placed

one above the other within the intervertebral discs between them and form the vertebral canal which lodges the spinal cord, its meninges and the blood vessels supplying it.

In dental radiology, the *cervical vertebrae* are mainly of concern. There are total 7 cervical vertebrae. C_3 to C_6 are typical cervical vertebrae while C_1, C_2 and C_7 vertebra are atypical vertebrae. All the cervical vertebrae are identified by presence of foramen transversarium (a foramen that transmits vertebral arteries, vertebral veins and inferior cervical ganglion).

The specific features of atypical vertebrae are:

C_1 *(Atlas):* It is ring shaped vertebra without body and spine.

C_2 *(Axis):* It is identified by presence of odontoid process called as dens, which is a strong tooth like structure having bifid tip terminating into two rough tubercles.

C_3 to C_6 are typical vertebrae

C_7: It has most prominent spinous process, therefore known as 'vertebra prominens'.

Clavicle/Collar Bone

It is a subcutaneous bone that lies horizontally in front of the root of the neck. It is a long curved bone, that somewhat resembles the letter 'f'. It differs from other long bones viz. it has no medullary cavity and ossifies in membrane.

Clavicle is divided into following three parts:
- *Shaft:* It is the elongated, cylindrical part of clavicle.
- *Acromian end:* This is the flattened end that articulates with the acromian process of scapula.

15

- *Sternal end:* This is an expanded, quadrangular end that articulates with manubrium sterni.

B. SOFT TISSUES

Various soft tissues, which are of interest in radiographic interpretation, are as follows:

1. *Scalp:* The soft tissues covering the cranial vault form the scalp. They extend anteriorly till supraorbital margins; posteriorly till external occipital protuberance and superior nuchal lines and on each side till temporal lines.

2. *Nose:* The prominent ridge separating the right and left halves of nose is called the dorsum of the nose. The upper narrow end of the nose that is attached to forehead is its root and the rounded lower end of the dorsum is its tip. At the lower/anterior end, we see right and left openings known as nostrils/anterior nares that are separated by soft median partition called columella. Columella is continuous with the nasal septum. Lateral boundary of each nostril is called as 'ala'.

3. *Eye and palpebral fissure:* The palpebral fissure is an elliptical opening present between the upper and lower eye-lids that form the soft tissue counterpart of the bony orbit; forming a protective covering on the contents of orbit or eye.

   Through palpebral fissure following structures are seen:

   i. Sclera/white of eye

   ii. *Cornea:* A transparent circular structure

   iii. *Pupil and Iris:* seen through transparent cornea.

4. *External ear:* It is made up of two parts:

   i. *Auricle/pinna:* This is the superficial, projecting part of external ear. It consists of a thin plate of yellow, elastic fibro-cartilage covered with skin, except in the lobule and in the parts between tragus and helix, where fibrocartilage is absent.

   ii. *External acoustic meatus:* This is a deep S-shaped canal, 24 mm long of which 16 mm (medial 2/3rd) is bony and 8.0mm (lateral 1/3rd) is cartilaginous.

5. *Lips:* The lips are fleshy folds, composed of muscle and fat; lined externally by skin and internally by mucous membrane. Lips bound the oral fissure or mouth (formed by upper and lower lips).

   Each lip has a red margin (mucocutaneous junction) and a black margin with non hairy skin present between these two margins. Upper lip has a median vertical groove-known as philtrum, which extends from the centre of upper lip to the centre of nose.

6. *Cheeks:* These are fleshy flaps, composed of muscles and fat, lined externally by skin and internally by mucous membrane, that form the lateral boundary of vestibule on the sides of face.

7. *Tongue:* The tongue has following parts:

   a. *The root:* It is attached to mandible and soft palate superiorly and to hyoid bone inferiorly.

   b. *The tip:* It is the anterior, free, mobile end of tongue that rests behind the incisor teeth.

   c. *The Body:* The body consists of:

      i. *Dorsum:* It is a curved superior surface of tongue that is having two parts separated by V-shaped sulcus (sulcus terminals)—an oral part anterior 2/3rd) that lies in the oral cavity and a pharyngeal part (posterior 1/3rd) that lies in the pharynx.

15

ii. *Ventral surface:* It is the inferior surface of tongue.

  d. The posterior most part of tongue is connected to the epiglottis by three folds—right and left lateral epiglottic folds and a median epiglottic fold.

8. *Pharynx:* It is a wide muscular tube, about 12 cm long that extends from base of the skull to the level of body of sixth cervical vertebrae (C_6); from here it continues downwards into oesophagus. It has three parts:

  a. *Nasopharynx:* This is the upper part of pharynx, situated behind the nose and above the lower border of soft palate.

  b. *Oropharynx:* It is the middle part of the pharynx that is situated posterior to the oral cavity.

  c. *Laryngopharynx:* It is the laryngeal part of pharynx that is situated posterior to the larynx and extends from upper border of epiglottis to lower border of cricoid cartilage.

9. *Larynx (Voice box):* It is a cartilaginous structure, lying in the anterior midline of neck that extends superiorly from the root of the tongue to the trachea inferiorly. It is concerned with production of voice/phonation, acts as a passage for air, and as a sphincter at the inlet of lower respiratory passage.

10. *Trachea:* It is about 10 to 15 cm long, non-collapsible wide tube forming the beginning of lower respiratory passages that begins at the lower border of cricoid cartilage opposite the C_6 vertebrae and enters thorax in the median plane. It has C-shaped cartilaginous rings that keep its opening patent during passage of air. These rings are deficient posteriorly and are closed by trachealis muscle.

11. *Muscles:* A variety of muscles are present in the region of head and neck. Some important ones are enumerated below:

  a. *Muscles of facial expression:* Orbicularis oris, Orbicularis Oculi, Frontalis, Procerus, Nasalis, Zygomatics Major, Zygomatics Minor, Mentalis, Levator anguli Oris, Depressor anguli Oris, Risorius

  b. *Muscles of mastication:* Masseter, Temporalis, Medial and Lateral Pterygoids.

  c. *Muscles in region of floor of mouth:* Mylohyoid and Genioglossus.

  d. *Suprahyoid muscles:* Digastric, geniohyoid, Hyoglossus and Mylohyoid

  e. *Infrahyoid muscles:* Sternohyoid, Sterno-thyroid, Thyrohyoid, Omohyoid.

  f. *Prominent muscles of neck:* Sternocleido-mastoid and Trapezius.

IMAGE EVALUATION PROTOCOL

Roger Windle in early 80's devised a protocol to determine whether a film radiograph is of diagnostic value or not. The technique helps other radiographers and students to critically evaluate radiographic images. It is being widely used under the acronym PACEMAN.

PACEMAN implies the following:
- **Position**
- **Area**
- **Collimation**
- **Exposure**
- **Markers**
- **Aesthetics**
- **Name**

The summary of the qualities that are needed for each letter of PACEMAN are:

(P) Position
- Is the patient in correct position?

- Is the patient rotated?
- Does the image correctly show any needed joint space?

(A) Area
- Is enough of the area being filmed covered? For example, in an occlusal film, is the arches from left to right covered?
- Has any area exposed which is not required?

(C) Collimation
- Is the image properly collimated? For example, is collimation seen on an extremities film?

(E) Exposure
- Were the exposure factors set correctly?
- Does the image show the correct contrast and density?
- Are there any factors that need to be changed to produce a better image?

(M) Markers
- Have markers been placed on the image?
- Are they correctly identified left and right?

(A) Aesthetics
- Is the image nice to look at?
- Is it centered on the film?
- Is the image properly collimated?

(N) Name
- Does the image correctly identify the patient?
- Does it have any other relevant identification details? For example, department labels or identification number?

Landmarks in Oral Radiology

A landmark is a structure, or any consistent point on the structures, which is to be studied in a radiograph. It can be used for any quantitative analysis or measurement carried out for a particular radiograph.

The landmarks can be classified as follows:

1. On the basis of their location
   a. *Intraoral landmarks:* These are the points or structures that are present inside the oral cavity and are seen in intraoral radiographs e.g. in Intraoral periapical view, Occlusal view etc.
   b. *Extraoral landmarks:* These are the points or structures that are present outside the oral cavity and are seen in extraoral radiographs, e.g. in Posterior-anterior view, Lateral oblique view, etc.

2. On the basis of the nature of tissues involved
   a. *Hard tissue landmarks:* These are the bony structures or the points that are present on the bony structures e.g. anterior nasal spine, vertebrae, etc.
   b. *Soft tissue landmarks:* These are the structures or points present on the structures that do not have any ossification or have minimal ossification within them e.g. shadow of lips, nose, trachea etc.

3. On the basis of anatomical consi-derations:
   a. *Anatomical landmarks:* These are the structures or points that represent the actual anatomical structures present in the body e.g. sella turcica, zygomatic arch, teeth etc.
   b. *Derived landmarks:* These are the points or structures that have been obtained secondarily from actual anatomical structures, e.g. in cephalogram—Pterygomaxillary (ptm) point and Broadbent registration point are the derived landmarks.

15

Requirements

The landmarks are required to have the following features:

- *Visibility:* It should be directly, clearly and easily visible on the radiograph.
- *Reproducibility:* It should be uniform in outline and easily reproducible when required so.
- *Validity:* These landmarks should permit valid quantitative measurements of the lines and angles projected from them.

The landmarks that are important for radiographic interpretation and are commonly visible on the radiographs are as follows:

I. Extraoral Landmarks

The extraoral landmarks that are visible on different extraoral views are described below:

1. Posterior-Anterior (PA) View of Mandible

The different landmarks visible in this view (Fig. 15.9) are:

Hard tissue landmarks

The **radiopaque landmarks** of **skull** visible in PA view of mandible are:

a. *Crista galli:* It is a small, thick, triangular process projecting from the midline of cribriform plate of ethmoid bone.

b. *Superior border of orbit:* It has supraorbital notch and is formed by supraorbital margin of frontal bone.

c. *Inferior border of orbit:* It is formed by the zygomatic bone and maxilla; has infra orbital ridge with infraorbital notch on it.

d. *Zygomatic process of maxilla:* It is a short process that projects upwards and laterally from the junction of anterior, posterior and orbital surfaces of maxilla; forms the anterior part of zygomatic arch and is palpable through cheek.

e. *Medial pterygoid plates:* These are one of the pterygoid processes of sphenoid bone that is medial in its location and is longer than the lateral pterygoid plate.

f. *Lesser wing of sphenoid:* These are two triangular plates projecting laterally from upper and anterior parts of body of sphenoid and are connected to body by two roots which harbor the optic canal.

g. *Vomer:* also known as plowshare bone; it is thin flat bone almost trapezoidal in shape situated in mid plane and forms the postero-inferior part of septum of nose.

h. *Middle nasal concha:* This is a part of ethmoid bone that is visible in the lateral wall of nose in radiograph.

i. *Inferior nasal concha:* It is an oval plate that forms a part of lateral wall of nasal cavity.

j. *Floor of posterior cranial fossa* (Not demarcated in Fig.15.9)

k. *Occipital condyles:* These are structures, oval/kidney shaped convex articular surfaces which articulate with the superior concave articular facet of atlas forming atlanto-occipital joint (Not demarcated in Fig.15.9).

The **radiolucent landmarks** of **skull** visible in PA view of mandible are:

a. *Frontal sinus:* These are paired structures, roughly triangular in shape that are situated behind the superciliary arches between outer and inner tables of frontal bone.
  - Each sinus extends upwards above medial part of the roof of the orbit.
  - It is underdeveloped at birth, appears during 2nd year of life and

15

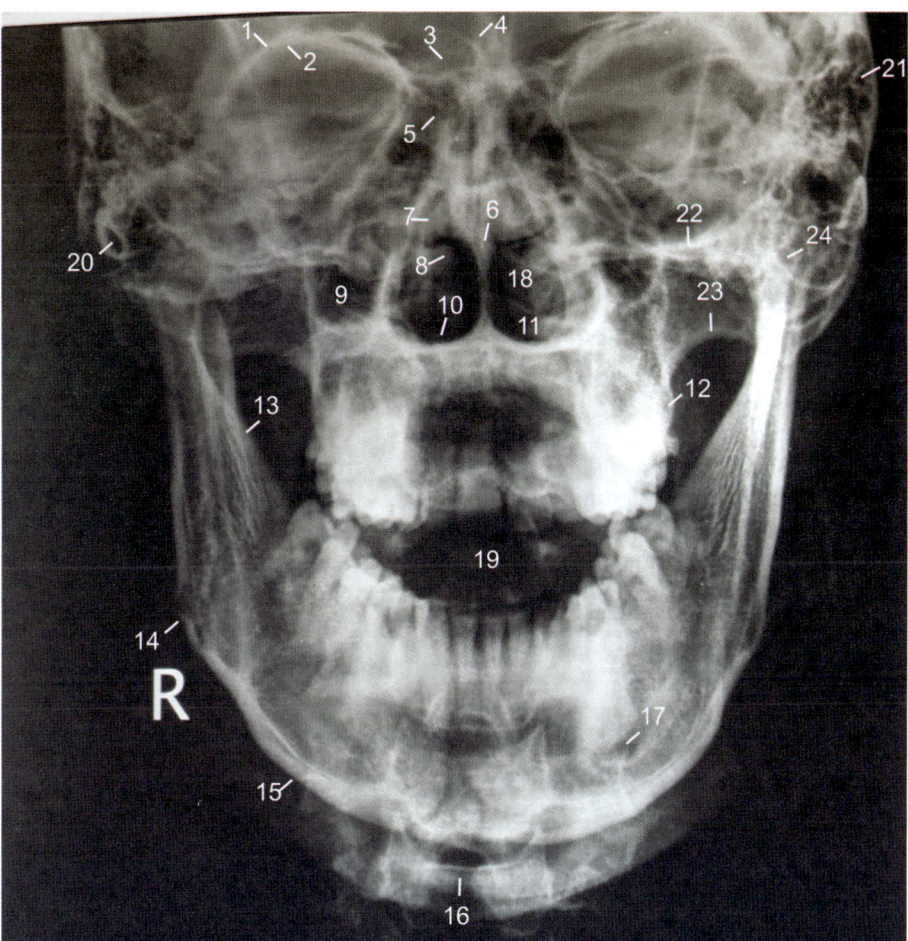

Fig. 15.9: PA View of mandible: (1) Superior border of orbit (2) lesser wing of sphenoid (3) frontal sinus (4) crista galli (5) ethmoid air cells (6) vomer (7) middle nasal concha (8) medial pterygoid plate (9) maxillary sinus (10) inferior nasal meatus (11) inferior nasal concha (12) maxillary tuberosity (13) anterior border of ascending ramus (14) angle of mandible (15) inferior border of mandible (16) cervical vertebra (17) mental foramen (18) nasal cavity (19) oral cavity (20) external auditory meatus (21) mastoid air cells (22) inferior border of orbit (23) zygomatic process of maxilla (24) condyloid process

reaches full size after puberty. Its configuration is 3.15 cm × 2.5 cm × 1.8 cm.

b. *Sphenoid sinus:* These are two in number, situated behind the upper part of nasal cavity on each side, within the body of sphenoid. These two sinuses may be unequal in size due to deviated nasal septum (Not clearly visible in Fig.15.9).

Each sinus opens into spheno-ethmoidal recess, which opens into superior meatus of nose. Its configuration is 2.0 cm × 1.8 cm × 2.0 cm.

c. *Ethmoid air cells:* These are small, thin walled cavities or cells which occupy the labyrinth of ethmoid bone. They are made up of incomplete walls, that are completed with the help of following bones:
- Frontal
- Maxilla
- Palatine
- Sphenoid
- Lacrimal

These cells vary in size and numbers from three large sinuses to 18 small sinuses. These are arranged into three groups:

Number of groups	Opening in lateral wall of nose
Anterior (about 11–12 in number)	Middle meatus
Middle (3 in number)	Superior meatus
Posterior (1 to 7 in number)	Superior meatus

d. *Maxillary sinus*
- It is a large pyramidal cavity present in the body of maxilla. It is the largest of all other paranasal sinuses.
- Its apex is directed laterally, into zygomatic process of maxilla.
- Its base faces medially and is formed by lateral wall of nasal cavity.
- The roof is formed by the floor of orbit and the floor is formed by the alveolar process of maxilla and lies about 1.25 cm below the level of floor of nose.
- It opens into middle meatus of nose in the lower part of hiatus semilunaris.

e. *Mastoid air cells*

f. *External auditory meatus*

g. *Nasal cavity*

h. *Oral cavity*

The **radiopaque landmarks** of **mandible** visible in PA view of mandible are:

a. *Neck of condyle:* The constriction below the head of the condyle is known as neck of condyle.

b. *Anterior border of ascending ramus:* This is the thin border of ramus, which is visible on radiograph.

c. *Inferior border of mandible:* The backward continuation of base of the mandible forms the inferior border of mandible.

d. *Angle of mandible:* The point where inferior border of mandible ends by becoming continuous with the posterior border of mandible is known as angle of mandible.

The **radiolucent landmarks** of **mandible** visible in PA view mandible are:

a. *Mental Foramen*

A foramen present below the interval between first and second premolar teeth or below the second premolar tooth.

Apart from these landmarks, certain **other landmarks** visible in this view are:

a. Cervical Vertebrae

i. *Transverse process of atlas:* These are radiopaque processes, two in number and project laterally from pedicle and lamina. These have a foramen (foramen transversarium).

ii. *Odontoid process of axis:* It is a strong tooth like process, about 0.5 inch long that is attached to the body of the axis. It is also a radiopaque process with a pointed apex that projects in an upward direction. It acts as a pivot for the rotation of skull.

iii. *Atlanto-occipital joint:* The joint present between occipital condyles of occipital bone and atlas vertebrae is known as

15

atlanto-occipital joint. The 'yes' movement, that is, up and down movement of neck occurs around this joint.

Soft tissue landmarks

The soft tissue **radiolucent landmarks** visible in PA view of mandible are:

a. *Inferior nasal meatus:* This is a passage present beneath the inferior nasal concha in which nasolacrimal duct opens.

2. Lateral Oblique View of Mandible

The different landmarks visible in this view (Fig. 15.10) are:

Hard tissue landmarks

The **radiopaque landmarks** of **skull** visible in Lateral oblique view of mandible are:

a. *Zygomatic process of maxilla:* A short process that projects upwards and laterally from the junction of anterior, posterior and orbital surfaces of maxilla; forms the anterior part of zygomatic arch and is palpable through cheek.

b. *Zygomatic bone:* This bone lies on the upper and lateral part of face and forms the bony prominence of cheek.

c. *Articular eminence:* It is a ramp-shaped prominence of temporal bone that extends forwards and downwards from temporal fossa.

d. *Maxillary tuberosity:* It is a rounded eminence at the lower and posterior part of the infra-temporal surface of maxilla.

e. *Mastoid process:* It is the conical projection from the antero-inferior part of the external surface of base of the skull.

f. *Styloid process:* A slender, thin pointed process, about 2.5 cm long, projecting downwards and forwards from the under surface of petrous part of temporal bone (Not clear in Fig.15.10).

g. *Inferior border of orbit* (Not visible in Fig. 15.10).

The **radiolucent landmarks** of **skull** visible in Lateral oblique view of mandible are:

a. *Maxillary sinus*
b. *Nasal cavity.*

The **radiopaque landmarks** of **mandible** visible in Lateral oblique view of mandible are:

a. *Coronoid process:* It is a flat and triangular process of mandible that has an apex that points upwards and a base that is fused with the upper and anterior part of mandible.

b. *Condylar process:* It is a flat triangular process of mandible that has an apex that points upwards and a base that is fused with the upper and anterior part of mandible.

c. *External oblique ridge:* An elevation present on the external surface of the body of the mandible which runs upwards and backwards from mental tubercles.

d. *Inferior border of mandible:* The backward continuation of the base of the mandible forms the inferior border of mandible.

e. *Contra-lateral inferior border of mandible*

The **radiolucent landmarks** present in the **mandible** are:

a. *Sigmoid notch:* A wide concave notch in the upper border of ramus of mandible that is present between the coronoid and condylar processes.

b. *Mandibular foramen and canal:* A canal that runs within the substance of bone from the mandibular foramen in the ramus and body of mandible.

c. *Mental foramen.*

15

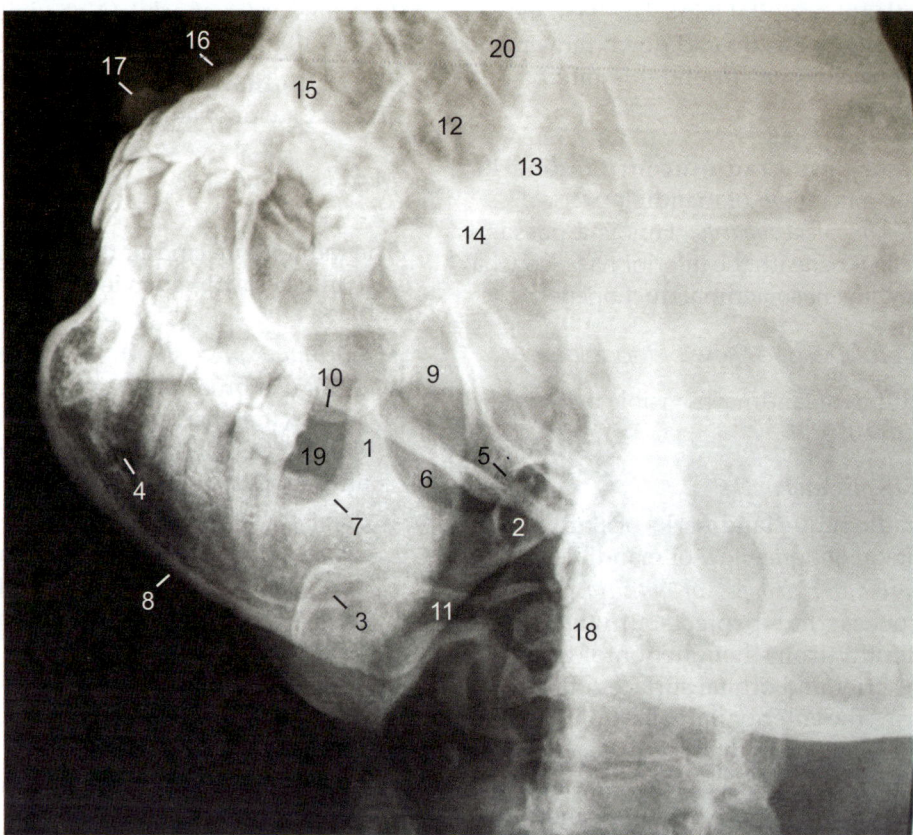

Fig. 15.10: Lateral oblique view of mandible (1) Coronoid process (2) condyloid process (3) mandibular canal (4) mental foramen (5) articular eminence (6) sigmoid notch (7) external oblique ridge (8) inferior border of mandible (9) contralateral inferior border of mandible (10) maxillary tuberosity (11) hyoid bone (12) maxillary sinus (13) zygomatic bone (14) zygomatic process of maxilla (15) nasal cavity (16) shadow of nose (17) shadow of lips (18) mastoid process (19) shadow of tongue (20) orbital cavity

Apart from these landmarks, certain **other landmarks** visible in this view are:

Hyoid bone: It is a radiopaque, u-shaped bone located anterior to the spinal column between the mandible and larynx. It is suspended between mandible above and the clavicle below by suprahyoid and infrahyoid groups of muscles.

Soft tissue landmarks

The soft tissue landmarks commonly visible are:

a. *Shadow of superior border of tongue:* It is the dorsal surface of the tongue that is visible on the radiograph.
b. *Shadow of lips and nose*
c. *Pharyngeal walls of oropharynx and nasopharynx* (Not clearly visible in Fig.15.10)

d. The muscular fold that forms the posterior part of the roof of oral cavity (*soft palate*) (Not clearly demarcated in Fig. 15.10).

3. Waters' View (PA view of skull)

The different landmarks visible in this view (Fig. 15.11) are:

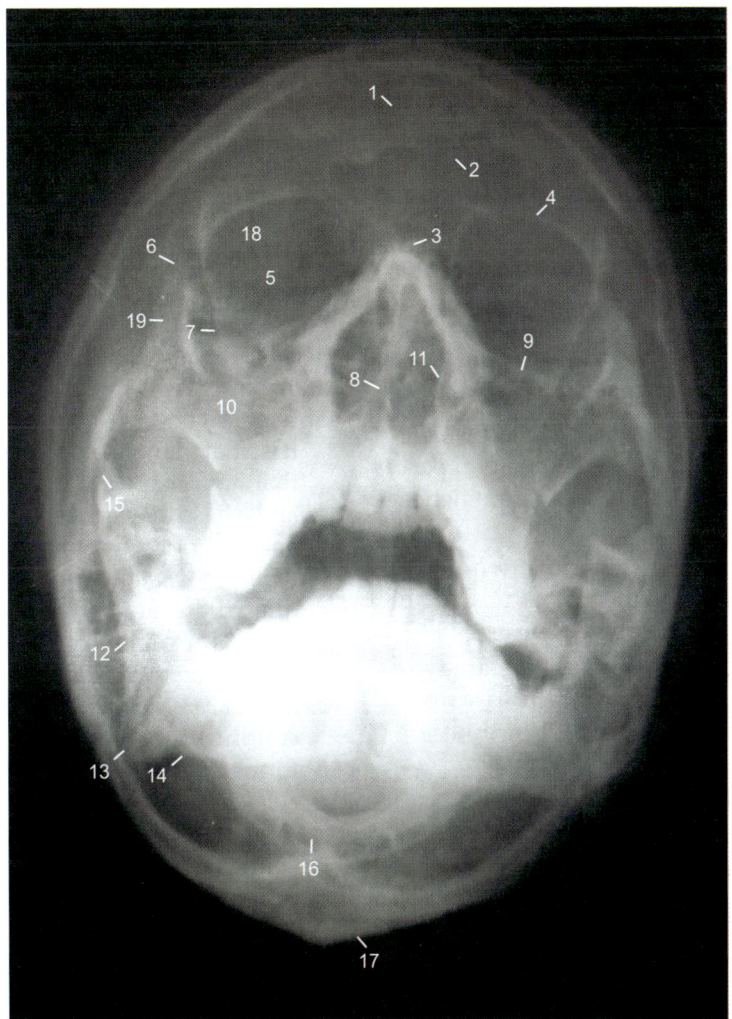

Fig 15.11: PA View of skull (Water's view): (1) Frontal bone (2) frontal sinus (3) crista galli (4) superior border of orbit (5) orbit (6) zygomatic process of frontal bone (7) zygomatic bone (8) nasal septum (9) infraorbital ridge (10) maxillary sinus (11) sphenoid sinus (12) border of ascending ramus (13) angle of mandible (14) inferior border of mandible (15) coronoid process (16) arch of atlas (17) inferior aspect of base of skull (18) lesser wing of sphenoid (19) frontal process of zygomatic bone

15

The **radiopaque landmarks** of **skull** visible in Waters' view are:

a. *Frontal bone:* It is a bone in the skull that resembles cockshell and forms the forehead in human beings.

b. *Zygomatic process of frontal bone:* It originates from the supraorbital margin of the frontal bone and ends by articulating with the frontal process of the zygomatic bone.

c. *Frontal process of zygomatic bone:* It is a thick, three sided process of frontal bone that projects in an upward direction from it.

d. *Crista galli:* It is a small, thick, triangular process projecting from the midline of cribriform plate of ethmoid bone.

e. *Zygomatic bone (Zygoma):* The zygomatic bone lies on the upper and lateral part of face and forms the bony prominence of cheek.

f. *Nasal septum:* It separates two nasal cavities and is formed by vertical plate of ethmoid and vomer bone.

g. *Lesser wing of sphenoid:* These are two thin triangular plates which arise from upper and anterior part of body of sphenoid bone.

h. *Superior border of orbit*

i. *Infraorbital ridge/Inferior border of orbit*

j. *Inferior aspect of base of skull*

k. *Floor of middle cranial fossa*

The **radiolucent landmarks** of **skull** visible in Water's view are:

a. *Supra-orbital notch:* It is a notch present on the supra-orbital margin at the junction of lateral 2/3rd and medial 1/3rd.

b. *Infra-orbital foramen and canal:* The end of infra-orbital canal above the canine fossa presents as infra-orbital foramen (not demarcated in the presented X-ray).

c. *Frontal sinus:* These are paired structures, roughly triangular in shape, that are situated behind the superciliary arches between outer and inner tables of frontal bone.

• Each sinus extends upwards above medial part of the roof of the orbit.

• It is underdeveloped at birth, appears during 2nd year of life and reaches full size after puberty. Its configuration is 3.15 cm × 2.5 cm × 1.8 cm.

d. *Maxillary sinus*

e. *Ethmoid air cells*

The **radiopaque landmarks** of **mandible** visible in this view are:

a. *Coronoid process (Processes coronoideus):* It is a flat triangular process of mandible that has an apex that points upwards and a base that is fused with the upper and anterior part of mandible.

b. *Ramus of mandible:* It is the flattened, quardilateral part of mandible that projects upwards from the posterior end of body on each side of mandible.

c. *Inferior border of mandible:* The backward continuation of the base of mandible forms the inferior border of mandible.

d. *Angle of mandible:* The inferior border of mandible ends by becoming continuous with the posterior border of mandible at an angular point known as angle of mandible.

Apart from these, **other radiopaque landmarks** are:

a. *Arch of atlas*

b. *Odontoid process of axis:* It is a strong tooth like process, about 0.5 inch long that is attached to the body of the axis. Its apex projects upwards and is pointed. It acts as a pivot for the rotation

15

of skull (not visible in the presented radiograph).

4. Submentovertex View

The different landmarks visible in this view (Fig. 15.12) are:

The **radiopaque landmarks** of **skull** visible in this view are:

a. *Lateral wall of orbit:* It is formed by the greater using of sphenoid and frontal process of zygomatic bone.

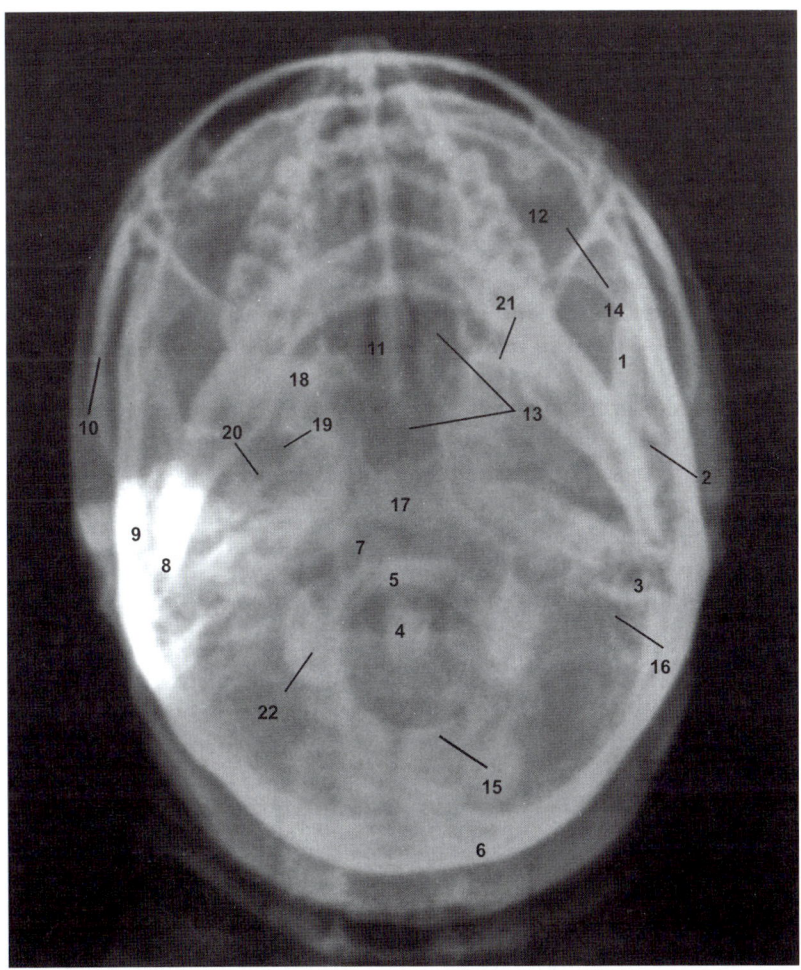

Fig. 15.12: Submentovertex view: (1) Coronoid process (2) condyloid process (3) mastoid air cells (4) dens (5) anterior arch of atlas (6) base of skull (7) hyoid bone (8) angle of mandible (9) ramus of mandible (10) zygomatic arch (11) nasal septum (12) maxillary sinus (13) sphenoid sinus (14) lateral wall of orbit (15) foramen magnum (16) external acoustic meatus (17) clivus (18) anterior wall of middle cranial fossa (19) foramen ovale (20) foramen spinosum (21) pterygoid plate complex (22) occipital condyle

15

b. *Zygomatic arch:* Zygomatic arch is formed by the zygomatic process of temporal bone and temporal process of zygomatic bone. It forms the prominence of the cheek so is also called 'cheek bone'.

c. *Nasal septum:* It is a midline structure that separates two nasal cavities and is formed by vertical plate of ethmoid and vomer bone.

d. *Anterior wall of middle cranial fossa.*

The **radiolucent landmarks** of **skull** visible in this view are:

a. *Maxillary sinus*

b. *Sphenoid sinus:* These are two in number, situated behind the upper part of nasal cavity on each side, within the body of sphenoid. These two sinuses are usually unequal in size due to deviated nasal septum (Not clearly visible in Fig.15.12).

c. *Mastoid air cell:* These are the number of air filled spaces present in the mastoid process of temporal bone.

d. *Foramen magnum:* It is an oval aperture in the base of skull in the occipital bone through which medulla oblongata enters and exits from the skull vault.

The **radiopaque landmarks** of **mandible** visible in this view are:

a. *Coronoid process*

b. *Condyle of mandible:* This is a strong upward projection from the posterior-superior part of the ramus of mandible whose upper end is expanded from side to side to form the head of condyle that articulates with temporal bone to form Temporomandibular joint.

c. *Ramus of mandible:* It is the flattened, quardilateral part of mandible that projects upwards from the posterior end of body on each side of mandible.

d. *Angle of mandible:* The inferior border of mandible ends by becoming continuous with the posterior border of mandible at an angular point known as angle of mandible.

Apart from these the **other radiopaque landmarks** are:

a. *Anterior arch of atlas*

b. *Dens/Odontoid process of axis*: It is a strong tooth like process, about 0.5 inch long and is attached to the body of the axis. The apex is pointed and projects upwards. It acts as a picot for the rotation of skull.

c. *Hyoid bone:* It is a radiopaque, u-shaped bone located anterior to the spinal column between the mandible and larynx. It is suspended between mandible above and the clavicle below by suprahyoid and infrahyoid groups of muscles.

5. Ortho-pantomogram

The different landmarks visible in this view (Fig. 15.13) are:

The **radiopaque landmarks** of **skull** in panoramic radiograph are:

a. *Hard palate:* It forms the roof of oral cavity proper and is formed by the fusion of palatine shelves or horizontal plates of palatine bone.

b. *Maxillary tuberosity:* It is a rounded eminence at the lower and posterior part of the infratemporal surface of maxilla.

c. *Nasal spine*

d. *Articular eminence:* It is a ramp-shaped prominence of temporal bone that extends forwards and downwards from temporal fossa.

e. *Zygomatic process of maxilla (Malar process):* It is a rough projection from

15

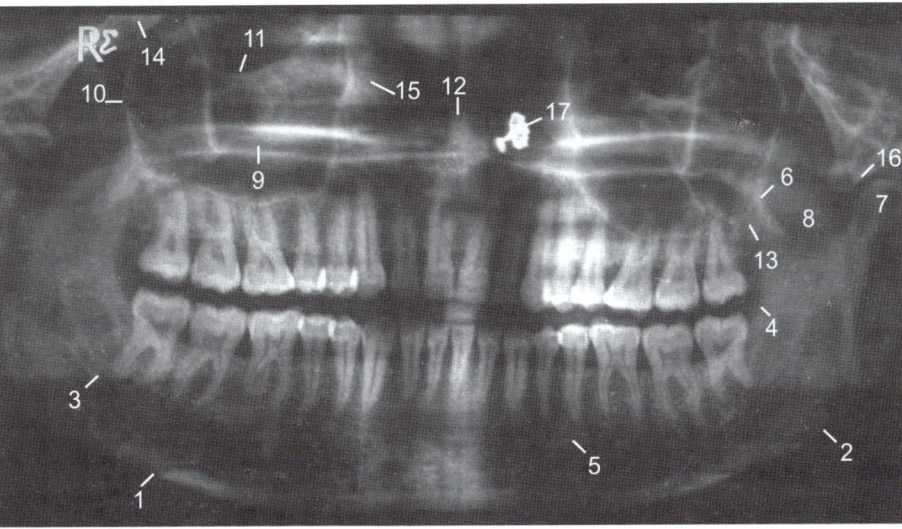

Fig. 15.13: Orthopantomogram (1) Inferior border of mandible (2) angle of mandible (3) mandibular canal (4) external oblique ridge (5) mental foramen (6) coronoid process (7) condyloid process (8) sigmoid notch (9) hard palate (10) wall of maxillary sinus (11) inferior border of orbit (12) Anterior nasal spine (13) maxillary tuberosity (14) zygomatic process of maxilla (15) inferior nasal concha (16) articular eminence (17) nose pin

maxilla that articulates with the zygomatic bone.

f. *Zygomatic process of temporal bone:* It is a long arched process projecting from the lower part of squamous portion of temporal bone (not visible in Fig. 15.13).

g. *Inferior border of orbit:*

The **radiolucent landmarks** of **skull** in panoramic radiograph are:

i. *Inferior nasal meatus:* This is a passage present beneath the inferior nasal concha in which nasolacrimal duct opens.

ii. *Maxillary sinus*

The **radiopaque landmarks** of **mandible** in panoramic radiograph are:

a. *Coronoid process:* It is a flat triangular process of mandible that has an apex that points upwards and a base that is fused with the upper and anterior part of mandible.

b. *Condyle:* This is a strong upward projection from the posterior-superior part of the ramus of mandible whose upper end is expanded from side to side to form the head of condyle that articulates with temporal bone to form Temporomandibular joint.

c. *External oblique ridge:* This is an elevation present on the external surface of the mandible which runs downwards and forwards towards mental tubercles.

d. *Angle of mandible:* The inferior border of mandible ends by becoming continuous with the posterior border of mandible at an angular point known as angle of mandible.

e. *Inferior Border of mandible:* The backward continuation of base of the mandible is the inferior border of mandible.

15

The **radiolucent landmarks** of **mandible** in this view are:

a. *Mental foramen*
b. *Mandibular canal*
c. *Sigmoid notch:* A wide concave notch in the upper border of ramus of mandible that is present between the coronoid and condylar processes.

Others landmarks visible are:

Hyoid bone: It is a radiopaque, u-shaped bone located anterior to the spinal column between the mandible and larynx. It is suspended between mandible above and the clavicle below by suprahyoid and infrahyoid groups of muscles.

6. Transpharyngeal View of Temporomandibular joint

This view mainly shows mandible and temporomandibular joint. The landmarks visible in this view (Fig. 15.14) are:

Radiopaque landmarks of **Mandible** visible in this view are:

• *Condyloid process*
• *Coronoid process*
• *Inferior border of mandible*
• *Angle of mandible*
• *External oblique ridge.*

Radiolucent Landmarks of **Mandible** visible are:

• *Mandibular canal*
• *Sigmoid notch.*

Radiopaque landmark of **skull** visible in this view is:

• *Articular eminence.*

Radiolucent landmark of **skull** visible in this view is:

• *Glenoid fossa/Mandibular fossa.*

II. Intraoral Landmarks

The landmarks (both radiolucent and radiopaque) visible in intraoral radiograph

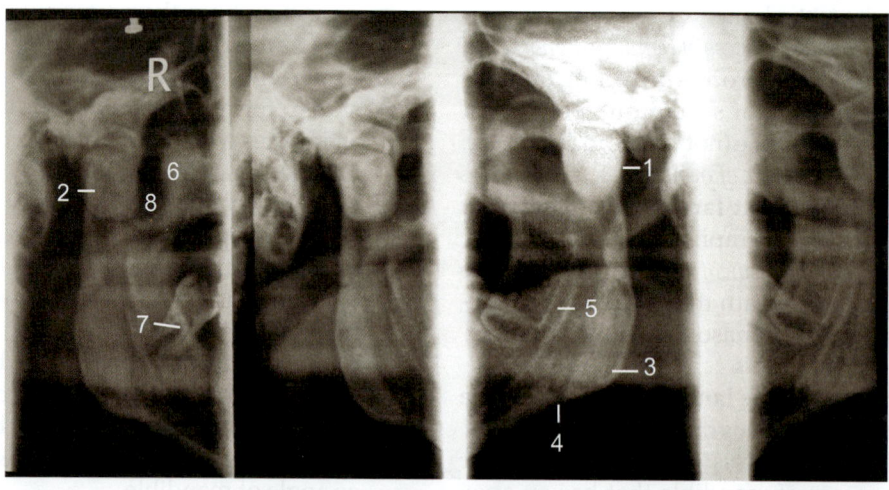

Fig. 15.14: Transpharyngeal view of TMJ: (1) Ankylosed left TMJ (Condyle ankylosed with glenoid fossa and articular eminence) (2) ankylosed right TMJ (condyle ankylosed with glenoid fossa and articular eminence) (3) angle of mandible (4) inferior border of mandible (5) mandibular canal (6) coronoid process (7) external oblique ridge (8) sigmoid notch

15

are discussed area wise for both maxillary and mandibular radiographs.

1. Maxillary occlusal view (Fig. 15.15)
2. Mandibular occlusal view (Fig. 15.16)
3. Maxillary incisors (Fig. 15.17)
4. Maxillary canines (Fig. 15.18)
5. Maxillary premolars (Fig. 15.19)
6. Maxillary molars (Fig. 15.20)
7. Mandibular incisors (Fig. 15.21)
8. Mandibular canines (Fig. 15.22)
9. Mandibular premolars (Fig. 15.23)
10. Mandibular molars (Fig. 15.24)

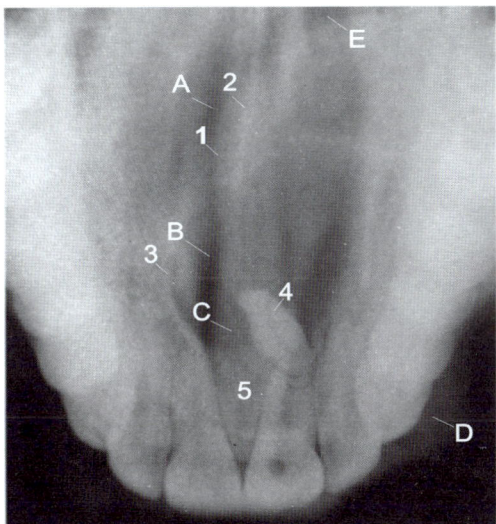

Fig. 15.15: Maxillary occlusal view

Radiopaque	Radiolucent
1. Nasal septum (bony)	A. Maxillary sinus
2. Median palatine suture	B. Common nasal meatus
3. Anterior and lateral border of nasal fossa	C. Nasal septum (cartilagenous)
4. A supernumerary tooth	D. Soft tissues of lips
5. Anterior nasal spine	E. Orbital entrance of nasolacrimal canal

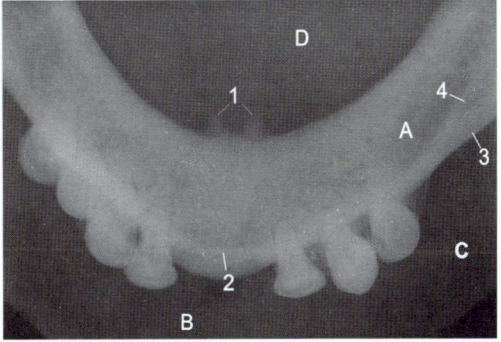

Fig. 15.16: Mandibular occlusal view

Radiopaque	Radiolucent
1. Genial tubercles	A. Submandibular fossa
2. Mental ridge	B. Soft tissues of lips
3. External oblique ridge	C. Soft tissues of cheeks
4. Internal oblique ridge	D. Shadow of tongue

15

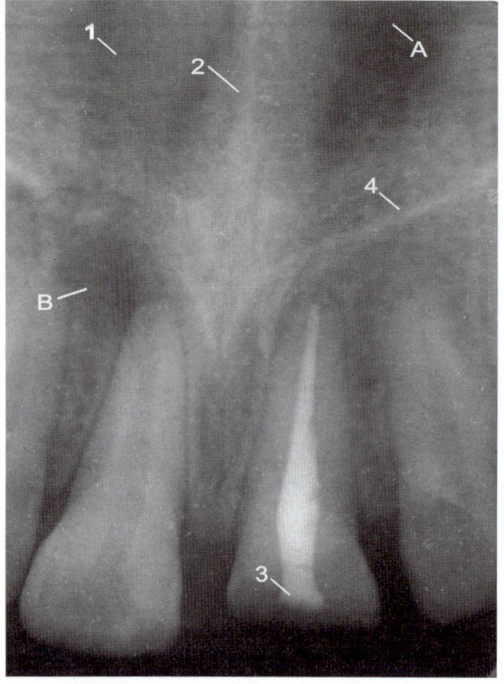

Fig. 15.17: Maxillary incisors

Radiopaque	Radiolucent
1. Inferior nasal concha	A. Nostril (shadow)
2. Nasal septum	B. Periapical
3. Obturated root canal	granuloma
4. Anterior and lateral	
border of nasal fossa	

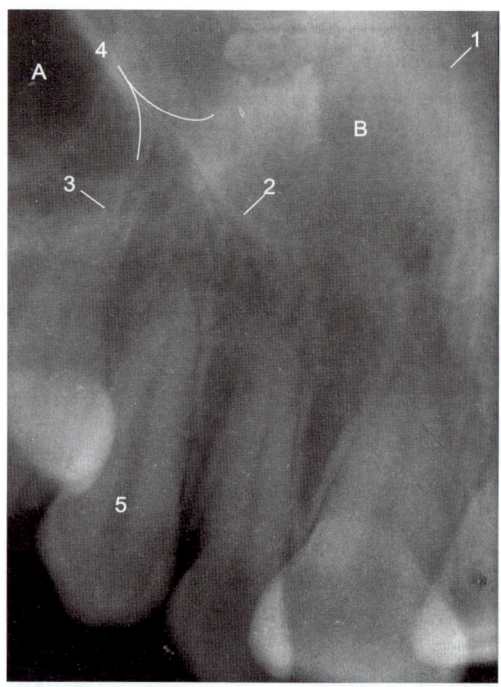

Fig. 15.18: Maxillary canine

Radiopaque	Radiolucent
1. Nasal septum	A. Maxillary sinus
2. Anterior lateral border	B. Nasal cavity
of nasal fossa	
3. Wall of maxillary sinus	
4. Inverted Y-line of	
Ennis	
5. Canine tooth with	
incomplete root	

15

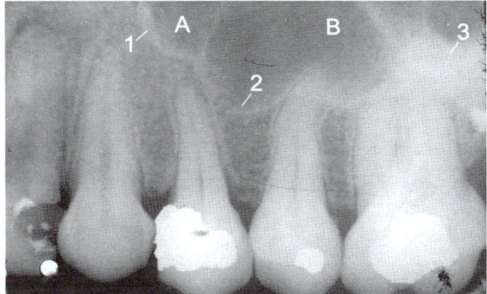

Fig. 15.19: Maxillary premolars

Radiopaque	Radiolucent
1. Wall of nasal fossa	A. Nasal fossa
2. Wall of maxillary sinus	B. Maxillary sinus
3. Zygomatic process of maxilla	

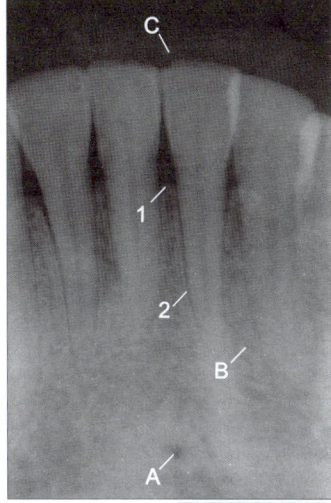

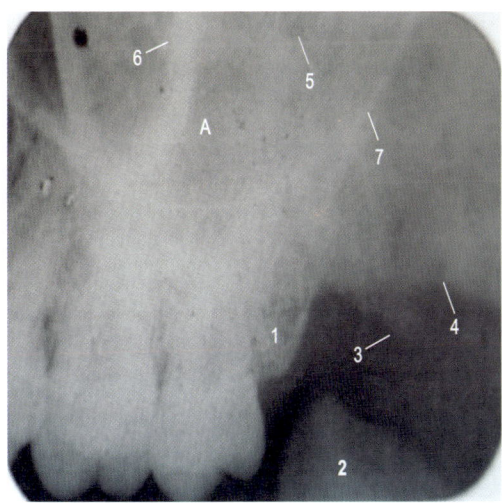

Fig. 15.20: Maxillary molars

Radiopaque	Radiolucent
1. Maxillary tuberosity	A. Maxillary sinus
2. Coronoid process of mandible	
3. Pterygoid plate complex	
4. Inferior border of zygomatic bone	
5. Zygomatic process of maxilla	
6. Inferior aspect of lateral wall of nasal fossa	
7. Wall of maxillary sinus	

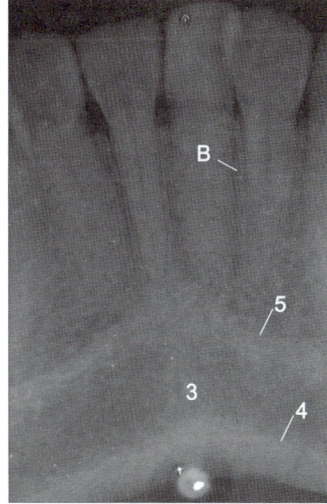

Fig. 15.21: Mandibular incisors

Radiopaque	Radiolucent
1. Crest of alveolar ridge	A. Lingual foramen
2. Lamina dura	B. Nutrient canal
3. Genial tubercle	C. Shadow of lower lip
4. Inferior border of mandible	
5. Mental ridge	

15

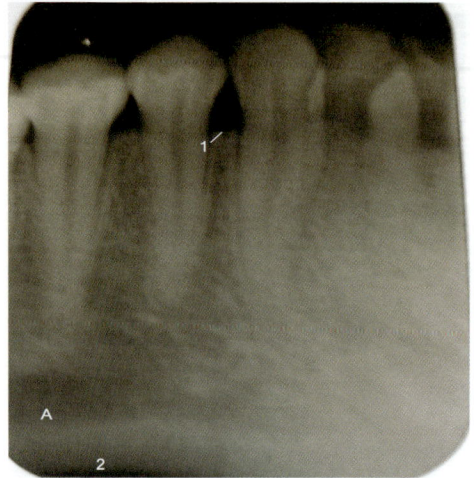

Fig. 15.22: Mandibular canine

Radiopaque	Radiolucent
1. Crest of alveolar ridge	A. Mandibular canal
2. Inferior border of mandible	

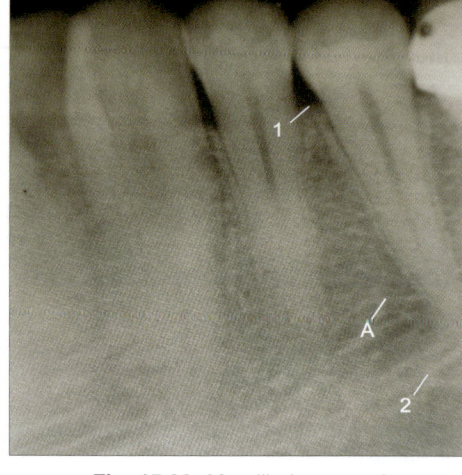

Fig. 15.23: Mandibular premolars

Radiopaque	Radiolucent
1. Crest of alveolar ridge	A. Mental foramen
2. Internal oblique ridge	

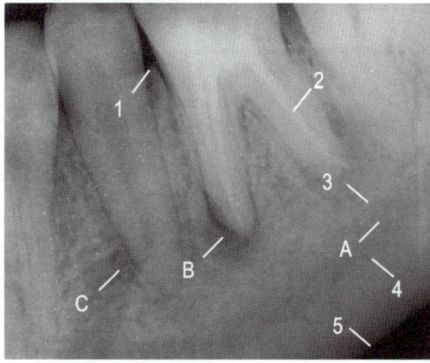
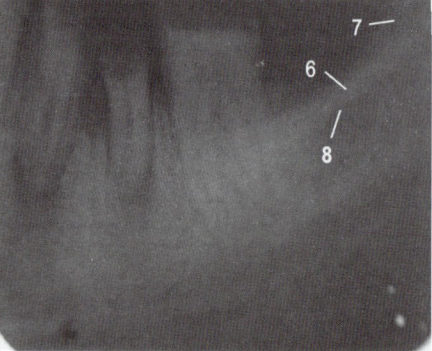

Fig. 15.24: Mandibular molars

Radiopaque	Radiolucent
1. Crest of alveolar ridge	A. Mandibular canal
2. Obturated root canals	B. Periapical pathology
3. Superior border of mandibular canal	C. Mental foramen
4. Inferior border of mandibular canal	
5. Inferior border of mandible	
6. External oblique ridge	
7. Ramus of mandible	
8. Internal oblique ridge	

15

The landmarks are described as follows:

RADIOLUCENT LANDMARKS OF MAXILLA

1. Incisive Foramen or Incisal Foramen or Anterior Palatine Foramen

It is the oral terminal of the nasopalatine canal, transmitting nasopalatine nerves and vessels. Present palatally between the central incisors, it can be of various shapes viz., mere slit, rounded, oval, rhomboid, heart shaped, etc. (Figs 15.25A and B).

Margins of the foramen are also variable. Some foramina have a well defined cortical plate around them while others have a partial covering of the cortical plate. The size of the foramen also varies. It can be 2.0 mm to 6.0 mm in diameter. Its average dimensions are 3.0 mm × 3.0 mm. Sometimes a root is projected beyond the foramen, making it appear similar to localized periodontal problems. The great variability of its radiographic image is primarily as a result of the different angle at which the X-ray beam may be directed for the radiograph. The lateral wall of the nasopalatine duct is rarely visible.

The incisive foramen is a potential site for an incisive canal cyst. The cyst causes enlargement of the foramen. The presence of a cyst can be suspected when the size of the lesion is around 1.0 cm.

Also, its presence over the central incisors may be mistaken for a periapical lesion. The points of differentiation can be:
  i. Intact lamina dura
  ii. Tooth would be vital
  iii. Shadow would shift from its original position by the change in angulation of the X-rays in case of normal appearance.

2. Intermaxillary Suture

The intermaxillary suture is also known as the median palatine suture, premaxillary suture and post-palatine suture. It appears between the two portions of the pre-maxilla

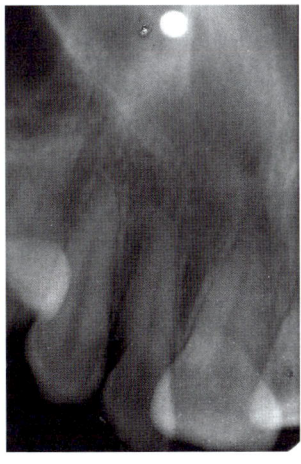

A

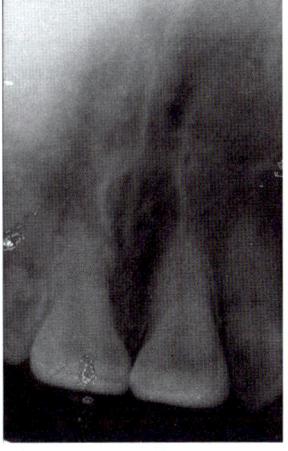

B

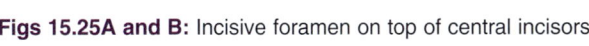

Figs 15.25A and B: Incisive foramen on top of central incisors

15

as a thin radiolucent line extending from the middle of the central incisors to the posterior aspect of the palate. This is visible usually in young children. The width of the suture is almost uniform; only in very young patients it may terminate as a funnel-shaped widening at the anterior end. Its margins are lined by cortical bone, and appear radiopaque. The cortical margins may or may not be uniform.

The appearance of this radiolucent line is sometimes mistaken for a fracture in the alveolar process on periapical films or a fracture of the palate on occlusal films.

Normal anatomical landmarks can be differentiated from pathological landmarks by changing the angulation of X-radiations. In case of fractures, the radiolucent line or width would be increased or there might be overlapping of the radiopacities, whereas in normal landmarks, the radiolucent appearance would be obscured. Secondly, in case of a fracture, the continuity of the radiopaque margin would be disturbed.

3. Nasal Fossae or Nostrils

These appear as dark shadows over the lateral incisors. The nasal cavities are air-filled, therefore, appear as radiolucent areas on periapical radiographs of anterior teeth. The nasal septum, a dark radiopaque line, divides the two fossae (Fig. 15.26).

The margins of the fossae are lined with compact bone. Therefore, on a radiograph, the dark shadows of the cavities are lined by narrow white lines.

The nasal septum frequently deviates from the midline and the vomer bone is usually curved. The cavity, which appears as a dark radiolucent area, contains a hazy shadow of the inferior concha extending from the right and left lateral walls. The floor

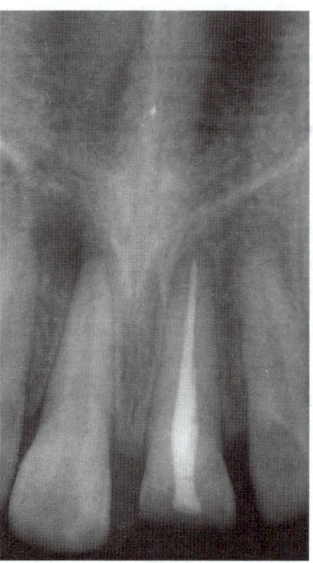

Fig. 15.26: Upper black area is nostrils. In the centre is the nasal septum (radiopaque)

of the nasal fossa appears radiopaque at the margin. Sometimes the nasal floor extends posteriorly, superimposed over the maxillary sinus. This may falsely convey the impression of the septum being present in the sinus or a limiting superior sinus wall.

Normal bone pattern is to be seen before finally making the diagnosis of pathological conditions.

4. Nasopalatine Canals

The nasopalatine canals are rarely seen on a periapical film but can be viewed on occlusal films. This canal originates at two sites at the floor of the nasal cavity. The openings are on either side of the nasal septum. Each branch of the canal passes downward, and joins the other canal from the other side to form a common opening, the incisive foramen. Depending upon the angle of projection, the superior border of

15

the foramen may appear oval or round on radiographs. On occlusal films it appears Y-shaped.

5. Maxillary Antrum or Sinus

The maxillary sinuses appear as dark shadows over the posterior teeth—usually from the second premolar to the tuberosity region (Figs 15.27A and B). Their appearance is quite dark because they contain air. The maxillary sinus is the largest of the paranasal sinuses. The two sinuses, right and left, can be of similar or different shapes. The maxillary sinus communicates with the nasal cavity via an aperture about 3–6 mm in diameter under the posterior

aspect of the middle turbinate. The inner antral wall, which forms the outer surface of nasal fossae, is variable in thickness; this factor leads to variations in the appearance of the sinus. The soft tissue of the cheeks too has its influence over the relative darkness of the radiograph.

The antrum is usually covered with a continuous, thin cortical plate but some small interruptions may be present because of anatomical variations.

In a normal individual with intact teeth, the antral floor is over the roots. Very rarely the roots extend into the sinus. In such cases, a lamina dura is always present (Figs 15.28A and B).

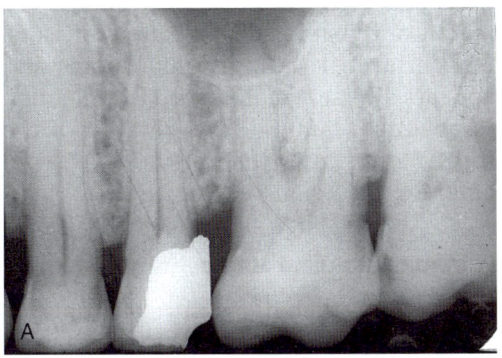
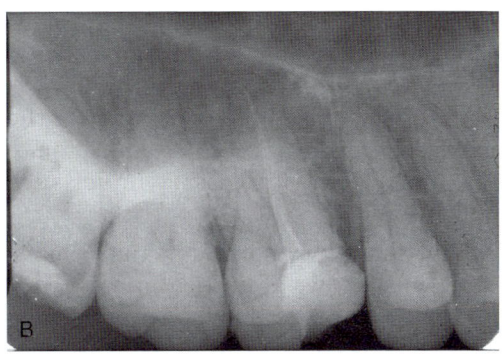

Figs 15.27A and B: Maxillary antrum

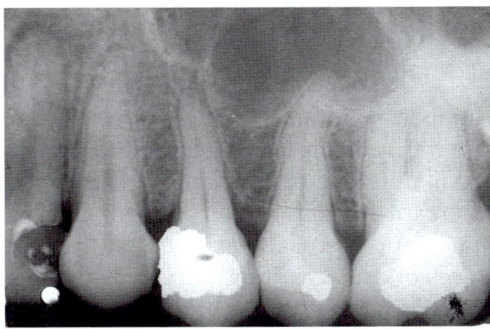
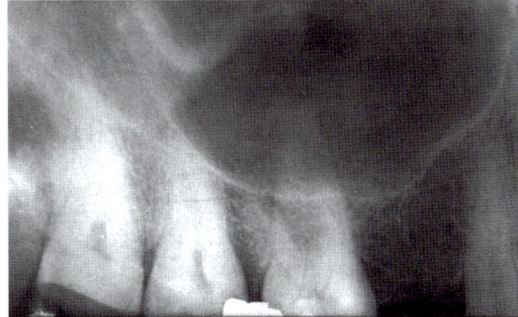

Fig. 15.28A: Maxillary antrum over the roots of maxillary molars

Fig. 15.28B: Maxillary molar roots extending into the maxillary sinus

15

15

The antrum sometimes dips down between the buccal and palatal roots of the first molar.

Following extraction of teeth, the antrum may extend to the alveolar crest. A very thin lining remains between the remaining roots and the antrum wall, so care should be exercised while extracting the residual roots.

In many cases, sinuses are divided by septae into various compartments. The division may be partial or complete. Usually one septum and occasionally 2–3 septa may be present, which arise from the medial and lateral walls of the sinus.

The intimate relationship of the teeth and maxillary sinus poses the possibility that clinical symptoms originating in the sinus can be perceived in the teeth and also vice versa. Acute inflammation in the sinus is usually accompanied by pain in the maxillary teeth. So, careful examination of maxillary teeth is necessary under such circumstances.

Sometimes, the maxillary sinus exhibits uniform shadows of nutrient canals. They can follow any direction; however, usually the course is convex towards the alveolar process.

The floor of the sinus may exhibit bony nodules appearing radiopaque on the radiograph. They are well-defined, diffuse, and can be differentiated from roots by the absence of root canals and a lamina dura.

6. Nasolacrimal Duct

The nasolacrimal duct is not seen on periapical films, but may be visible on occlusal films. It runs from the medial aspect of the anteroinferior border of the orbit inferiorly. If at all it is visible on periapical

films, it is seen above the canine region. It can be mistaken for cysts or the infraorbital foramen.

7. Posterior Palatine Foramen

The posterior palatine foramen is seen only on occlusal films and very rarely on periapical films. This is a round or oval radiolucent area over the roots of the first molar and may be slightly mesial or distal to it. It can be superimposed over the apices of either the second bicuspids or the first and second molars.

8. Lateral Fossa

The lateral fossa is also known as incisive fossa. It is a depression in the maxilla in the region of the apices of the lateral incisors. On periapical radiographs, this region appears diffusely radiolucent. Examination of an intact lamina dura, vitality of the tooth, etc. can differentiate it from pathological lesions.

9. Median Palatine Suture

The medium palatine suture can only be seen on occlusal films as a thin radiolucent line in the centre of the palate. Usually, it is visible in young patients.

10. Aberrant Foramen

The aberrant foramen, though rarely visible, may be seen in the anterior portion of maxilla. Its size varies from 1.0 to 3.0 mm. Aberrant foramina are round or oval in shape, and are usually present at the root apices of canines. These vary considerably in their configuration. If present around the root apices, they may be mistaken for pathological lesions.

RADIOPAQUE LANDMARKS OF MAXILLA

1. Zygomatic Bone and Zygomatic Process

On the periapical radiograph, the zygomatic process appears as a U-shaped radiopaque line with its open end directed superiorly. Depending upon the angulation of X-rays, the size and width of the process can vary (Fig. 15.29).

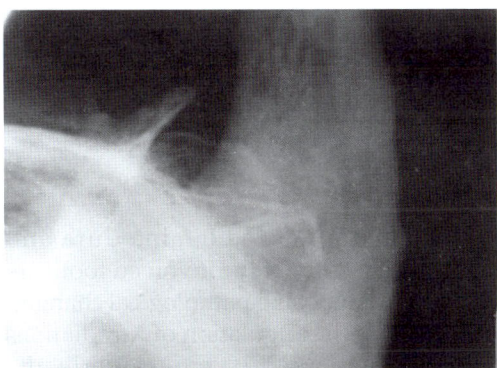

Fig. 15.29: Zygomatic bone and zygomatic process

It can be seen projecting into the maxillary sinus. By changing the angulation of X-radiations the exact position can be noted.

The inferior border of the zygomatic bone can be seen extending posteriorly from the inferior border of the zygomatic process of the maxilla. This is identified as a uniform gray or white radiopacity over the apices of the molars.

2. Zygoma or Malar Bone

It appears as an irregular radiopaque shadow covering the third molar apices, which may extend upto the apices of second molars. In cases where the palatal vault is low, this shadow of the malar bone may be interpreted as hypercementosis or sometimes even ankylosis of second and third molars.

To overcome this, Le-master's technique is employed, so that the shadow of the malar bone may not superimpose over the apices of molar teeth.

3. Hamular Process of Sphenoid Bone

This is seldom visible on intraoral films. On extraoral films this appears as a thick radiopaque line terminating just below the region of the maxillary tuberosity. It can be overshadowed by the maxillary tuberosity.

4. Nasal Septum

It is seen as a pear-shaped radiopaque area extending backwards from the incisive foramen in between the two central incisors (Fig. 15.26).

5. Coronoid Process of Mandible

This is a triangular gray area of radiopacity seen on the radiograph of upper molars. This is sometimes wrongly perceived as an impacted third molar (Fig. 15.30).

RADIOLUCENT LANDMARKS OF MANDIBLE

1. Lingual Foramen

The foramen contains the termination of the incisive branch of the mandibular canal. It is seen as a radiolucent dot slightly above the inferior border of the mandible (Fig. 15.31).

2. Mental Foramen

It is present under the roots of the first and second bicuspids. It is visible mostly in youngsters because with age the mental

15

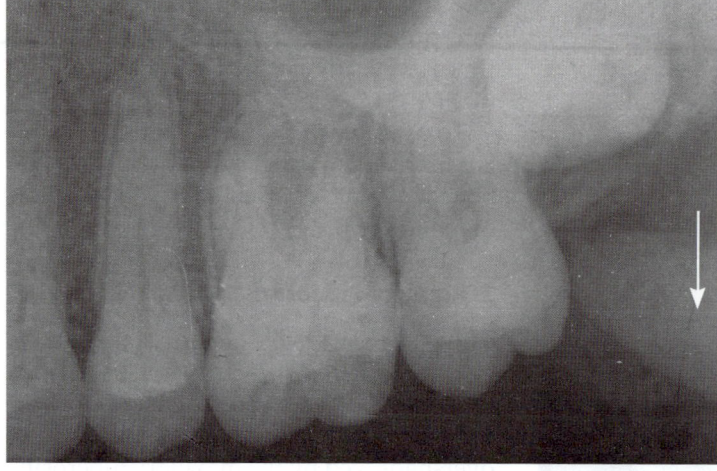

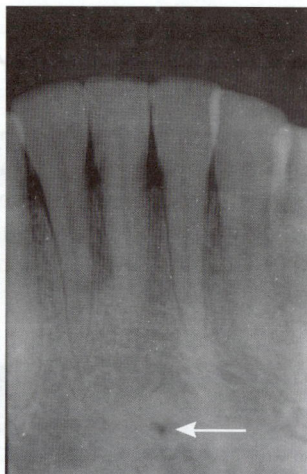

Fig. 15.30: Coronoid process of mandible

Fig. 15.31: Lingual foramen

canal is directed superiorly and posteriorly. The shape of the foramen may vary from round, oblong, slit-like or very irregular. Its size can vary from 1.0 mm to 1.0 cm. Usually the opening is partially or completely corticated (Fig. 15.32).

Occasionally, the anterior portion of the mandibular canal is visible as a funnel-shaped radiolucent area. If the image of the mental foramen is projected over the roots of any of the premolar teeth, periapical pathosis can be suspected by mistake.

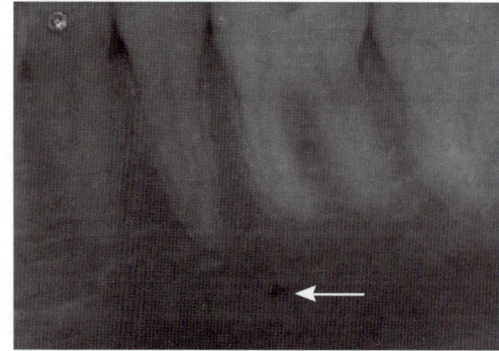

Fig. 15.32: Mental foramen

Examination of the lamina dura and testing the vitality of the involved tooth are helpful in diagnosing pathological changes. By changing the angulation of X-radiations the foramen would move while the periapical pathosis would remain at the root apex.

3. Mandibular Foramen

This is only visible on lateral jaw films. It is a small rounded or funnel-shaped black shadow over the ramus of the mandible. This is guided by the lingula.

4. Mandibular Canal

It commences from the mandibular foramen in the ascending ramus. It appears as a radiolucent area covered superiorly and inferiorly by a radiopaque margin. The borders are either only partially visible or may be absent. The position of the canal varies; it lies below the roots of the molars and a little below the bicuspids (Fig. 15.33). The apices of the molars may appear to be

15

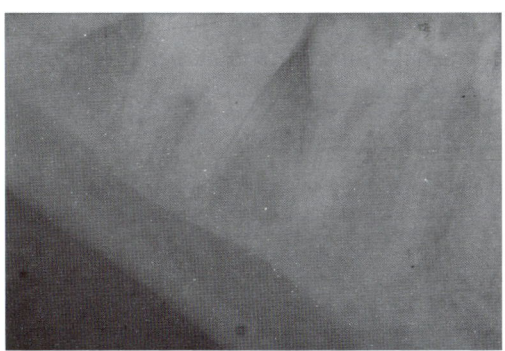

Fig. 15.33: Mandibular canal

superimposed over it. Anatomically, the mandibular canal lies buccal to the molars and premolars. The width of the canal varies from 3.0 mm to 1.0 cm. To confirm the soundness of the tooth, vitality tests, etc. should be performed. A change in the angulation of the X-ray beam does not cause much difference.

5. Mental Fossa

The mental fossa is a depression found on the labial aspect of the mandible in the anterior region. This may be mistaken for periapical pathology of the mandibular anterior teeth.

6. Nutrient Canals or Interdental Canals

These are often seen on mandibular periapical radiographs. They carry neurovascular bundles traversing the jaw bones and supply the teeth and gingival tissue. The width of a nutrient canal may vary from 100 micron to 1.0 mm. The margins of the canal may reveal a thin cortical plate, which may be slightly irregular. Very rarely, a nutrient canal is perpendicular to the cortex and can appear as a small, round radiolucency.

7. Pharyngeal Space

The pharyngeal space is seen as a radiolucent area, only on lateral jaw films, as a broad, dark region extending vertically on the ramus. It is caused by the patient's swallowing when the film is being exposed. Care must be taken to see the area and to differentially diagnose it from pathological lesions.

8. Physiological Thinning of Bone

The body of the mandible anterior to the angle is thinned down physiologically in most cases. The thinness which appears radiolucent over the radiograph must be differentially diagnosed from the following pathological lesions.

a. *Ameloblastoma*: The bony cavity is divided into compartments, which may the give the false appearance of trabeculae. The mandible shifts towards the affected side and there is swelling of the side. Roots are resorbed and teeth become mobile.

b. *Osteomyelitis*: Multiple sinuses are present, which open intra or extra-orally. The cavity is well defined in contrast to the irregular outline in physiological thinning of bone.

c. *Fibrous dysplasia*: A radiolucent mass is traversed densely by radiopaque lines in different directions. The interior of the cavity does not follow a trabecular pattern as in physiological thinning of bone. The outline of a lesion of fibrous dysplasia does not merge with peripheral bone.

d. *Resorption of bone:* This appears as a completely radiolucent mass. The periphery of the resorbed area shows a thick radiopaque line.

15

RADIOPAQUE LANDMARKS OF MANDIBLE

1. External Oblique Ridge

It is observed as a white line on the anterior portion of the ascending ramus. Sometimes the radiopacity is so heavy that it is mistaken for the roots of molars.

2. Genial Tubercle

These are four in number, two on either side of the median line on the internal surface of the mandible in the region of the incisors. This is usually seen on occlusal films. This appears as a white ring with a dark centre immediately beneath and between the lower central incisors. These are sometimes mistaken for condensed bone (Fig. 15.34).

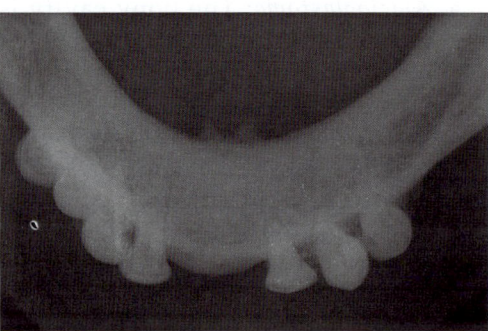

Fig. 15.34: Occlusal view mandible showing genial tubercles

3. Mental Ridge

The mental ridge appears as a dense line extending from the symphysis to the bicuspid region. Sometimes the radiopacity is superimposed by apices of lower anterior teeth.

4. Mylohyoid Ridge

This appears as a white line beginning at the lower border of the symphysis and continuing upwards in the molar region toward the ramus. It sometimes overlaps the molar apices.

5. Border of Mandible

This appears as a heavy white line on the radiograph. This line is a definite proof of intact margins of the mandible (Figs 15.35A and B).

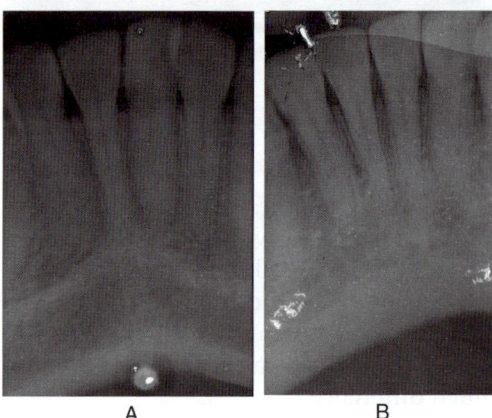

A   B

Figs 15.35A and B: Border of the mandible

In addition, the shadows of teeth and pulp cavities appear as radiopaque and radiolucent respectively in both the maxilla and mandible. The radiopacity of enamel, dentin and cementum varies but the radiolucency of pulp cavities is uniform. Occasionally, pulp stones are present in the pulp, which appear radiopaque (Figs 15.36A and B).

Bibliography

1. Baumrind S, Frantz RC: The reliability of head film measurements. I. Landmark Identification. *Am J Orthod* 1971;60:111.
2. Benn DK: A review of the reliability of radiographic measurements in estimating alveolar bone changes. *J Clinic Periodontol* 1990;17:14.

15

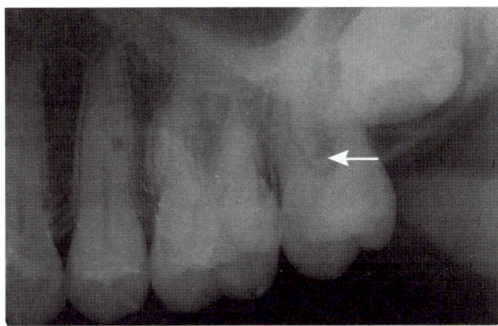

Fig. 15.36A: Pulp stones in maxillary second molar (crown)

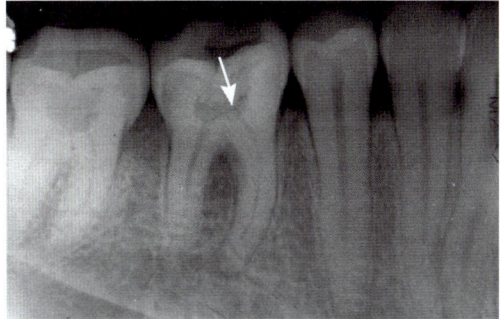

Fig. 15.36B: Pulp stones in mandibular first molar (crown)

3. Bragger U: Radiographic parameter: Biologic significance and clinical use. *Periodontol 2000*: 2005;39:73.
4. Britte G: A study of human mandibular nutrient canals. *O Surg, O Med, O Path*: 1977;44: 635.
5. Burch JG, Hulen S: The relationship of the apical foramen to the anatomic apex of the tooth root. *O Surg, O Med, O Path* 1972;34:262.
6. Hollender L: Decision making in radiographic imaging. *J Dent Educ* 1992;56:834.
7. Lovelle CL, Wu CJ. When will be the excellent radiographic image available to the dental office? *Dentomaxillofacial Radiology* 1994;23:183.
8. Manson JD: The lamina dura. *O Surg, O Med, O Path* 1963;16:432.
9. Palmer MJ, Weine FS, Healy HJ: Position of apical foramen in relation to endodontic therapy. *J Can Dent Assoc*: 1971;8:305.
10. Patel J, Wuerhman A: A radiographic study of nutrient canals. *O Surg, O Med, O Path*. 1976;42: 693.
11. Smith CJ, Fleming RD: A comprehensive review of normal anatomic landmarks and artifacts as visualized on panorex radiographs. *O Surg, O Med, O Path* 1984;37:291.
12. Turp JC, Vach W, Harbish K, Alt KW, Sturb JR: Determining mandibular condyle and ramus height with the help of an orthopantomogram a valid method ? *J Oral Rehab* 1996;23:395.
13. White SC, Pharvah MJ: Oral Radiology–principles and interpretation. The C.V. Mosby Co., Toronto, Fifth edition, 2004.
14. Wuehrman AH: Evaluation criteria for intraoral radiographic film quality. *JADA*. 1974;89:345.
15. Williams FL, Richtsmeier JT: Comparison of mandibular landmarks from computed tomography and 3D digitizer data. *Clinic Anat* 2003;16:494.

15

Radiological Appearances of Pathological Lesions

After having studied the normal radiolucent and radiopaque anatomical landmarks in both maxilla and mandible, the radiographic appearance of pathological lesions associated with teeth, their surrounding structures, periapical areas and other miscellaneous conditions are to be studied and differentiated.

RADIOGRAPHIC APPEARANCE OF CARIES

Caries, in very simple terms, can be classified into occlusal caries, proximal caries, buccal/lingual caries and cemental caries. The caries usually progress along the enamel rods or cementum. Their initiation, progress and pathogenesis is described in textbook of operative dentistry. Here, we are concerned mainly with their radiographic appearances.

a. Occlusal Caries

Occlusal caries can be detected by mirror and explorer before it becomes observable radiographically. It is seen only when the lesion has reached dentino-enamel junction (Fig. 16.1). As the caries progress along the

enamel rods, a triangle is formed, the base being the dentino-enamel junction. Further progress of the caries towards the pulp visualizes as inverted triangle with base at dentino-enamel junction and apex at the pulp floor.

Usually the appearance of occlusal caries is obscured because of the presence of enamel all round. Radiographs are of importance when pulpal involvement is to be decided. Caries of the crown before eruption has also been reported in the literature, though it is a rare phenomenon.

b. Buccal and/or Lingual Caries

Caries on the buccal and lingual surfaces start, either from the anatomical pits or from the cervical surfaces. Caries progress as usual along the enamel rods. Caries at the pits are usually rounded initially but soon become semilunar. The underlying enamel retains its integrity thereby providing fairly definite periphery of the lesion. This clear cut outline differentiate this lesion from the occlusal caries. The depth of these lesions is difficult to be ascertained and usually gives

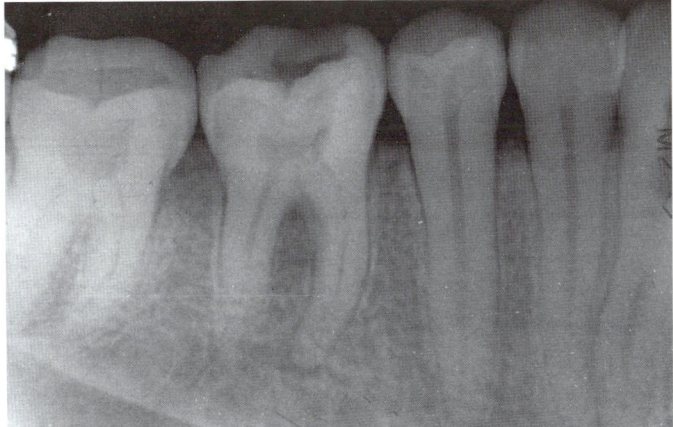

Fig. 16.1: Occlusal caries. Mandibular first molar

a false impression. Large lesions look like the one where pulp exposure has occurred (Figs 16.2, 16.3). Even a fracture of a tooth from one corner may appear radiographically at the same site as buccal or lingual caries. Clinical examination is more important to diagnose the depth, etc.

c. Proximal Caries

Bitewing radiographs are the method of choice in detecting the proximal caries at early stages. Proximal caries may start anywhere between the contact point and the proximal cervical lines (Figs 16.4A, B). Radiographs are of great importance especially while detecting secondary caries below amalgam fillings and under gold inlays (Figs 16.5A, B, C). The carious lesion appears as a notch or irregularity on the proximal surface, which otherwise appears smooth. The initial lesion is wide and due to the direction of enamel rods, taper at the dentino-enamel junction. The lesion again widens in the dentin and taper towards the pulpal wall. A tooth with pit and fissure caries must always be radiographed to check the proximal caries.

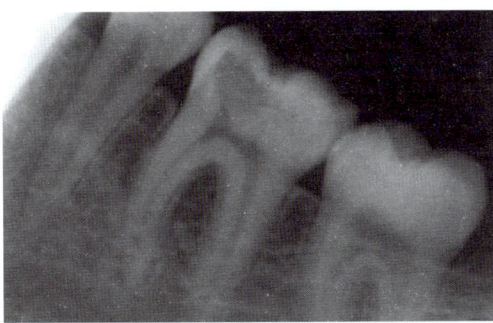

Fig. 16.2: Buccal caries as evident radiologically

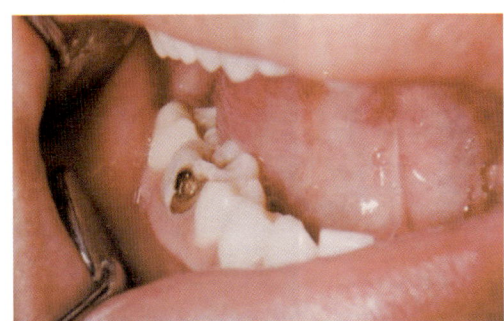

Fig. 16.3: Buccal caries (clinical appearance)

16

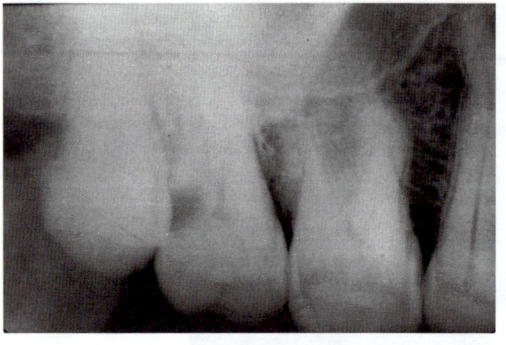

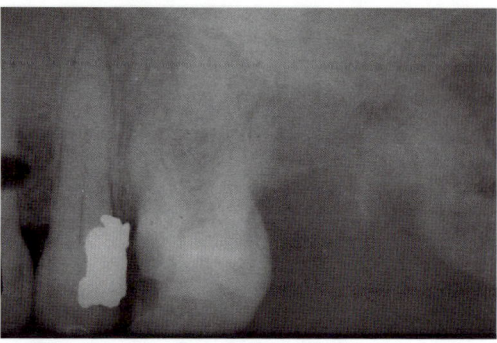

A   B

Figs 16.4A and B: Proximal caries. (A) Maxillary second molar; (B) Maxillary first molar

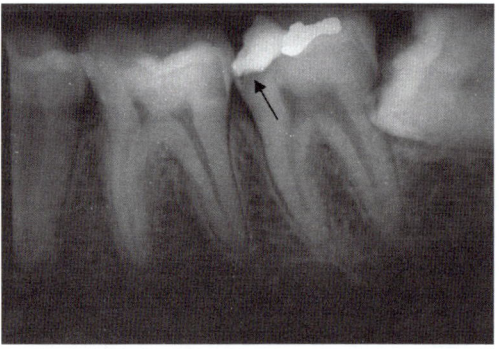

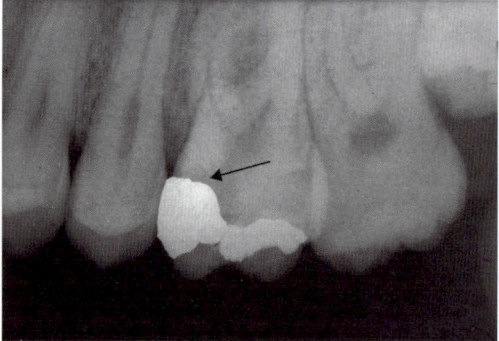

Fig. 16.5A: Secondary caries below amalgam filling in mandibular second molar

Fig. 16.5B: Secondary caries below amalgam filling in maxillary first molar

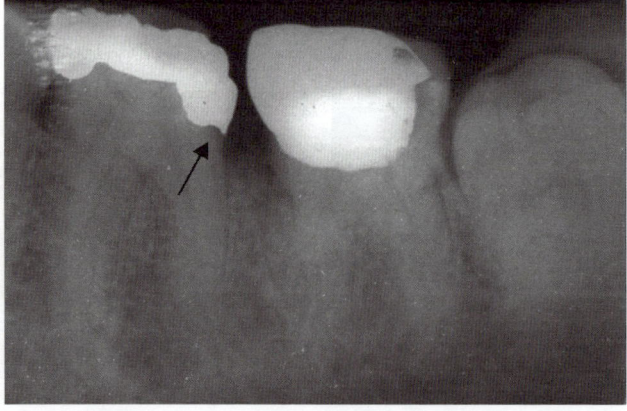

Fig. 16.5C: Secondary caries below gold inlay (mandibular first molar)

16

d. Cemental Caries (Root caries)

Cemental caries is more common in the elderly where a reasonable amount of recession has occurred. The lesion starts at the free gingival margin either in cementum or enamel or both (Figs 16.6A to D). Radiologically, these appear as saucer shaped lesions. They can appear on any tooth surface, but mesial surfaces are thought to be more susceptible. These lesions are to be differentially diagnosed from caries under class II preparations and even erosions of these surfaces. The neck of

the tooth, i.e. the area between the crown and root, absorbs less X-ray photons and appears radiolucent, either uniformly or more consistently so on the proximal surfaces. This is known as *cervical burn out* (Fig. 16.7). Careful examination of the patient clinically along with careful 'reading' of the radiographs is important. Many a times, the tilt in maxillary lateral incisors appears radiolucent on radiographs, giving an impression of proximal caries (Fig. 16.8). These shadows are generally long inciso-gingivally and do

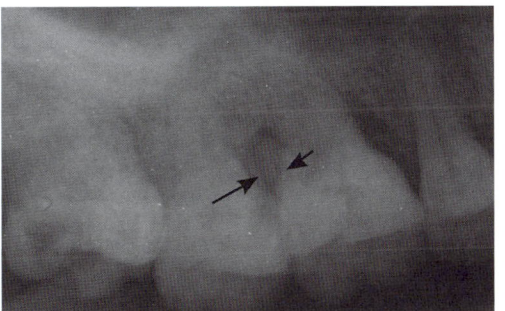

Fig. 16.6A: Cemental caries (maxillary molars)

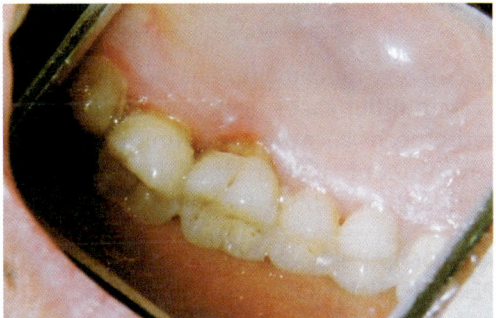

Fig. 16.6B: Cemental caries (clinical appearance)

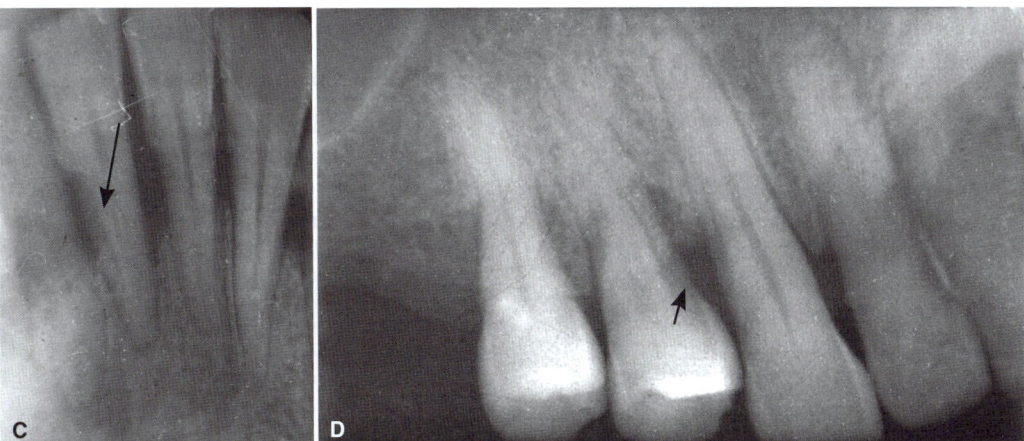

C D

Figs 16.6C and D: (C) Cemental caries (mandibular incisor) (D) Cemental caries (maxillary first premolar)

16

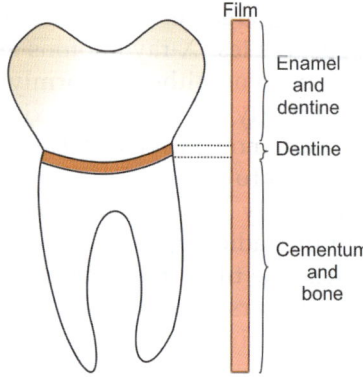

Fig. 16.7: Cervical burnout (diagrammatic)

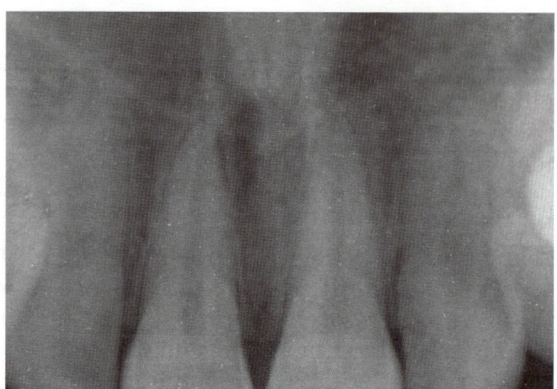

Fig. 16.8: Tilt in lateral incisors appear as caries

not involve the cemento-enamel junction. In certain other cases, restored teeth appear radiolucent because the filling material is radiolucent. Such teeth should be thoroughly examined clinically.

RADIOGRAPHIC APPEARANCE OF PERIAPICAL LESIONS

In radiographs of periapical region, the bone surrounding the teeth and the configuration of root canals are of paramount importance in detecting many pathological lesions. Diagnosis of periapical lesions is complex and must be seconded by auxiliary diagnostic procedures.

The radiographic appearance of periapical lesions varies greatly. The first sign would be the loss of continuity of the lamina dura. The shape of the lesion can be rounded, spherical or having irregular periphery. Usually the periapical rarefaction is the result of periapical infection, mostly by *Streptococci* and *Staphylococci* bacteria. Depending upon the virulence of bacteria, resistance of the patient and so on, the lesion becomes the *epitheliated type* if epithelial cells

predominate; *granulomatous* or *fibrous type* if granulation tissue predominates or simply a *chronic periapical abscess* if polymorphonuclear cells and lymphocytes predominate.

The early change(s) observable on radiographs in any periapical pathology is/ are :

a. Periodontal space thickening
b. Interruptions of the continuity of the lamina dura
c. Change in bony pattern.

a. Periodontal Space Thickening

It can be either pathological or non-pathological. In pathological thickening, the reasons can be root resorption, trauma from occlusion or extrusion of the tooth. The most common of all the reasons is the progressive destruction of the lamina dura due to infection (Fig. 16.9). A widening of periodontal ligamentum space, also called *Garrington sign*, is seen in several mesenchymal malignancies as an early finding but is most commonly seen in osteosarcoma.

16

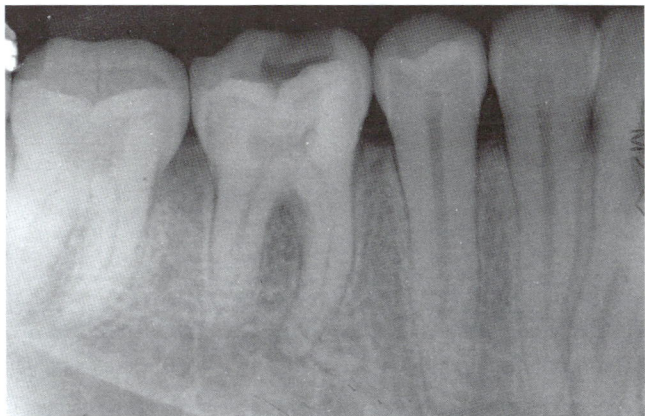

Fig. 16.9: Periodontal space thickening

It is important to emphasize that the periodontal space varies among individuals with site and age. Any periapical pathology, the shadow of which may be overlapped by the other radiolucent areas, will reveal thickening of periodontal ligament at the apex. Orthodontic tooth movement is another cause of periodontal space thickening.

b. Interruptions in the Continuity of Lamina Dura

A break in the continuity of the lamina dura is considered the first sign in periapical pathosis (Figs 16.10A, B, C). In case of a normal tooth, its thickness remains constant. Superimposition of the lamina dura on an anatomical entity also produce an apparent break in its continuity. Root apices extending into the maxillary sinus usually demonstrate a continuity of lamina dura.

c. Change in Bony Pattern

In case of acute clinical manifestation, no change is seen radiologically. It is established that at least two weeks are taken by a pathological process to be interpreted on radiographs. And also, root ends curved buccally or lingually do not show the pathological changes on radiographs. The pattern of bone changes is to be evaluated thoroughly. Early changes can be due to trauma from occlusion and/or periodontal problems (Figs 16.11A and B). Therefore, a thorough clinical examination should be carried out alongwith the assessment of radiographs.

The **radiographic appearance** of a cyst, granuloma and abscess is described below, since these lesions are routinely encountered by students.

THE CYSTS

The cyst appears as a circumscribed radiolucent area, bounded by thin radiopaque lining (Figs 16.12A and B). Clinically, the cyst, if not infected secondarily, is an intact sac containing straw-coloured fluid. If infection invades it, breakdown of the cyst wall results giving rise to chronic abscesses. Very few cysts, such as the traumatic bone cyst (Fig. 16.13) lack a radiopaque lining. Histopathological

16

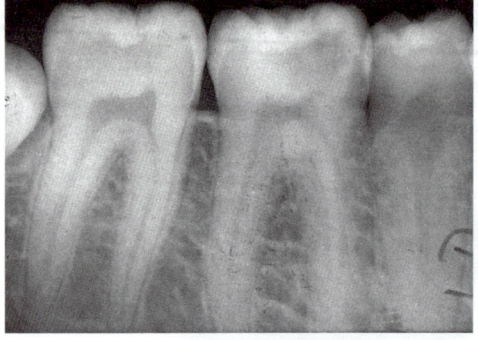

A. Normal appearance (lamina dura)

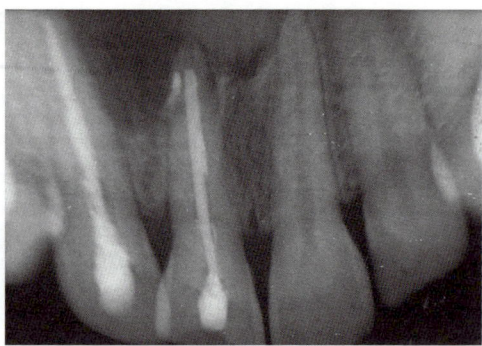

B. Break in lamina dura

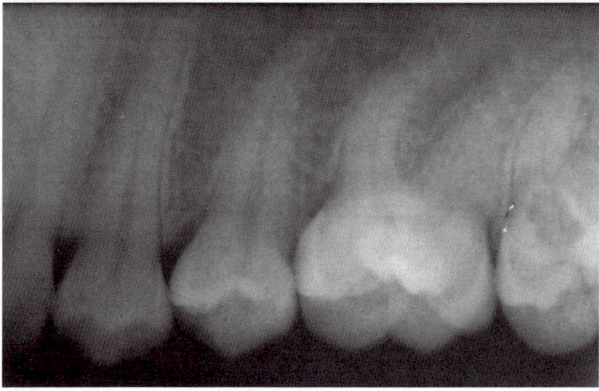

C. Thickening of lamina dura

Figs 16.10A to C: Lamina dura

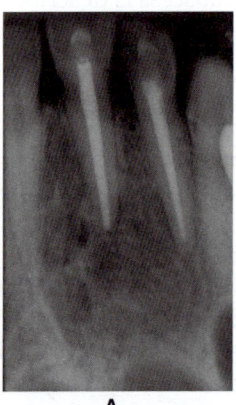

A

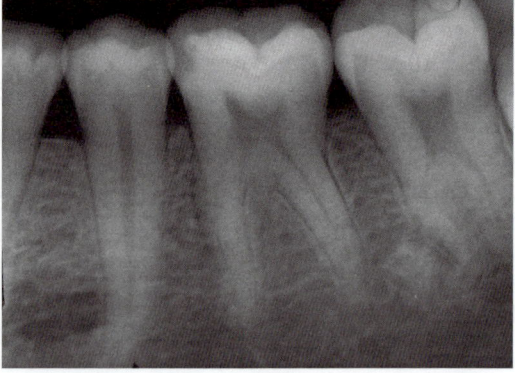

B

Figs 16.11A and B: Change in bony pattern

16

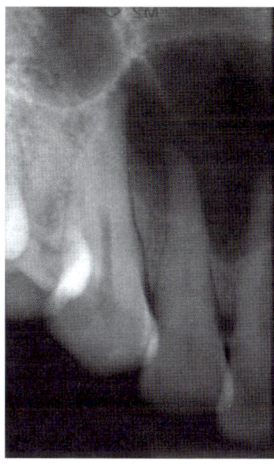

Fig. 16.12A: Periapical cyst

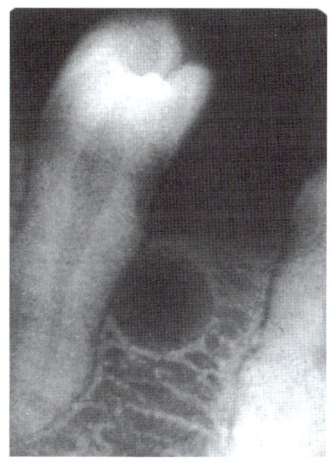

Fig. 16.12B: Lateral periodontal cyst

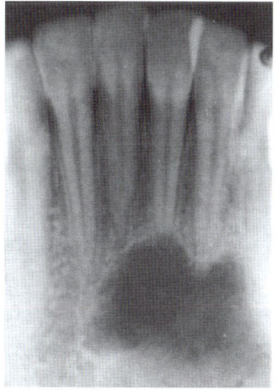

Fig. 16.13A: Traumatic bone cyst

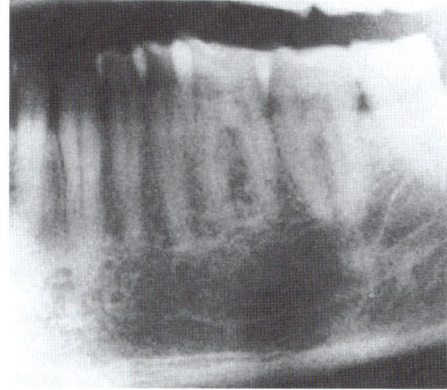

Fig. 16.13B: Hemopoietic bone marrow space

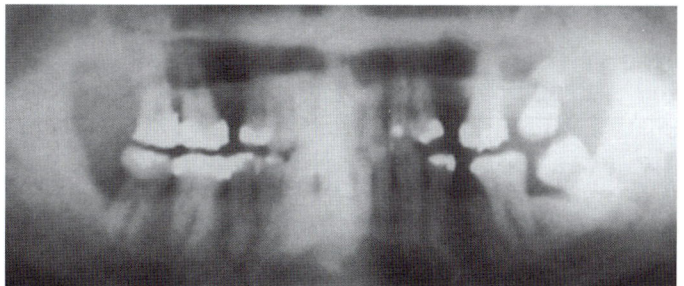

Fig. 16.13C: Median mandibular cyst

16

examination is the most reliable method to diagnose a cyst.

Classification of Cysts

The cysts are classified as shown in Flow Chart 16.1.

RADIOGRAPHIC FINDINGS OF ODONTOGENIC CYSTS

DENTIGEROUS CYST (FOLLICULAR CYST)

The dentigerous cyst typically manifests as a unilocular or multilocular radiolucent area, usually surrounded by a well-defined sclerotic radiopaque border, and is associated with the crown of an unerupted tooth. An infected cyst may show an illdefined border rather than a sclerotic one.

Radiographic variation according to the cyst-to-crown relationship can be of the following types.

- **Central variety**: The central variety is the most common, in which the cyst symmetrically surrounds the crown of tooth.

Flow chart 16.1: Classification of cysts

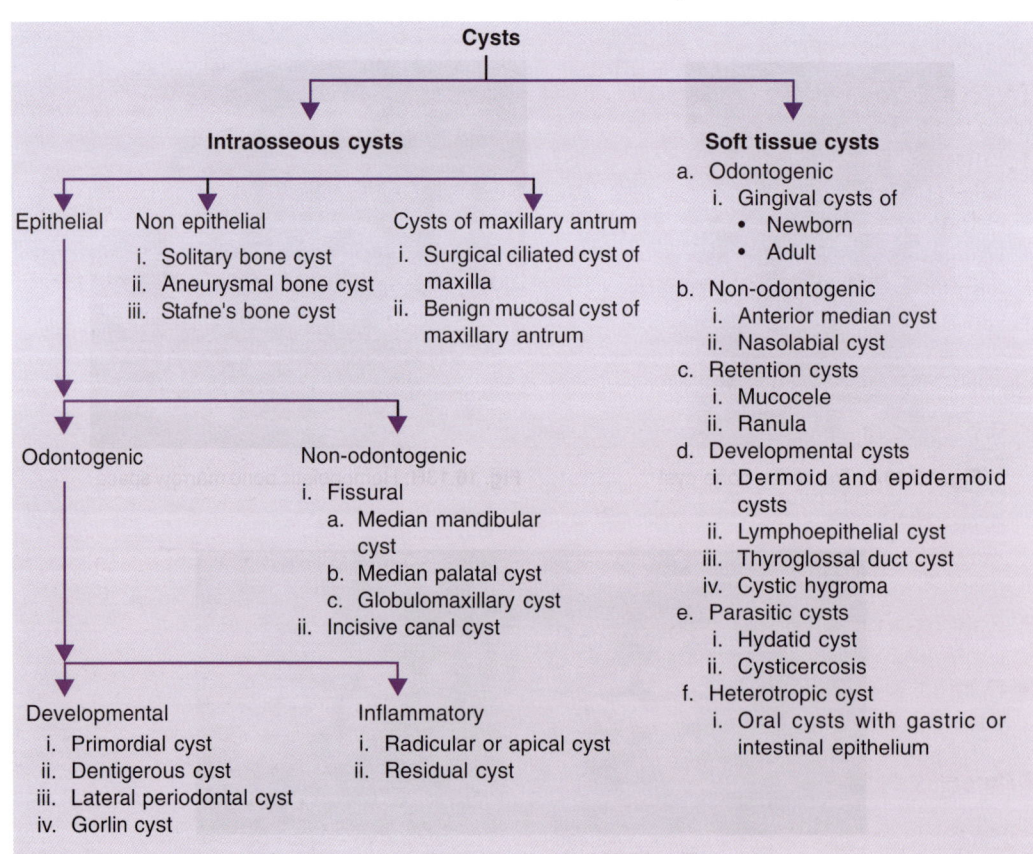

- **Lateral variety:** The lateral variety cyst grows laterally and partially surrounds the crown. This is mostly seen with teeth which are partially erupted with only the upper aspect exposed.
- **Circumferential:** In the circumferential variety, the entire tooth with the exception of the occlusal surface appears to be surrounded by the cyst.

A dentigerous cyst may displace the involved tooth for a considerable distance, like up to lower border of mandible, high in the ramus, floor of the nose or orbit. It may cause resorption of the involved tooth or an adjacent erupted tooth.

Differential Diagnosis

The cyst is to be differentially diagnosed from the following lesions:
- Enlarged follicle (normal follicle size is 3.0–4.0 mm)
- Odontogenic keratocyst
- Unilocular ameloblastoma
- Adenomatoid odontogenic tumor
- Calcifying odontogenic cyst.

ODONTOGENIC KERATOCYST (OKC)

- It presents as a well-defined unilocular radiolucent area surrounded by corticated margins, particularly in the posterior body and ramus of the mandible. A multilocular character is more common in larger lesions.
- Root resorption of adjacent teeth is less common than dentigerous cyst.
- Diagnosis of odontogenic keratocyst is based on histopathological findings.

Differential Diagnosis

The cyst is to be differentially diagnosed from the following lesions:

- Dentigerous cyst, radicular cyst and ameloblastoma.
- Multiple odotogenic keratocyst may be associated with Gorlin and Goltz syndrome.

LATERAL PERIODONTAL CYST/BOTRYOID ODONTOGENIC CYST

- It presents as a well circumscribed radiolucent area located lateral to the root/roots of a vital tooth. The lamina dura of the involved tooth is destroyed. It is usually less than 1.0 cm in the area of its greatest diameter.
- A polycystic, *grape bunch* like multilocular radiographic appearance is characteristic of botryoid odontogenic cyst.

Periapical Cyst

It is present as a small periapical radiolucent area encircling the affected non-vital tooth; however, it may show significant growth to the extent of involving an entire quadrant.

Residual Periapical Cyst

It presents as a round to oval radiolucent area of variable size with well-defined borders located in the alveolar process and/or body of jaw bones.

Simple Bone Cyst (Traumatic bone cyst/solitary bone cyst/haemorrhagic bone cyst /idiopathic bone cavity)

It appears as a well-defined radiolucent area with ill-defined or sharply demarcated margins. The radiolucent area often shows dome-like projections that scallop upward between the roots of teeth. Teeth are less frequently displaced/undergo resorption (Fig. 16.13A).

16

Differential Diagnosis

The lesion is to be differentially diagnosed from Stafne's cyst, as the latter is always present below the inferior alveolar canal and the former is present above the canal.

Periapical Granuloma

It manifest as a radiolucent area of variable size, may be circumscribed or ill-defined, surrounding the apex of the tooth (Fig. 16.14).
- Root resorption is not uncommon
- The affected tooth is non-vital
- Difficult to distinguish it from periapical cyst radiographically.

Periapical Abscess

It may present as a thickening of the apical periodontal ligament, an ill-defined radiolucency or both because of significant bone destruction occurring in a too short duration to appear on radiograph. (Figs 16.15A, B).

Periapical changes can remain restricted to the apex of the root as seen in cases of root resorption and hypercementosis.

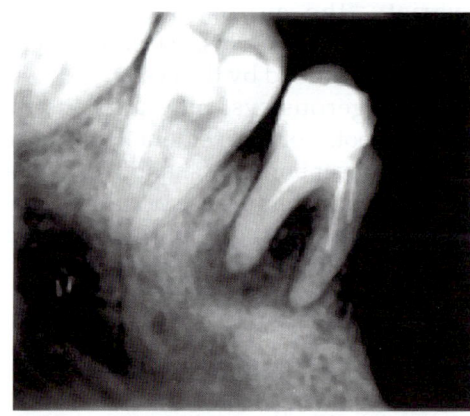

Fig. 16.15A: Periapical abscess (mandibular first molar)

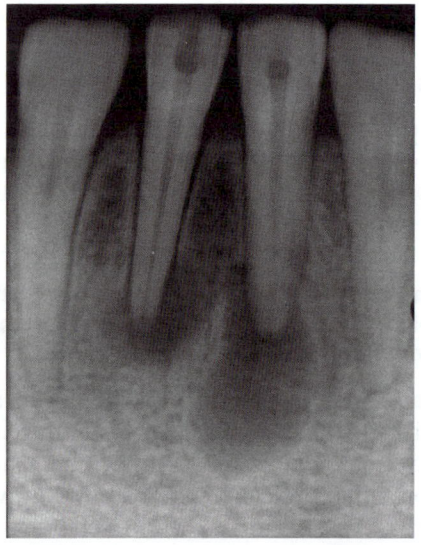

Fig. 16.14: Periapical granuloma (mandibular central incisors)

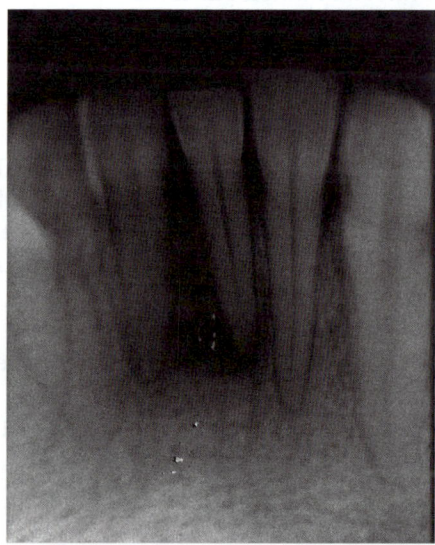

Fig. 16.15B: Periapical abscess (mandibular incisors)

16

ROOT RESORPTION

Root resorption is usually pathological but physiological root resorption during shedding of deciduous teeth does occur (Fig. 16.16). Physiological root resorption always occurs uniformly. Retained roots of deciduous teeth call for a radiographic examination. Deciduous root resorption is associated with the growth of permanent successors. Very rarely, resorption in deciduous tooth occurs even when the permanent successor is missing (Fig. 16.17).

Pathological root resorption can be:
  i. Internal
 ii. External.

  i. *Internal root resorption* occurs as a result of local irritation with the resulting inflammation of pulp (Fig. 16.18). Any trauma resulting in a

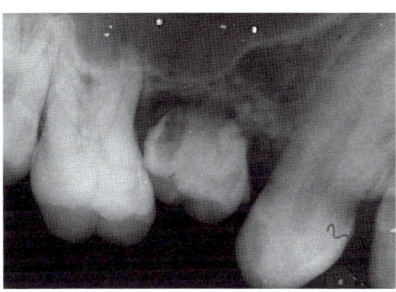

Fig. 16.17: Root resorption of deciduous tooth even when permanent tooth is missing

disturbance of blood circulation within the pulp may lead to resorption of the tooth. This process, if allowed to continue, may lead to perforation of the root. Root resorption has also been reported after pulpotomy. Occasionally, deciduous molars show internal resorption.

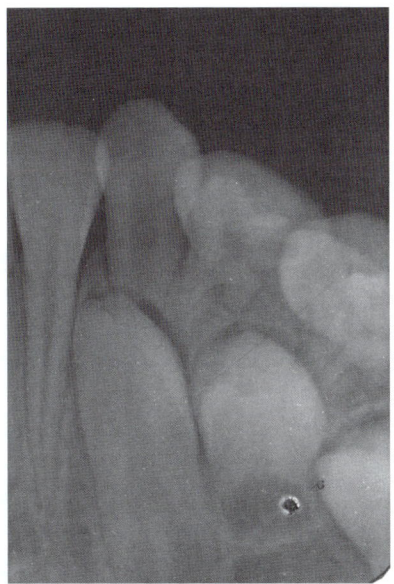

Fig. 16.16: Resorption during shedding of deciduous teeth

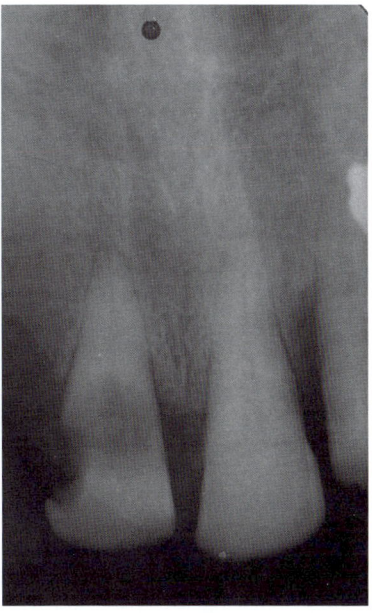

Fig. 16.18: Internal root resorption

16

ii. **External root resorption** occurs because of following reasons:

- Inflammation of periodontal ligament resulting from trauma or due to root canal infections (Fig. 16.19).
- Pressure from an impacted tooth (Figs 16.20A, B, C).
- Adjacent to tumors or cysts.
- Root resorption after reimplantation (Figs 16.21A, B, C).
- Concomitant internal and external root resorption can occur (Fig. 16.22).
- Idiopathic root resorption is also common (Fig. 16.23).

HYPERCEMENTOSIS

It is an excessive deposition of cementum either along the entire length of the root or only in the apical region. It may be due to systemic effects or because of mild infection,

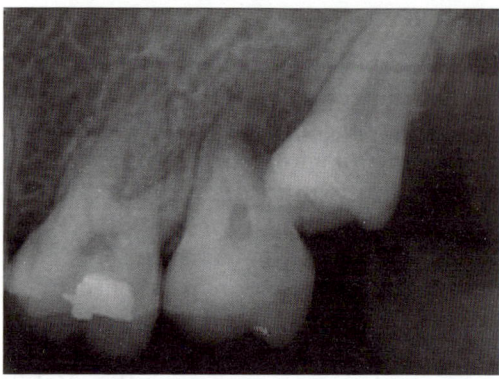

Fig. 16.20A: External root resorption because of impacted third molar

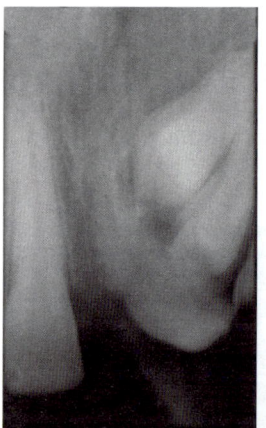

B

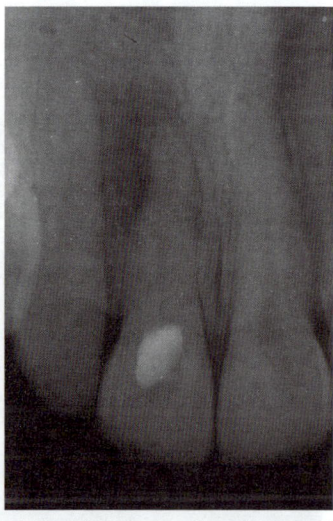

Fig. 16.19: External root resorption due to root canal infection

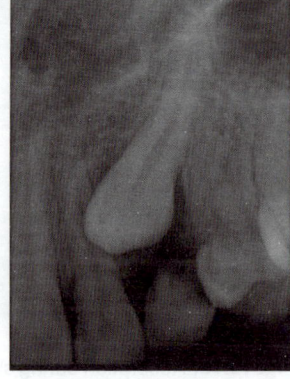

C

Figs 16.20B and C: Resorption with impacted teeth

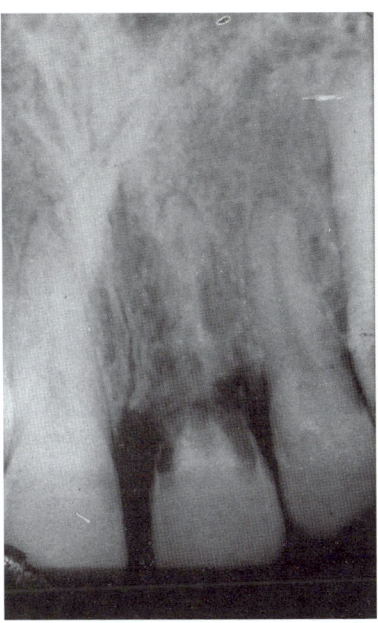

Fig. 16.21A: External root resorption due to re-implantation

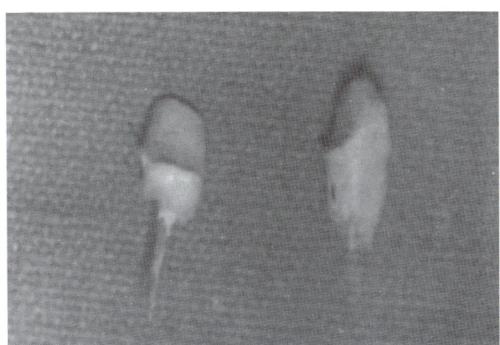

Fig. 16.21C: Same teeth after extraction

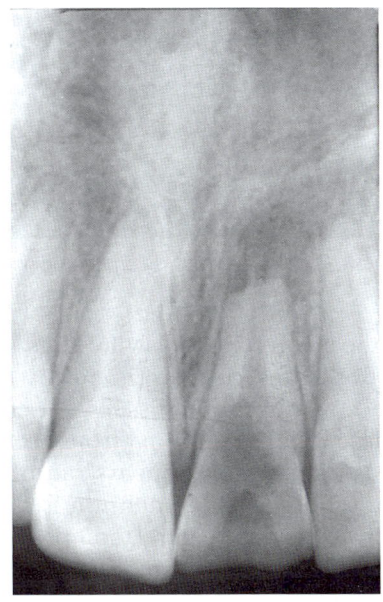

Fig. 16.22: Concomitant internal and external root resorption

which causes depositional rather than destructive activity.

PERIAPICAL OSTEOFIBROSIS (CEMENTOMA)

In the early stages, it resembles a granuloma and can be differentiated from it by the fact

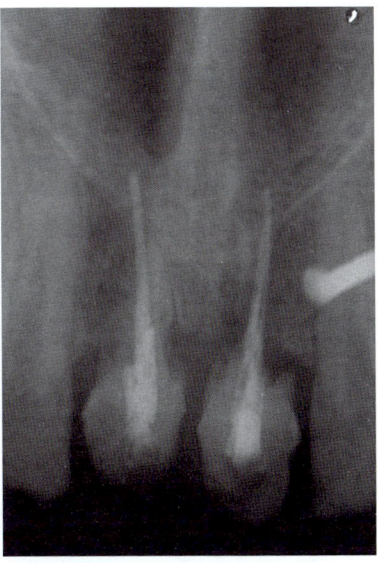

Fig. 16.21B: Complete root resorption after re-implantation

16

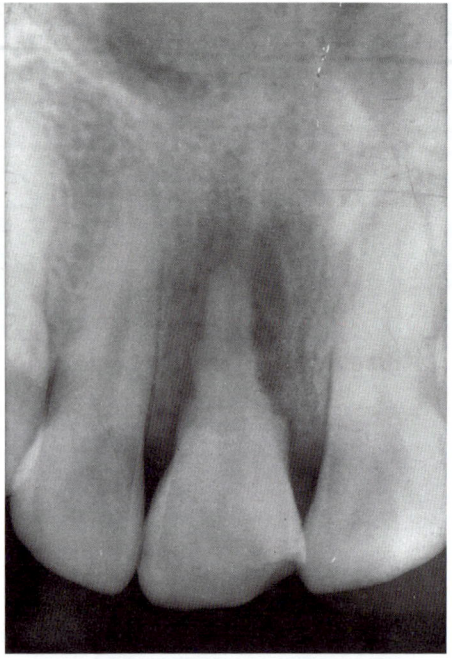

Fig. 16.23: External root resorption (idiopathic)

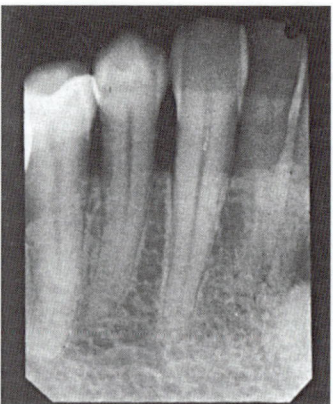

Fig. 16.24A: Periapical osteofibrosis

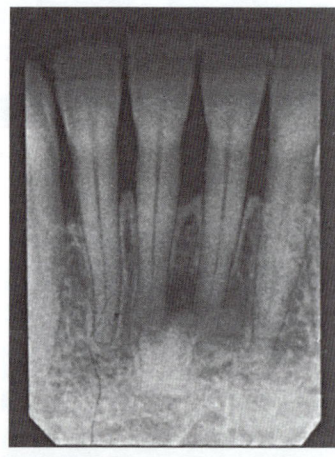

Fig. 16.24B: Cementoma

that the involved tooth is vital (Figs 16.24A, B). Bone destruction is followed by replacement by fibrous tissues. The etiology of these lesions is trauma from occlusion. Initially the lesion appears radiolucent. Later on however, cementum is formed, which appears as a central radiopaque mass resembling bone (Fig. 16.24C). That is why it is also known as *cementoma*. Its presence is more common in the mandible, than the maxilla. Usually, the lesion remains inactive and may disappear if the causative factor is removed. Only in some circumstances surgery is indicated.

16 RADIOGRAPHIC APPEARANCE OF PERIODONTAL DISEASES

Periodontal disease being the most prevalent, needs extra attention as regards

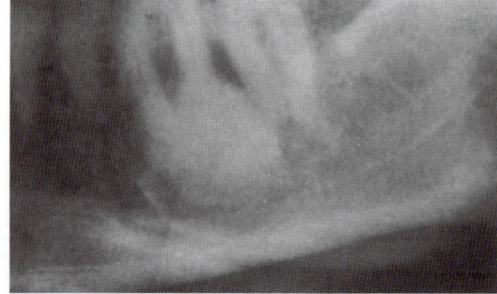

Fig. 16.24C: Lateral view of mandible showing cementoma

to its radiographic appearance. It is considered to be the disease of the middle aged, although even children may suffer from it.

Regular follow-up visits alongwith bitewing radiographs of patients are mandatory to detect the initiation of periodontal disease. Radiographs have definite value in diagnosing this disease.

- The first sign, thickening of the periodontal ligament space can be registered (Figs 16.9, 16.25).
- Root resorption may be evident.
- Bone loss, both horizontal (Figs 16.26A to C) and vertical (Figs 16.27A, B) can be easily detected.
- Radiographs are also important in diagnosing certain periodontal endodontal lesions (perio-endo relations) (Figs 16.28A to C).

Full mouth radiographs are preferred to locate the site and extent of bone loss.

Pattern of Bone Loss

Bone loss can be generalized or restricted to a few areas. It is estimated by assuming the normal alveolar crest as being 1.0 mm from the cemento-enamel junction. Bone loss is usually present in all the four sides of a tooth, but radiologically buccal and lingual sides are not appreciable. There are certain methods to locate these sides, which are beyond the scope of this book.

The amount of bone loss observed radiologically is kept in mind while evaluating the prognosis of periodontal disease.

Bone loss can be horizontal (Fig. 16.26) or vertical (Fig. 16.27). Horizontal bone loss is usually found in chronic periodontitis, may be generalized or localized, and vertical bone loss is evident where there is trauma from occlusion. If bone loss is parallel with the plane drawn from one cemento-enamel junction to another, this is called horizontal bone loss and if there occurs greater bone loss proximally on one tooth, than on the adjacent tooth, it is called vertical bone loss. Certain systemic diseases may also effect generalized bone loss. Certain specific types of bacteria are responsible for aggressive periodontitis viz.

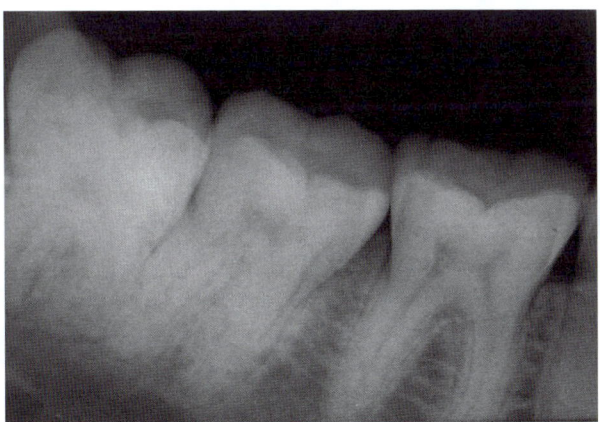

16

Fig. 16.25: Periodontal ligament thickening in maxillary premolars, cause is trauma from occlusion

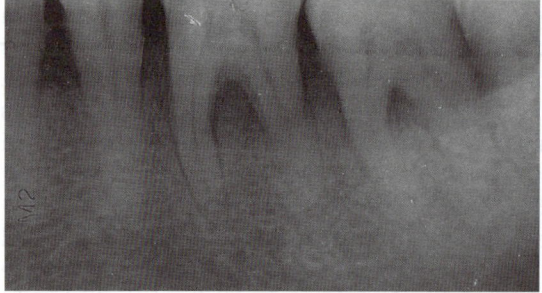

A. Mandibular molars

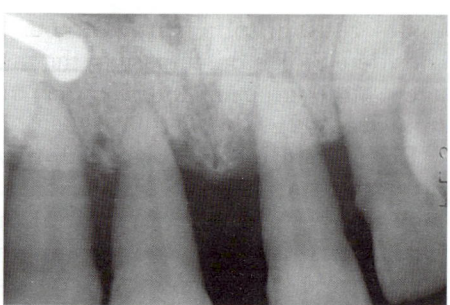

B. Maxillary incisors

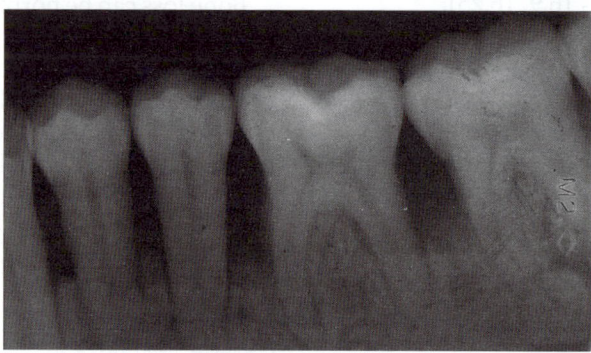

C. Mandibular molars

Figs 16.26A to C: Horizontal bone loss

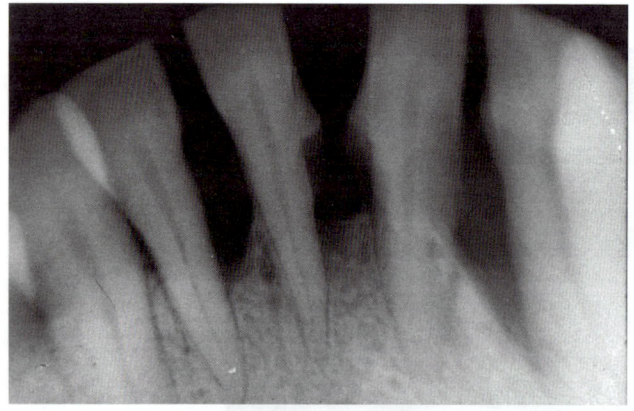

A. Mandibular incisors

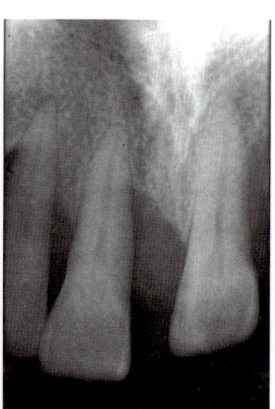

B. Maxillary incisors

Figs 16.27A and B: Vertical bone loss

16

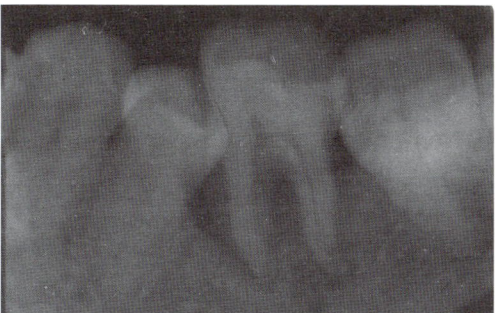

A. Infrabony resorption of bone in mandibular first molar led to endodontic problem

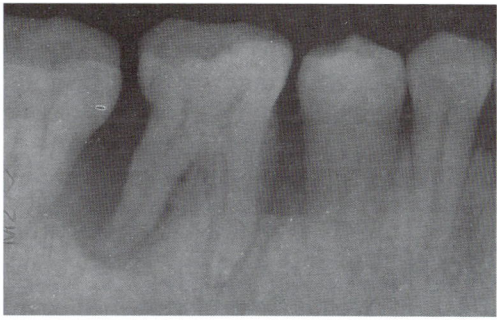

B. Total resorption of bone around distal root of first molar and infrabony bone loss around second premolar

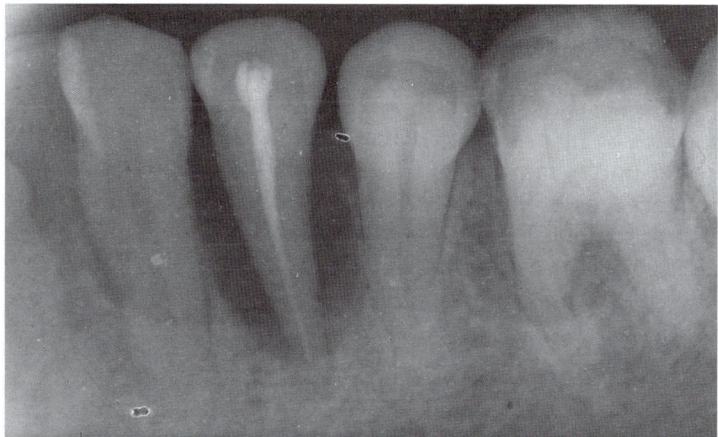

C. Endodontic problem in mandibular first premolar led to periodontal inflammation

Figs 16.28A to C: Periodontal endodontal lesion

- *Capnocytophaga*
- *Actinobacillus actinomycetem comitans*
- *Eubacterium saburreum*

All the three groups of organisms are more prevalent in patients suffering from this form of periodontitis, though they are present in routine in other individuals also. In aggressive periodontitis, all the first molars show semilunar bone loss and anterior teeth exhibit severe bone loss (Figs 16.29A to F).

Local irritating factors such as calculus, overhanging margins and carious lesions etc. predispose an individual to periodontal problems. Their radiographic detection followed by correction improves periodontal condition.

16

Radiographs are also of importance in follow-up examination, especially to observe bone-formation after grafting of infrabony defects with natural or synthetic bone grafts. Radiographic data is a must to decide the prognosis of any periodontal disease.

ORAL LESIONS

There is a plethora of lesions which could possibly be seen in the soft and hard tissues of the oral and para-oral structures. These lesions can range from simple tissue hyperplasias to life-threatening malignant lesions. An alert dentist, who is armed with a thorough knowledge of the appearance of such lesions, can play a vital role in the early diagnosis. Early diagnosis of such lesions may prove to be a life-saving event in dental practice. For better understanding of the radiological appearances of various oral lesions, a brief description of the clinical features of these lesions is also described.

For convenience, the common oral lesions are as follows:

TUMORS

a. Odontogenic

  i. Ectodermal (epithelial)
   • Ameloblastoma
   • Adenomatoid odontogenic tumour (adenoameloblastoma)
   • Calcifying epithelial odontogenic tumor (Pindborg tumor)
  ii. Mesodermal (connective tissue)
   • Odontogenic myxoma/odontogenic fibromyxoma
   • Benign cementoblastoma
 iii. Mixed tumors (ectodermal-meso-dermal)
   • Odontoma (complex and com-pound)

   • Cementifying or ossifying fibroma
   • Periapical cemental dysplasia
   • Ameloblastic fibroma

b. Non-odontogenic

  i. Ectodermal
   • Neurilemmoma/schwannoma
   • Neuroma (traumatic amputation neuroma)
  ii. Mesodermal
   • Osteoma
   • Central haemangioma
   • Central giant cell granuloma
   • Chondroma
   • Gardner's syndrome

c. Malignant Lesions

  i. Carcinomas
   • Squamous cell carcinoma
   • Metastatic carcinoma
  ii. Sarcomas
   • Osteosarcoma
   • Chondrosarcoma
   • Fibrosarcoma
   • Ewing's sarcoma

d. Hematologic Neoplasms

   • Leukemia
   • Lymphomas

e. Immunologic Neoplasms

   • Burkitt's lymphoma
   • Multiple myeloma

f. Bony Hyperplasias

   • Torus palatinus (maxillary tori)
   • Torus mandibularis (mandibular tori)
   • Exostoses
   • Endostoses

g. Bony Pathologies

   • Paget's disease

16

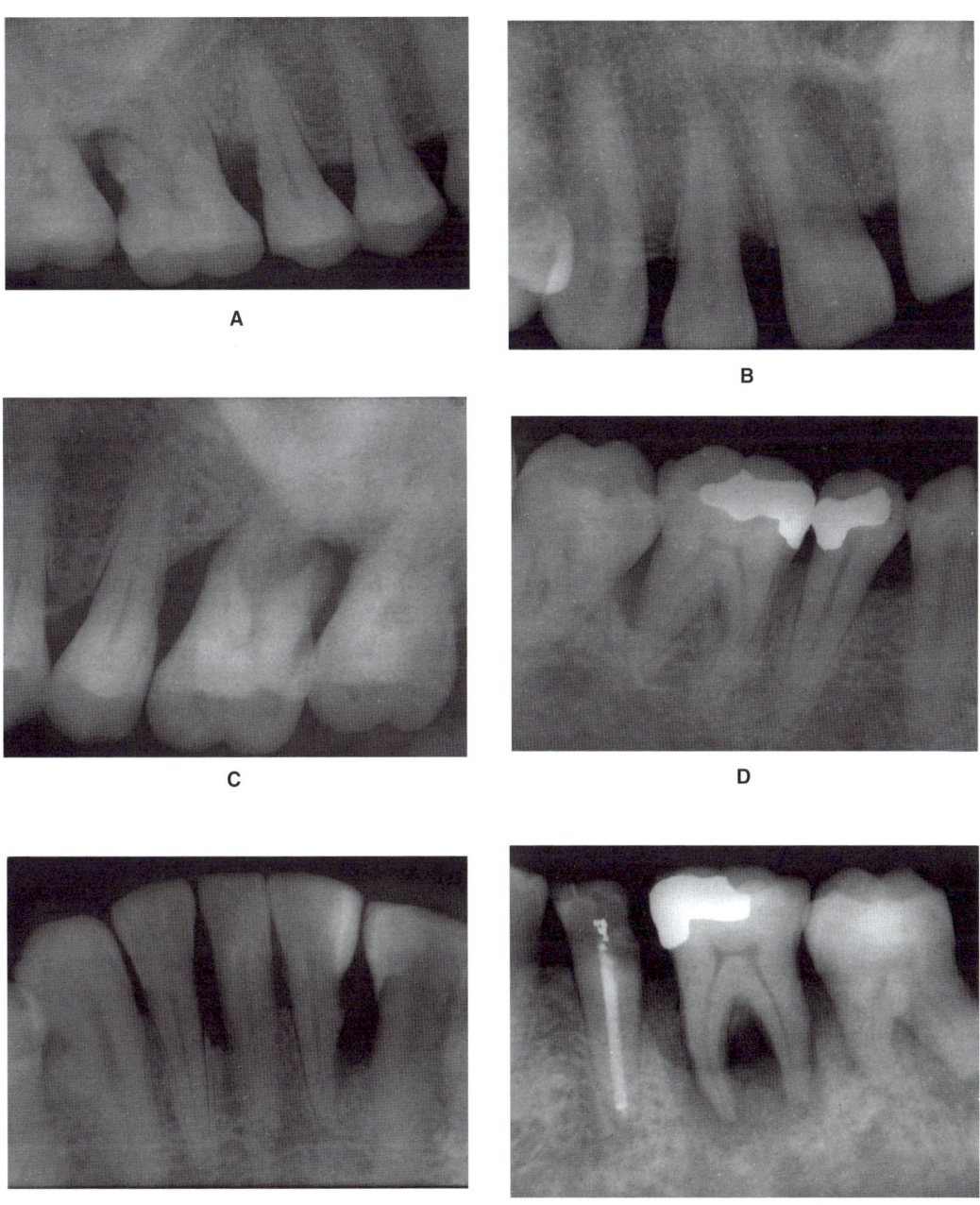

Figs 16.29A to F: A case of aggressive periodontitis. Note the semilunar bone loss in all first molars and near total bone loss in anteriors

16

- Fibrous dysplasia
- Ossifying/cementifying fibroma
- Osteomyelitis

a. Odontogenic tumors

These tumors arise from the odontogenic tissues. On the basis of their origin these can be classified as :

- i. Ectodermal (epithelial)
- ii. Mesodermal (connective tissue)
- iii. Mixed (ectodermal-mesodermal).

ECTODERMAL (EPITHELIAL) TUMORS

AMELOBLASTOMA

It is a locally aggressive neoplastic lesion arising from the remnants of the dental lamina and dental organ, i.e. the odontogenic epithelium. The malignant variety of ameloblastoma may rarely metastasize (1–5%) via haematogenous route (Fig. 16.30).

Clinical Features

- It has a predilection for males and is more often seen in blacks.
- Most probable age is 20–50 years.
- Mostly in the molar/ramus region of the mandible.
- In the maxilla, it occurs most frequently in the third molar region, gradually progressing to involve the maxillary sinus and the floor of the nose.
- Teeth may be displaced or resorbed with gradual increase in size. Facial asymmetry may occur. Intraorally, it is covered by healthy normal mucosa.
- Palpation of the site may elicit a bony hard feeling or crepitus.

Ameloblastoma (Intraosseous Variety)

The radiographic appearance has the following features:

- Unilocular/multilocular radiolucency in different forms and shapes.
- Typically, it appears to be a multilocular radiolucent area, often described as *soap-bubble* appearance when radiolucent loculations are large. If loculations are small, it is described as *honey-comb appearance*.
- It frequently shows both buccal and lingual plate expansions. Lesions in dentulous areas may cause root resorption and tooth displacement.
- Many cases are associated with unerupted teeth giving the appearance of a dentigerous cyst. But, the unilocular variety may resemble any type of cyst.
- One of the variants, desmoplastic ameloblastoma appears radiopaque because of its dense connective tissue content.

Differential Diagnosis

When the lesion is small and unilocular, it resembles a cyst but most of the cysts, namely residual cyst, traumatic bone cyst and keratocyst tend to occur in patients in their mid-twenties whereas ameloblastoma occurs in older persons. Ameloblastoma is also to be differentiated from giant cell granuloma and the lateral periodontal cyst, both of which generally occur anterior to the molars.

When the lesion grows in size and is multilocular, it is most likely to be confused with odontogenic myxoma. In odontogenic myxoma, the tooth is generally missing or fails to erupt. The *tennis racquet* appearance of odontogenic myxoma is different from the honeycomb appearance of ameloblastoma.

16

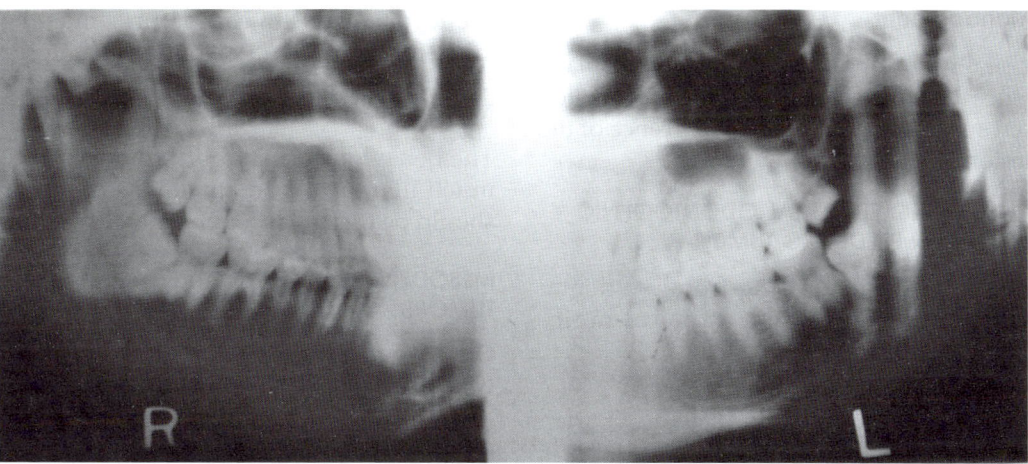

Fig. 16.30: Ameloblastoma (right mandible) panoramic view

Management

For small lesions an intraoral approach is preferred with en bloc resection of jaw.

In advanced lesions with extensive proliferation segmental resection is advocated. For lesions which are inoperable, megavoltage radiotherapy is carried out which gradually reduces the size of the lesion.

ADENOMATOID ODONTOGENIC TUMOR (ADENOAMELOBLASTOMA)

It is a developmental overgrowth of odontogenic tissues which is not related to ameloblastoma as its treatment requires only localized removal of the growth rather than extensive removal as in the case of an ameloblastoma.

Clinical Features

The lesion has a predilection for females (2 : 1) and is more frequently found in the maxilla. The clinical features are that of ameloblastoma. The usual site are the canine and first premolar areas with some tendency for occurrence in the incisor region also.

Radiographic Features

The adenomatoid odontogenic tumor is a well defined unilocular radiolucency associated with unerupted teeth. This appearance is similar to that of dentigerous cyst with the exception that the outline of an adenomatoid odontogenic tumor may attach well beyond the crown of the impacted tooth. The border of the radiolucency is frequently sclerotic and there may be radiopacities in the substance of the lesion. The size, number, and density of these radiopacities vary from lesion to lesion. Displacement of roots may be seen but resorption is rarely present.

Differential Diagnosis

The adenoameloblastoma is to be differentiated from dentigerous cyst.

16

Management

Usually the tumor expands the cortical plate. Since it is not invasive, it can be easily shelled out surgically. There is no recurrence of the lesion.

CALCIFYING EPITHELIAL ODONTOGENIC TUMOR OR PINDBORG TUMOR

It is a rare lesion arising from the dental epithelium and present a typical radiographic appearance.

Clinical Features

It is locally aggressive tumor with a high rate of recurrence. It has a propensity of being present in males like ameloblastoma and has a definite predilection for the mandible and mostly develops in the premolar, molar region. The expansile nature of the lesion may result in expansion of buccal and the lingual cortical plates, which is the only symptom. On palpation, the lesion feels like a hard swelling.

The tumor represents a variable number of radiographic patterns. It may appear to be well circumscribed or diffuse, unilocular or multilocular, radiolucent or mixed radiolucent/radiopaque. The scattered flecks of calcification throughout the radiolucency give the lesion a 'driven snow' appearance (Fig. 16.31).

It may sometimes be associated with an impacted/embedded tooth, resembling a dentigerous cyst.

Differential Diagnosis

Radiographically, the tumor may be very similar to the calcifying odontogenic cyst, adenomatoid odontogenic tumor and ameloblastic fibroodontoma. All radiolucent lesions with radiopaque foci must be considered in the differential diagnosis of the lesion. The clinical features must be taken into consideration for final diagnosis.

Management

The behaviour of Pindborg tumor is very much like that of an ameloblastoma and should be treated as for an ameloblastoma.

MESODERMAL (CONNECTIVE TISSUE) TUMORS

Odontogenic Myxoma (Odontogenic Fibromyxoma)

It is a relatively uncommon lesion, which is locally aggressive and non-metastasizing. It arises from a developing tooth's primitive mesenchymal tissue and appears only in the facial skeleton. It usually affects young persons and is related with teeth that fail to erupt or are missing.

Clinical Features

The lesion has a sex predilection favouring females and it occurs more frequently in the age group of 10–30 years. It more commonly affects the mandible than the maxilla (3 : 1).

In the mandible it occurs in the molar and premolar regions and rarely involves the condyle and the ramus area, i.e. non-tooth bearing areas. In the maxilla it may also involve the maxillary sinus causing exophthalmos. Usually it involves the alveolar processes of premolar and molar regions.

Its rate of growth is slow and may result in the displacement of teeth. Upto 25% cases may recur.

Radiographic Appearance

As the lesion is aggressive and destructive, the picture is very well apparent radiographically. It may give a typical

16

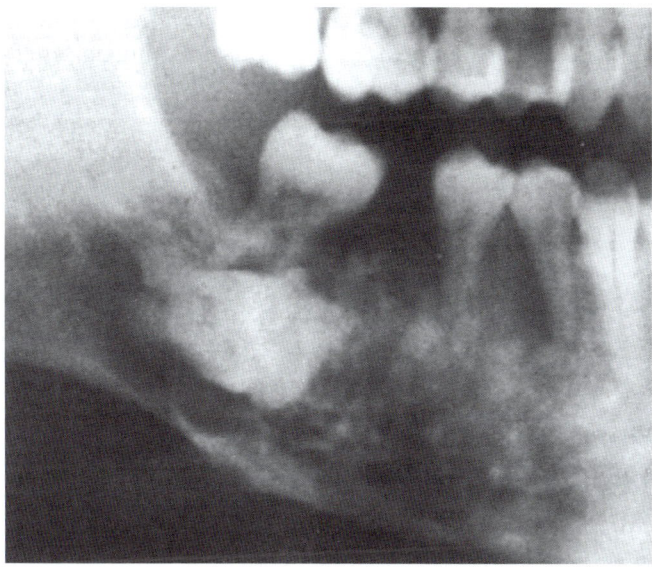

Fig. 16.31: Lateral oblique mandible showing Pindborg tumor (calcifying epithelial odontogenic tumor) ('snow driven' appearance)

picture of a honeycomb or a tennis racquet; occasionally a soap bubble appearance may also be present.

The radiolucent area is usually well-defined and has a corticated margin. At times the outline is poorly defined. The lesion scallops around the roots of the teeth and rarely results in the resorption of roots of the teeth.

CT scan and MRI enhance the knowledge of the anatomic extent of the lesion and help in planning the surgical treatment of the lesion.

Differential Diagnosis

- *Ameloblastoma:* It is seen more often in the older age group. Honey comb appearance with trabeculae in loculi is less likely to be seen in an ameloblastoma when compared to odontogenic myxoma.

- Central giant cell fibroma is usually located anteriorly.
- *Central giant cell lesion of hyper-parathyroidism:* The patient has a history of kidney disease and abnormal serum chemistry.
- *Cherubism:* It is seen in the younger age group and is bilateral. It has a familial tendency.
- Aneurysmal bone cyst is relatively rare. It is tender and painful.
- *Metastatic tumor of jaw (carcinoma) :* It is usually seen in the older age group and the primary tumor must be looked for.
- *Central haemangioma:* It has all the features of a myxoma as regards the site of radiographic appearance but it is not associated with young teeth. When aspiration is done, blood is revealed from the lesion in contrast to a myxoma which is not productive.

16

- Myxoid lipo-sarcoma secondarily invading the jaw.
- Fibrosarcoma with myeloid changes.
- Primary liposarcoma

⎫ These are some of the most difficult to differentiate. Histopathological evaluation is of prime importance ⎬

Management

It is treated by resection with a generous amount of the surrounding bone being sacrificed to ensure complete removal of the tumor that has infiltrated into the marrow spaces. Radiation therapy is of no value.

BENIGN CEMENTOBLASTOMA

It is a neoplasm of cementum and is a result of the activity of the cementoblasts in the periodontal ligament. It is commonly seen in association with permanent teeth and rarely with primary teeth.

Clinical Features

It is seen more often in males and the usual age group is 12–65 years. The lesion is solitary and there is a greater probability of finding it in association with the mandibular premolars or first molar. It is slow growing resulting in the formation of a bulbous mass at the root tip and may gradually displace the tooth. Rarely, it may cause expansion of the bone.

Radiographic Features

It is a well-defined radiopacity merging with the image of the root and usually has a radiolucent halo present at the border of the calcified mass. The outline of the root is generally obscured. If present, it always shows some resorption. Occlusal radiographs are quite helpful to demonstrate the extent of the lesion.

Differential Diagnosis

- Periapical cemental dysplasia
- Chronic focal sclerosing osteomyelitis
- Periapical osteosclerosis
- Hypercementosis (is smaller than cemento-blastoma)

⎫ The tumor cementoblastoma is associated with the root of the tooth and is separated from the surrounding bone by a radiolucent border ⎬

The lesion should be evaluated on the basis of both clinical and radiographic findings.

Management

It is self-limiting and does not recur after enucleation. Simple excision and extraction of the associated tooth is sufficient. Endodontic therapy after enucleation of the lesion is also helpful.

MIXED (ECTODERMAL-MESODERMAL) TUMORS

Odontoma (Complex and Compounds)

Odontomas are hamartomatous malformations of odontogenic tissues that demonstrate various stages of histological and morphological differentiation. These are formed by extraneous budding of the odontogenic epithelial cells of the dental lamina. The differentiation is quite variable hence giving a relative radiographic picture.

16

- **Complex odontoma:** These are non-descript masses of dental tissues.
- **Compound odontoma:** These are multiple, well-formed tooth-like growths (twice as common as complex odontoma).

Occasionally, however, differentiation might not take place at all. In such a case the lesion is known as ameloblastic odontoma (there is simultaneous occurrence of ameloblastoma and complex odontoma) (Table 16.1).

Symptoms of ameloblastic odontoma : The symptoms are bony expansion, destruction of cortex, displacement of teeth and mild pain.

Clinical Features

It is the most common odontogenic tumor interfering with the eruption of teeth. It has no sex predilection and the period of growth corresponds well with the period of development of the associated teeth. It mostly occurs in the second decade of life.

Impaction, malpositioning, diastema, aplasia, malformation and devitalization of adjacent teeth are other clinical features associated with 70% of the odontomas.

RADIOGRAPHIC FEATURES

A compound odontoma appears as a collection of tooth-like structures of different sizes and shapes surrounded by a narrow radiolucent zone (Fig. 16.34).

A complex odontoma appears as a calcified mass surrounded by a radiolucent rim resembling tooth structure in radiodensity but not in shape (Figs 16.32, 16.33).

Differential Diagnosis

The lesion has a typical appearance of a radiopaque structure in a well-defined radiolucent lesion.

CEMENTIFYING OR OSSIFYING FIBROMA

It is not associated with any tooth as is the case with complex odontoma, and is usually less radiopaque than the compound odontoma (Figs 16.35A, B). This lesion develops at a younger age.

PERIAPICAL CEMENTAL DYSPLASIA

It is a small lesion occurring in the mandibular anterior region of middle-aged adults (Fig. 16.36).

Table 16.1: Differences between complex and compound odontoma

	Complex odontoma	*Compound odontoma*
Age and sex	Second decade More in females	Second decade Same in males and females
Associated teeth	Permanent	Permanent
Occurrence	Half as that of compound odontoma	Twice as that of complex odontoma
Site	Mandibular first and second molars often associated with unerupted canine	Incisor and premolar regions
Bony expansion	May be associated with bone expansion	Bony expansion seldom present

16

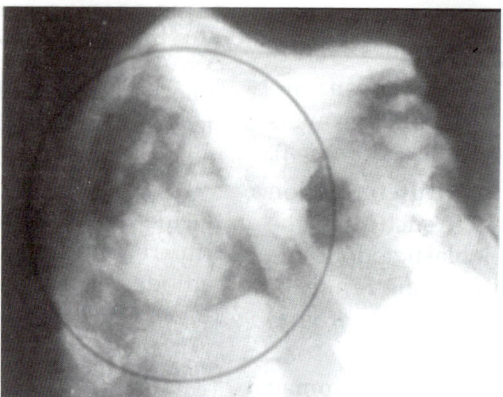

Fig. 16.32: Complex composite odontoma (lateral oblique)

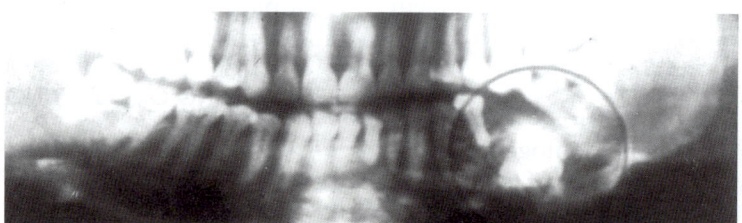

Fig. 16.33: Complex composite odontoma (panoramic view)

AMELOBLASTIC FIBROMA

It is a mixed odontogenic tumor arising from both epithelial and mesenchymal tissues of the tooth germ.

Clinical Features

It usually occurs in the age group of 5 to 20 years (i.e. during the period of tooth formation) and is completely benign. It has a predilection for the premolar and molar areas of the mandible. There is expansion of cortical plates and migration of involved teeth. It may also be associated with a missing tooth.

Radiographic Features

Radiographically, it resembles ameloblastoma. It may present itself as a unilocular or multilocular lesion associated with an unerupted tooth. It has well-defined borders. Cortical plate expansion can also be detected at times.

Differential Diagnosis

- Central giant cell granuloma
- Odontogenic myxoma
- Central haemangioma

(i) All these lesions have a fine trabecular pattern with honey comb or tennis racquet pattern

(ii) Association with tooth is not necessary

Central giant cell granuloma: It has a predilection for occurrence in the anterior regions of the jaws.

16

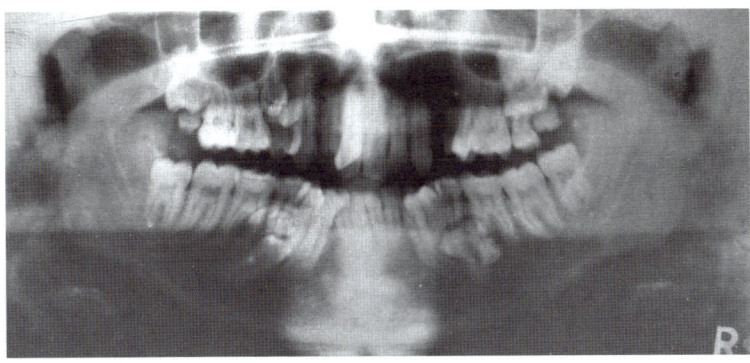

Fig. 16.34: Compound composite odontoma right mandible (panoramic view)

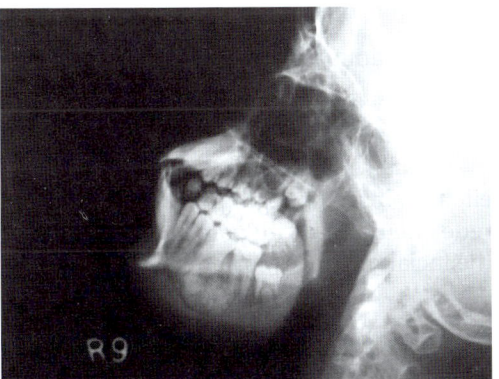

Fig. 16.35A: Lateral oblique mandible showing ossifying fibroma (fibroosseous lesion)

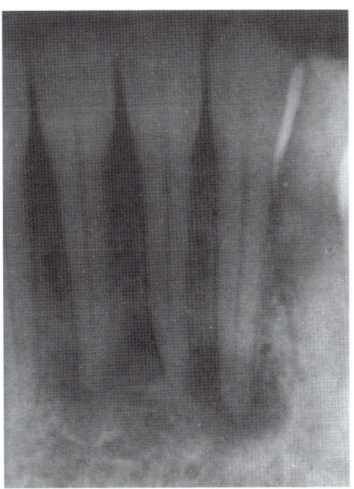

Fig. 16.36: Apical cemental dysplasia

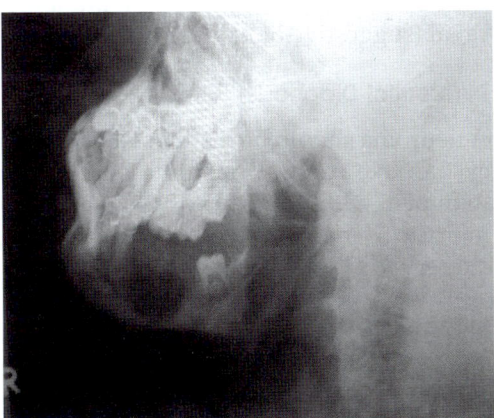

Fig. 16.35B: After surgery

A central haemangioma may show local gingival bleeding and rebound mobility of teeth.

- A keratocyst usually contains thick, yellowish granular fluid.
- Ameloblastoma is seen in a much older age group.

Management

As the lesion is benign and has a low rate of recurrence, excision is preferred.

16

b. Non-odontogenic Tumors

These are tumors in the oral cavity which arise from tissues other than those meant for the development of the tooth, e.g. nervous tissue, fibrous tissue, etc.

These tumors can be broadly classified as:
i. Ectodermal tumors
ii. Mesodermal tumors

Benign intraosseous non-odontogenic tumors arise from nervous tissue, i.e. nerve sheath, nerve fibres, and in combination with their supporting tissues. These tumors have a propensity to occur in the mandible (especially in the body) as the mandibular canal conveys a large neurovascular bundle (inferior alveolar) and that too over a reasonably large area.

ECTODERMAL TUMORS

NEURILEMMOMA (SCHWANNOMA)

It is a tumor of neuroectodermal origin arising from the Schwann cells. It is the most common of all the neural tumors.

Clinical Features

It is a slow growing tumor mostly involving the mandible. It shows no predilection for either sex. The usual complaint is that of a lump in the jaw. It is firm to palpation and non-productive on aspiration. Pain when present, is usually at the site of tumor with paraesthesia distal to it.

Radiographic Features

The tumor depicts itself as a radiolucent area in the jaw because of bone resorption, which is usually distal to the mental foramen.

There may be resorption of the roots of teeth and also loculization (as in ameloblastoma). The margins are well defined as they are hyperostotic.

Differential Diagnosis

The lesion when small, can be recognised by the expansion of the canal. As it grows in size, it gives an extremely varied picture and lacks any distinctive features.

NEUROMA
(TRAUMATIC AMPUTATION NEUROMA)

It is in fact proliferation of the nervous tissues after injury to the nerve, which is attempting to heal itself. The injury may be mechanical or chemical irritation, fractures or surgical procedures.

Clinical Features

It is a slow growing reactive hyperplastic tissue. Due to the over-growth of the tissue in a limited space, pressure is created which elicits pain in the region. There may also be reflex neuralgia with pain being referred to the facial region, eyes and head.

Radiographic Features

It manifests as a radiolucent area of reasonable size (depending on the extent of the lesion) and shape with well-defined borders. It usually forms in the mandibular canal (suggestive of neural origin).

Differential Diagnosis

A neuroma should be distinguished from a cyst. Unlike a cyst, an neuroma is associated with pain with a past history suggestive of injury to the nerve such as fracture or during surgery.

Management

Since neuromas tend to increase in size and cause persistent pain, excision is suggested. Recurrence is rare.

16

MESODERMAL TUMORS

OSTEOMA

The tumor arises from a cartilage or embryonal periosteum occurring almost exclusively in the skull and skeleton of the face. Structurally, it can be of three types :
- Compact bone
- Cancellous bone
- Combination of compact and cancellous bone

Clinical Features

It is usually located in the mandible. The most frequent site is the buccal side of ramus and lower border of the body of the mandible below the molars. Because of bony growth, it results in facial asymmetry. It generally occurs in patients who are more than 40 years of age. The nature of bone is dense, ivory-like, compact in males and cancellous in females.

Radiographic Features

Radiographically, an osteoma appears as a radiopaque mass with well-defined borders.

Mandibular lesions are *exophytic* (protruding out from the normal contour of the bone). The compact bone gives a picture of uniform radiopacity and the cancellous bone shows a trabecular pattern (Fig. 16.37).

Differential diagnosis

The lesion should be differentiated from:
- Mature ossifying fibroma
- Early osteogenic sarcoma
- Chondrosarcoma
- Exostoses or tori

Management

The management of the lesion depends upon:
- Any discomfort to the patient
- The functional and structural suitability of the prosthesis (when being planned)
- Cosmetic aspect

CENTRAL HAEMANGIOMA

It is benign proliferation of endothelium-lined vascular channels generally occurring in the vertebrae and the skull and rarely in the jaws.

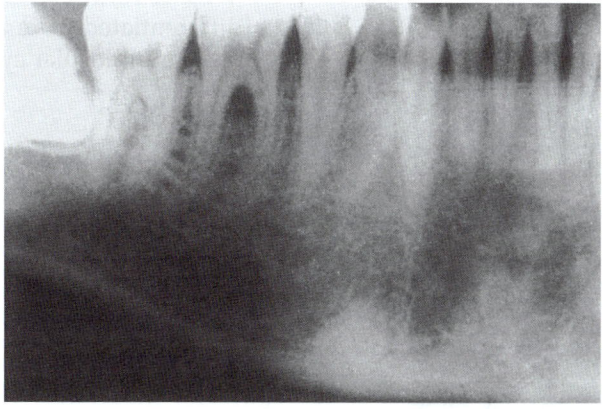

Fig. 16.37: Central osteoma (mental foramen area)

16

Clinical Features

Its occurrence is greater in females than males (2 : 1) and in the mandible than the maxilla (2 : 1). It is usually bony hard and may or may not be associated with pain. There may be loosening of teeth, which also show rebound mobility. Aspiration produces arterial blood.

Radiographic Feature

Radiologically, the lesion depicts a typical picture of an osteolytic lesion with enlargement of trabecular spaces. It may also give a soap bubble or honeycomb or at times even a sunburst or sunray appearance (Fig. 16.38). There may occur phleboliths (small areas of calcifications in the vein) which are of prime consideration of a central haemangioma, as the radiographic picture is much varied.

Differential Diagnosis

The radiographic picture of the lesion is like that of a multilocular lesion. For differential diagnosis, aspiration is helpful in establishing the nature of the lesion. If the test does not reveal the vascular nature of

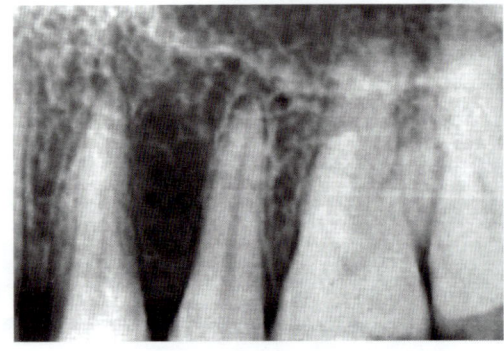

Fig. 16.38: Central haemangioma

the lesion, the possibility of other multilocular lesions, namely central giant cell granuloma, giant cell lesions of hyperparathyroidism, ameloblastic odontogenic myxoma, metastatic tumor and cherubism must be ruled out. The traumatic bone cyst and keratocyst have better defined borders.

Management

The management of the lesion is by en bloc resection with ligation of the external carotid artery as trauma may result in excessive bleeding. Management can also be accomplished by the introduction of inert materials to induce sclerosis.

CENTRAL GIANT CELL GRANULOMA

It usually presents as a multilocular or, less commonly, as a unilocular radiolucency with well-defined borders. Lesions in the maxilla may have ill-defined, malignant appearing borders.

Differential Diagnosis

- Unilocular tumors are to be differentiated from periapical granuloma/cyst.
- Multilocular lesions should be differentiated from ameloblastoma and other multilocular cysts.

CHONDROMA

It is a benign tumor of cartilaginous origin and is of rare occurrence in the jaws (Fig. 16.39).

Clinical Features

It is usually seen in the fifth and sixth decades of life and show predilection for the anterior maxillary region as the site of occurrence. In the mandible, it most often

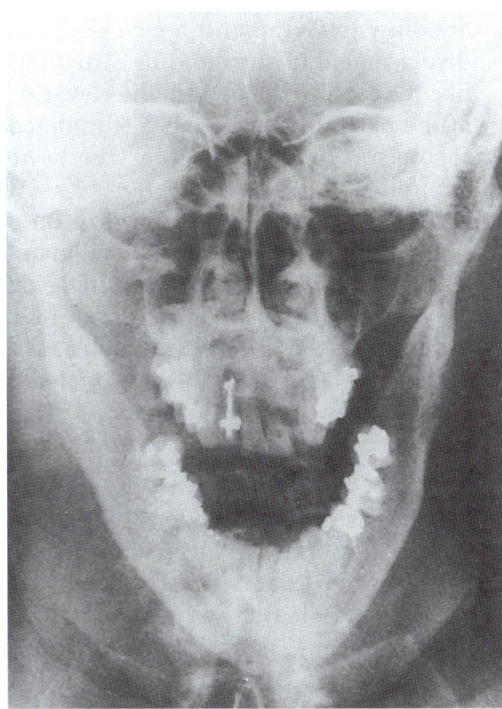

Fig. 16.39: Osteochondroma of left condyle (Reverse Towne's projection)

develops in the premolar-molar region. It usually presents itself as a painless swelling. There may be loosening and/or exfoliation of overlying teeth.

Radiographic Features

It appears as an irregular radiolucent area with or without a well-defined border. There may be resorption of teeth.

Differential Diagnosis

The radiographic picture is similar to that of:
• Chondrosarcoma
• Osteogenic sarcoma
• Osteoblastic metastatic carcinoma

• Ossifying subperiosteal haemangioma
• Fibrous dysplasia
• Peripheral fibroma

Management

A lesion suspected to be a chondroma should be considered as having potential for malignant change into chondrosarcoma. Hence it should be excised thoroughly along with a wide margin of normal tissues.

GARDNER'S SYNDROME

It is a hereditary condition characterised by multiple osteomas, sebaceous cysts, subcutaneous fibromas and multiple polyps of the small and large intestines.

Radiographic Features

The osteomas in this syndrome precede the intestinal polyps. Since the polyps have a tendency for malignant change, the detection of this syndrome on the basis of multiple osteomas is vital. Also, noteworthy from a dentist's point of view is the presence of supernumerary teeth (also detected with the help of radiograph). Early recognition of the syndrome may result in saving the life of the patient.

Management

The management is like any other osteoma but if Gardner's syndrome is suspected, the patient must be referred for procto-sigmoidoscopy and barium enema.

c. Malignant lesions

Characteristics of Malignant Lesions

As a result of a change in the nature of the lesion, it grows and disrupts normal anatomy, thereby causing obvious changes

16

in the anatomic and radiographic picture of the tissue and the surrounding structures. The nature of the metastatic lesion, the rate of its growth and that of surrounding tissues are factors, which ultimately elicit a radiographic picture specific (to some extent) to it. The various features, which are to be analysed, and the reasons for those features being so specific have been discussed below in comparison with benign lesions.

a. **Border of the lesion:** Benign lesions characteristically have well-defined borders, which is because of their inherent nature of being non-aggressive and slow growing. They grow gradually and hence have a rounded or oval shape.

   On the other hand, malignant lesions aggressively expand outwards and cause virtual erosion of the surrounding tissues. As a result, the borders are irregular, ragged and ill-defined. They have a mosaic form and blend with the normal tissue. For this reason, the radiographic extent of the lesion is difficult to define. At times, there may be superimposition of infection leading to the invasion of bone, thereby masking the actual picture of the lesion.

   Acute infection causes bony destruction, hence results in sclerosing osteitis and a conforming radiographic picture of well-defined radiopaque margin.

   It would not be out of place to mention that certain benign lesions of bony infection may elicit a radiographic picture resembling a malignant lesion. Hence, it is not the radiograph or the clinical picture alone, which is diagnostic of a pathology, but both acting as adjuncts to each other.

b. **Adjacent cortical bone:** Benign lesions are slow growing and hence result in displacement of surrounding structures like the cortical bone. With the elevation of the periosteum, there is a stimulated formation of layers of reactive bone termed *onion skin appearance* (as it resembles the peel of an onion on a radiograph). The growth of a malignant lesion occurs by destruction and invasion of the adjacent structures. Hence, expansion of the lesion causes destruction of the cortex and drags the bony material along its path of expansion. It forms a trail of bone, hence, giving a typical picture of *sunburst appearance*.

c. **Radiodensity:** The radiodensity of lesion varies depending upon the tissue involved. For example, an osteoma is a radiopaque lesion while a central haemangioma is radiolucent (both benign).

   Malignant lesions (carcinomas) are radiolucent except in the case of metastatic lesions (secondaries from carcinoma of prostrate gland). There is simultaneous resorption and deposition of bone in case of a sarcoma, a feature diagnostic of this lesion.

d. **Dental involvement:** Teeth are more calcified than the bone. When the lesion is expanding the response of teeth is recorded in the following two ways:

   i. *Displacement:* Usually benign lesions are slow growing and put slight, persistent pressure on the teeth resulting in their gradual displacement. In malignant lesions the expansion of the lesion occurs too rapidly for teeth to respond to the pressure. The roots are well within the border of the lesion. Therefore, in malignant lesions there is a typical picture of floating teeth; moreover, the teeth lie in their original position.

ii. *Resorption of roots* : So far as resorption of roots is concerned, benign lesions, because of their slow growth, have more time to be in contact with the surface of a tooth to cause resorption. In a malignant lesion, the contact period is relatively less, hence resorption is not a specific feature of a malignant lesion, which is observed in benign lesions.

e. **Radiographic features:** The lesion should be examined by at least two right angled radiographs so as to evaluate the extent and character of the lesion by evaluating its interaction with the surrounding bone. Since a radiograph is a two dimensional image of the tissues, superimposition of various structures occurs, thereby making it difficult for the observer to analyse the extent of the features of the lesion. Radiographic exposure at two angulations can solve this problem to some extent. CT scan or computerised tomography is a good answer to this problem. With CT scan, the invasion of the lesion into the soft tissue can also be analysed.

CARCINOMAS

SQUAMOUS CELL CARCINOMA

It is a tumor of epithelial origin arising mostly in the oral mucosa. It is the most common type of oral cancer spreading by invasion of soft tissues, neurovascular tissue and through the bone. A premalignant lesion is in the form of leukoplakia or erythroplakia or both. Early detection of this disease is of vital importance because, early it is detected and treated, better is the prognosis. Subsequent advancement brings

it in contact with bone resulting in bony involvement.

Etiology: There is no specific etiology but many factors have been implicated
- Spirits and alcohol
- Spices
- Smoking
- Sharp margins

Clinical Features

- Predominantly in men over 50 years of age.
- The most frequent site is the postero-lateral border of the tongue and lower lip, less frequently floor of the mouth, alveolar mucosa, palate and buccal mucosa.
- *Size and bony involvement*: Osseous involvement is most frequently in the third molar region of the mandible where it is closest to the bone. Small lesions, which are less than 1.0 cm in diameter are generally asymptomatic. It is only when the lesion enlarges that there is pain, anaesthesia or swelling. With the gradual increase in its size if a lesion lies close to a tooth, leads to loosening of the tooth with some root resorption or at times exfoliation.

Further, an increase in size may lead to metastasis through the lymphatic channels to submental and submandibular lymph nodes.

Radiographic Features

The appearance of the lesion is as similar that of a destructive lesion. There is gradual erosion of the bone resulting in ill-defined margins all along the tumor or at some specific points. In the mandible gradual growth of the lesion may lead to complete

16

erosion of the bone resulting in a pathological fracture (Fig. 16.40).

Usually a combination of posteroanterior occlusal and lateral oblique views is helpful in determining the extent of the lesion and in the demonstration of such pathological fractures.

Generally the lesion has an irregular border but at times the border of the tumor is lined by a radiopaque margin (as in condensing osteitis). There is no specific reason for it but it is probably due to the response of bone marrow cells to the advancing tumor cells. Also, sometimes specks of radiopaque material signifying pieces of left over bone by the rapidly advancing tumor (especially in central squamous cell carcinoma) may be seen.

Differential Diagnosis

Carcinomas have a typical feature of aggressive nature resulting in irregular borders. Hence, all lesions having ill-defined bony margins have to be differentiated from it, e.g. osteomyelitis.

In osteomyelitis the symptoms are entirely different. There is a definite infection and sequestration might also be detected. Also, osteomyelitis is a relatively slowly advancing pathology where reactive periosteal bone formation may occur giving a corresponding radiographic picture.

During treatment by radiotherapy, osteoradionecrosis may occur. In such cases it becomes difficult to distinguish between recurrence of carcinoma and radionecrosis. Other diseases to be considered for differential diagnosis with locally destructive bone loss are:

- Histiocytosis
- Periodontitis
- Aggressive periodontitis
- Papillon Lefevre syndrome.

16

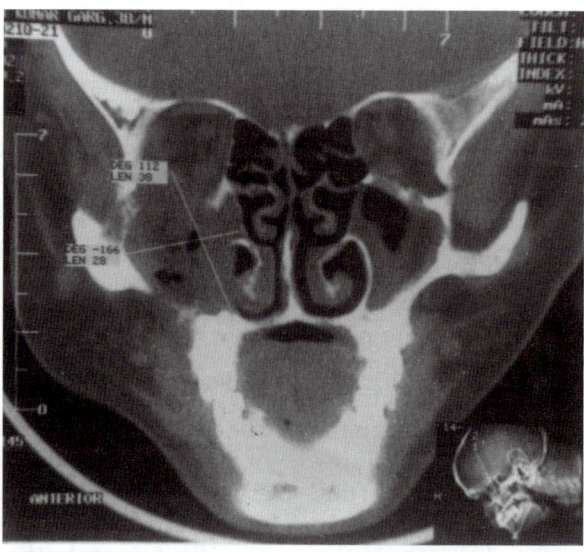

Fig. 16.40: Squamous cell carcinoma (coronal C.T.) (cross marked)

Management

The management is by radiotherapy, surgery or both.

METASTATIC CARCINOMA

It is the most common malignant tumor of the skeleton resulting from metastasis of primary carcinoma from a distant site to the bone. The metastatic carcinoma of the jaws however is relatively rare, accounting for only 1 to 8% of all malignant tumors of the oral region.

Clinical Features

The mandible is more susceptible to metastatic carcinoma than the maxilla. The most common site is premolar-molar region and age of occurrence varies from 40–60 years. Metastasis may occur from the breasts, lungs, kidneys, prostrate glands, colon, testis and stomach. Oral findings are usually the first indication of the disease. The lesion is asymptomatic. It is only when the mandibular nerve is involved by the lesion, that there is pain, paresthesia or anaesthesia. The teeth may become loose or get exfoliated with occasional evidence of root resorption. Prognosis for the patient with metastasis is poor.

Radiographic Features

The features of metastatic carcinoma are similar to those of primary carcinoma having a radiolucent picture with ill-defined margins. The lesions may be single or multiple or of variable size.

Differential Diagnosis

It is the same as that of primary carcinoma. If metastasis occurs in the alveolar bone, the picture of the lesion may resemble that of advanced periodontal disease. Identification will depend on histological examination and observation of advancement and growth of the lesion, especially when a primary carcinomatous lesion has not been detected.

SARCOMAS

OSTEOSARCOMA

It is the most common malignant tumor of bone, and arises from undifferentiated bone-forming mesenchymal tissue. Depending upon the nature of the lesion, sarcoma can be of three types :

- *Sclerosing*: This type forms neoplastic osteoid and bone.
- *Osteolytic*: This type does not form bone and elicits a picture of bone resorption only. The rate of growth of this type is greater than the sclerosing type.
- *Mixed*: It is one, which has both the components, i.e. resorption and formation of bone.

Clinical Features

The mean age of occurrence of an osteosarcoma is around 50 years. It involves the maxilla (antrum or alveolar ridge excluding the palate) and the mandible (body of mandible) equally and does not favour any sex. The incidence of this lesion is more in bones that have been irradiated, subjected to trauma or affected by *Paget's disease*.

The first sign of the disease is swelling, occasionally associated with pain having a fairly short history. Teeth may become loose and paresthesia may develop. The rate of growth of this lesion is very high; it doubles in size in about a month.

16

Radiographic Appearance

It often presents as a radiolucent lesion or shows mixed sclerosis or dense sclerosis with ill-defined irregular borders.

Typical *sun-burst* appearance is caused by bony spicules produced perpendicular to the bone and is best seen in the occlusal view. However, this *sun-burst* appearance is not pathognomic of osteosarcoma.

An important early finding is the symmetrical widening of the periodontal ligament space around a tooth or several teeth in the area of lesion. This is also seen in scleroderma (Fig. 16.41).

Differential Diagnosis

The osteolytic type must be differentiated from a carcinoma.

The mixed and sclerosing types manifest a sun-ray pattern hence they must be differentiated from lesions showing a similar radiographic picture. The lesions are:

• Myeloma
• Metastatic cancer
• Advanced benign carcinoma
• Tuberculosis

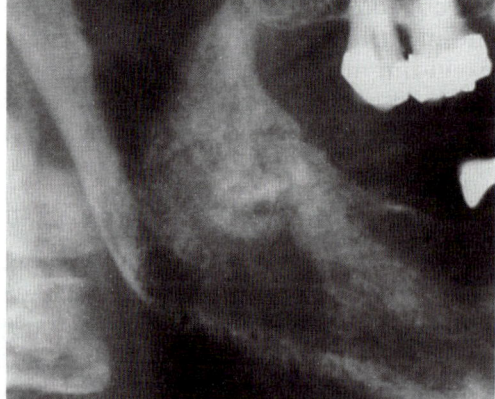

Fig. 16.41: Osteogenic sarcoma

• Inflammatory diseases other than tuberculosis

CHONDROSARCOMA

This tumor is a malignant lesion of cartilaginous origin. It may arise centrally in the bone, peripherally in the periosteum or in connective tissues containing cartilage. The origin is generally from bone and can be:

• *Central or medullary*: if arising from within the bone.
• *Peripheral*: if arising from cartilaginous caps on the bone.

Clinical Features

The lesion is rare in the jaws, but when present it is mostly in the maxilla. The average age of occurrence is 30 years (mean range 20–60 years). Males are more prone to this lesion and are affected twice as much as females. The first symptom is an innocuous hard swelling resulting in facial asymmetry. The affected tooth may get loosened, resorbed or even exfoliated. Irradiation can be one of the precipitating causes. Transition from a benign to malignant lesion is also common. The rate of growth of this lesion is relatively less than osteosarcoma and it seldom metastasizes. Recurrence of the lesion after surgery is common and death results by local aggressive nature.

Radiographic Features

Like osteosarcoma, the radiographic picture of the lesion is highly variable. There is resorption of the bone, which may or may not depict sclerosis. In addition, it may appear as a cystic lesion. The lobules of cartilage may give a soap-bubble appearance. There may also be a sun ray pattern (in one-fourth of the cases) or a ground-glass appearance. With the passage of time irregular, small, and dense foci of calcification may appear in the outer region. The widening of periodontal ligament space may also be evident as in osteosarcoma. As all these features are characteristics of a malignant lesion, the radiographic picture cannot be pathognomic but suggestive of a malignant lesion.

Differential Diagnosis

Osteosarcoma, fibrosarcoma, fibrous dysplasia and odontogenic cysts and tumor should be considered for differential diagnosis. Proper differential diagnosis is more dependent on histopathological examination than radiographic examination. Serious consideration of the nature of the lesion should be the line of approach till benign or inflammatory nature of the lesion is established histopathologically.

FIBROSARCOMA

It is a primary malignant fibroblastic tumor, which fails to exhibit bone or osteoid formation and also does not metastasize. It arises either from the periosteum or periodontal membrane or endosteal connective tissue.

Clinical Features

Mostly the lesion is central (arising in the bone) but it may also arise in the periosteal tissues. The usual age of occurrence is fifth decade, the range being 20–50 years. Clinical examination reveals a hard painful swelling with or without the covering of oral mucosa. Paresthesia is noted in one-third of the cases.

Radiographic Features

There are no specific radiographic features of the lesion, which helps to distinguish it from other lesions. The general features of a malignant lesion, namely osteolytic changes, ill-defined borders and displacement of teeth with or without root resorption may also be noted.

Management

The tumor is resistant to radiotherapy. The recurrence after surgery is common especially when removal of the lesion by surgical excision is limited. Prognosis depends upon analysis of the extent of the lesion and well-planned surgery.

EWING'S SARCOMA

It is a primary malignant tumor originating in the bone marrow from the mesenchymal connective tissues (Fig. 16.43).

Clinical Features

Although the lesion may occur at any age it is most common in the second decade of life, i.e. mostly below 30 years. Males are affected twice as more often as than females. It usually affects long bones and about 10% of the lesions affect the jaws. By nature, it is a fast-spreading and a highly invasive tumor. The involved bone is painful, tender to palpation, swollen and there is a feeling of warmth in the area. Metastasis may occur to other bones, lymph nodes and lungs. The teeth may become loose and there may be paresthesia of the soft tissue.

Radiographic Features

The radiograph shows osteolysis with ill-defined irregular borders. The picture is most likely to be confused with

16

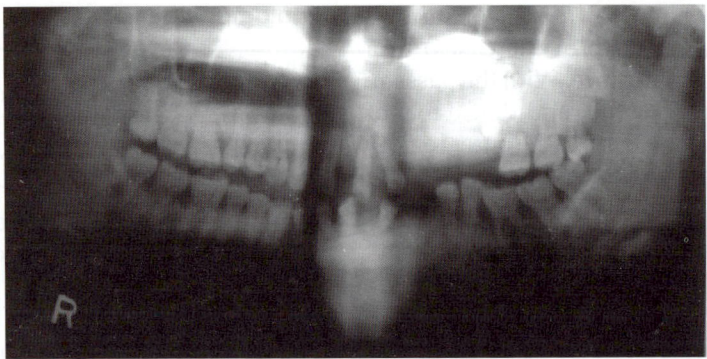

A. Orthopantomograph (fibrous dysplasia in midline mandible and left maxilla)

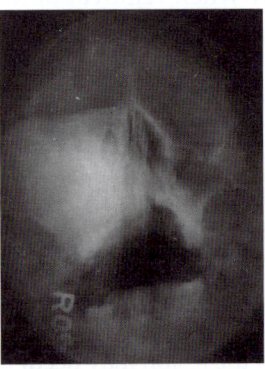

B. Waters' view (fibrous dysplasia in right maxilla)

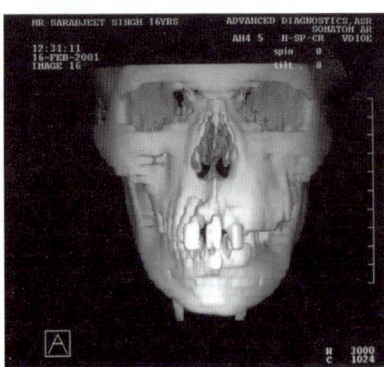

C. 3-D CT showing fibrous dysplasia in left maxilla and midline mandible

Figs 16.42A to C: Fibrous dysplasia

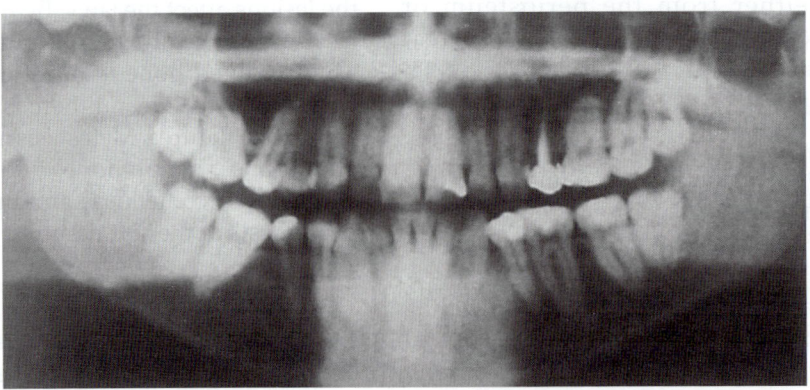

Fig. 16.43: Orthopantomogram showing Ewing's sarcoma of maxilla

16

osteomyelitis. Areas of sclerosis may develop at the border of the lesion. There may be expansion of the cortical bone and subsequent formation of new bone subperiostially. Hence, it may give an onion-peel appearance occasionally. Sunray pattern may be seen in advanced cases. But it may also be present in inflammatory conditions, malignant tumors and is not pathognomic for the same.

HAEMATOLOGIC NEOPLASMS

LEUKAEMIA

It refers to a set of diseases in which there is neoplastic proliferation of white blood cells (lymphoid, monocystic and myeloid stem cells). In acute leukaemia primitive blood cells (blast cells) are released into the blood whereas in chronic leukaemia the abnormal cells retain many of the morphological features of the normal cells.

Clinical Features

Acute leukaemia may occur in either sex and accounts for nearly 50 per cent of all the malignant diseases in children. Chronic leukaemia occurs in older people (50–70 years). Frequently, there is gingival hyperplasia particularly when gingival and periodontal disease is present. Oral manifestations are absent in very young and edentulous patients. Oral bleeding and petechiae are common findings. Other oral findings are swelling, paresthesia and extrusion of teeth. Fungal and herpetic infections may also be seen, which can occasionally be fatal.

Radiographic Features

Radiographic findings may include destruction of bone, which may be similar to those of periodontal disease. There is thinning or disappearance of the lamina dura, especially in the premolar and molar regions and also there is loss of crestal alveolar bone. With the infiltration of leukaemic cells, there may be bony destruction near the apices of teeth (generally mandibular molars) giving rise to a picture of periapical pathology. The lesion is reversible with chemotherapy. The cells may destroy the cortex and come to lie beneath the periosteum and result in reactive bone formation giving onion-peel effect.

Management

Acute leukaemia is managed with potent cytotoxic drugs and supportive care (e.g. control of infection, haemorrhagic tendencies, anaemia etc.).

In chronic leukaemia, no treatment is needed for asymptomatic patients. Otherwise treatment is carried out by cytotoxic drugs and radiotherapy.

Lymphomas

Lymphomas constitute a group of neoplasms of varying degrees of malignancy, which are derived from basic cells of lymphoid tissues, lymphocytes and histiocytes in any of their developmental stages. They are of two types, Non-Hodgkin's lymphoma and Hodgkin's lymphoma.

Non-Hodgkin's lymphomas are heterogenous group of lymphoproliferative malignancies, which can involve lymph nodes and lymphoid organs as well as extra nodal organs and tissues (Fig. 16.44).

Hodgkin's lymphoma is potentially curable malignant lymphoma with distinct histology and biological behaviour. The

16

characteristic malignant cells of this disease are called as *Reed-Sternberg* cells.

IMMUNOLOGIC NEOPLASMS

BURKITT'S LYMPHOMA

It is a malignancy of B-lymphocytes. The Epstein Barr virus (member of the herpes group) has been implicated as the causative organism for the disease.

Clinical Features

There are two varieties of this tumor; African and non-African. There is greater involvement of the jaws in the African form in young people alongwith abdominal manifestation with increasing age. In the non-African variety, it is the reverse (Table 16.2).

Clinically, both the varieties exhibit loosening, displacement or increased mobility of teeth. The mobility is usually the first sign of the tumor. There may be premature eruption of first molars leading to swollen and ulcerated gingiva and mucosa.

Radiographic Features

The lesion present itself as radiolucent patches randomly distributed in the affected area. With the passage of time, the radiolucent foci gradually increase in size resulting in the formation of bigger patches with poorly defined margins. There may be enlargement of the bony crypts containing tooth buds alongwith subsequent destruction of the cortex of the tooth germ. The gradual expansion of the lesion results in expansion or even perforation of the cortical plates. New bone formation may elicit a sunray pattern at its periphery. The teeth may get resorbed or shed prematurely.

16

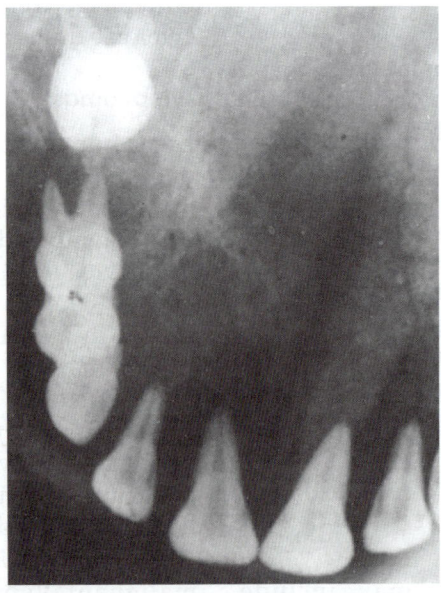

Fig. 16.44: Non-Hodgkin's lymphoma (diffuse nature of radiolucency)

Table 16.2: Clinical features of African and Non-African form of Burkitt's lymphoma

	African form	Non-African or American form
Primary involvement and subsequent change	Jaw involvement is more common than abdominal. Abdominal manitestations increase with age	Abdominal involvement manifests first
Jaw involvement	Affects all the four quadrants	Affects only one quadrant
Age of peak incidence	5–7 years	10–12 years
Prevalence	Both the varieties are two to four times more prevalent in boys than girls	

When the lesion involves the maxilla, it may spread rapidly to the floor of the orbit and the sinus. A CT scan is helpful in establishing the extent of the lesion.

Differential Diagnosis

Because of the apparent moth-eaten appearance, the possibility of an acute infection or osteomyelitis must be ruled out and supported by clinical examination and blood reports. Also, the rate at which the lesion advances should be analysed.

Management

Both forms of tumors, i.e. African and non-African, respond to chemotherapy and radiotherapy. In comparison to the non-African variety, the African variety is considered to be more aggressive and more difficult to manage and hence has a poor prognosis.

MULTIPLE MYELOMA

It is a neoplasm in which there is proliferation of a single clone of abnormal plasma cells in the bone marrow. With a gradual increase in the number of these cells,

replacement of the normal bone marrow occurs (Fig. 16.45).

Clinical Features

It affects adults in the age group of 40–70 years with a predilection for males (2 : 1). It may affect any part of the skeleton. With gradual growth of the lesion, discontinuity may ensue resulting in a pathological fracture. Laboratory tests reveal anaemia, elevated ESR and increased plasma protein levels. There is a high incidence of jaw involvement and oral manifestations may be one of the initial signs of systemic disease. It may cause pain, paresthesia, swelling, mobility and migration of teeth. Haemorrhage may also occur.

Radiographic Features

The usual roentgenographic picture of multiple myeloma presents as a multiple, well-defined radiolucent patches with sclerotic borders producing the typical picture of a punched out lesion. The radiolucencies are present bilaterally and gradually coalesce to form bigger defects. Cranial lesions are commonly present in addition to the involvement of other sites

16

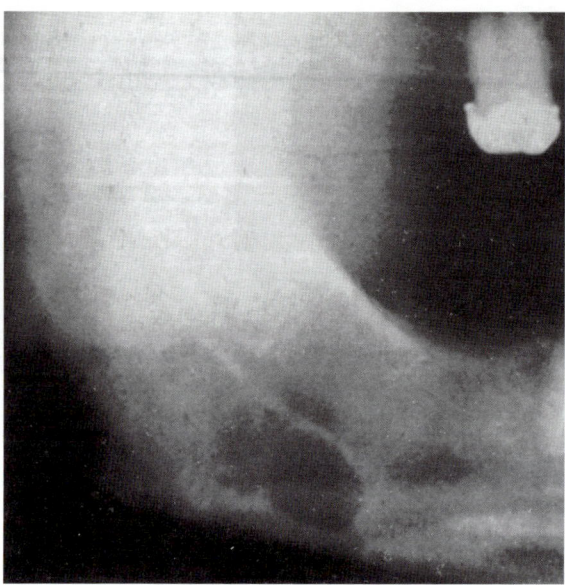

Fig. 16.45: Multiple myeloma

and a radiograph of the skull is advisable in suspected cases.

Differential Diagnosis

Although the punched out appearance is quite characteristic, however, other related skull lesions must be ruled out.

f. Bony Hyperplasias

These refers to growths of normal bone. They exceed the normal limits of the bone, which is of normal architecture and undergo spontaneous arrest in the increase in size; for example :
- Maxillary tori (Torus Palatinus)
- Mandibular tori (Torus Mandibularis)
- Exostoses
- Endostoses
These are usually slow growing with limited growth potential. The patients are usually unaware of their presence, because of their asymptomatic and innocuous nature.

TORUS PALATINUS (MAXILLARY TORI)

This is the most common of all exostoses and has a predilection for women. Its size and shape is highly variable and it usually goes unnoticed by the patient. Due to its prominence, the overlying mucosa is often traumatized.

Radiographic Features

On intraoral periapical radiographs, it may superimpose on the roots of the maxillary teeth. Occlusal radiographs are usually more explanatory regarding its extent. Depending on the angulation, the view of the tori may project with more or less sharply defined margins, or at times it may appear to be confluent with the normal picture of the surrounding bone.

16

TORUS MANDIBULARIS (MANDIBULAR TORI)

It is an outgrowth of the bone on the lingual surface of the mandible in relation to the first molar and premolar, and is often bilateral. It provides strength to the mandible (Fig. 16.46).

Radiographic Features

On intraoral periapical radiographs, it appears as a radiopaque shadow usually superimposing on the roots of premolars and the first molar. Its anterior extent is usually sharply defined as compared to the posterior (which is less dense).

On occlusal radiographs, it appears as a knobby projection on the lingual surface of the mandible.

EXOSTOSES

These are small nodular, pedunculated or sessile prominences on the surface of the bone. They are seldom of any clinical significance. They are present on the facial surfaces of alveolar processes and are rarely palpable.

Radiographic Features

They appear as uniform radiopaque masses, which are reasonably well-defined. The outline may merge with the surrounding bone. Large exostoses may present a picture simulating medullary bone.

ENDOSTOSES

It is the inward growth of the compact cortical bone into the medullary cancellous bone. It is seen more in the mandible and has a propensity for the premolar and molar region.

Radiographic features

It appears as a dense bony image with well defined irregular margins merging with the bony trabaculae. It has no radiolucent margins or capsule.

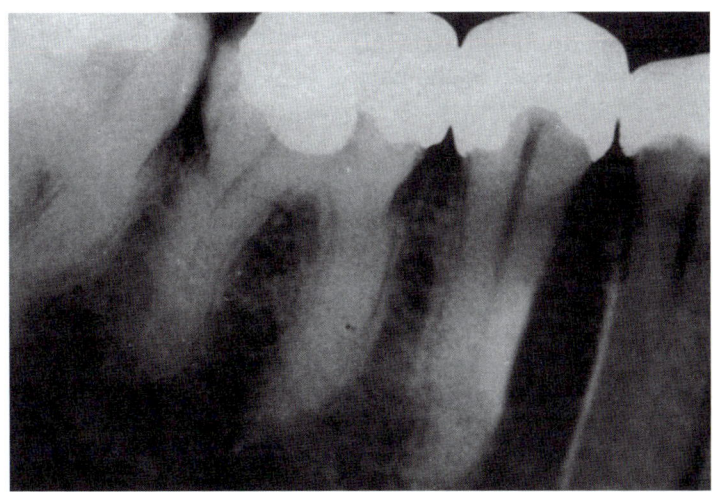

Fig. 16.46: Mandibular tori

16

Differential Diagnosis

Various lesions can have a similar picture of dense opacity e.g. :

i. Periapical cemental dysplasia

ii. Hyper-cementosis

iii. Cemento-blastoma

(These lesions have a radiolucent margin. They are present more or less around the roots of the teeth)

iv. Osteosarcoma

v. Chondro-sarcoma

vi. Osteoblastoma

vii. Metastatic osteoblastic carcinoma

(All these have a radiolucent component associated along with a predominantly radiopaque picture)

Management

All sclerotic lesions should have a periodic assessment to detect any increase/decrease in size. In case of any doubt, an excisional biopsy is preferred to rule out malignancy.

g. Bony Pathologies

PAGET'S DISEASE

The disease in its early stage presents as decreased radiodensity of bone with alteration of the trabecular pattern. This is known as the resorptive stage. The second stage has a ground glass or a granular, denser appearance; more radiopacity may present in later stages.

During the osteoblastic phase, patchy sclerosis is evident giving a typical 'cotton wool' appearance.

FIBROUS DYSPLASIA

It classically presents as homogeneous radiopacity with numerous trabeculae of woven bone giving a 'ground glass' appearance. Although it may also show a unilocular or multilocular radiolucency with or without irregular opacity giving a mottled appearance (Fig. 16.42).

OSSIFYING/CEMENTIFYING FIBROMA

It is either completely radiolucent or may present varying degrees of radiopacity with centrifugal type of cortical expansion. It may show downward bowing of the inferior border of the mandible. But its well-circumscribed mature with a sharply defined border between the lesion and normal bone makes it distinguishable from fibrous dysplasia.

OSTEOMYELITIS

It is of two types:

i. Chronic Osteomyelitis

It reveals a patchy, ragged, ill-defined radiolucency, which often contains central, radiopaque sequestra.

ii. Garre's Osteomyelitis

It presents as radiopaque duplication of cortical bone (extra-cortical bone deposition) and is better seen on an occlusal film.

Bibliography

1. Ahlfors E, Larsson A, Sjögren, S: The odontogenic keratocyst: A benign cystic tumor. *J Oral Max Surg* 1984;42:10.
2. Al-Dewachi HS, Al-Naib N, Sangal BC: Benign Chondroblastoma of the maxilla: a case report: A case report and review of chondroblastoma in cranial bones. *Br J Oral Surg* 1980;18:150.

16

3. Alexander WN, Lilly GE, Irby WB. Odontodysplasia: Report of a case and review of literature. *O Surg, O Med, O Path*. 1966;22: 814.

4. Anderson RA: Eruption Cysts—A retrograde study. *J Dent Child* 1990;57:124.

5. Archard HO, Carlson KP, Stanley HR. Leukoedema of the human oral mucosa. *Oral Surg*. 1968;25:717.

6. Austin LT Jr., Dahlin DC, Royer RQ. Giant cell reparative granuloma and related conditions affecting the jaw bones. *Oral Surg*: 1959;12:1285.

7. Axell T, Henriesson V: Leukoedema—an epidemiologic study with special reference to the influence of tobacco habits. *Oral Epidemiol*. 1981;9:142.

8. Azaz B, Ulmansky M, Lewin EJ: Dentinoma: report of a case. *O Surg, O Med, O Path*: 1967;66:659.

9. Baden E, Newman R: Liposarcoma of the oropharyngeal region. Review of the literature, and report of two cases. *Oral Surg*: 1977;44:889.

10. Ballard BR, Suess GR, Pickren JW, Greene GW and Jr. Shedd DP: Squamous cell carcinoma on the floor of the mouth. *Oral Surg*. 1978;45:568.

11. Basden E, Saroff SA: Periapical cemental dysplasia and periodontal disease. *J Periodontol* 1987;58;187.

12. Bender IB, Freedland JB: Adult root fracture. *JADA*: 1983;107:413.

13. Benn DK: A review of the reliability of radiographic measurements in estimating alveolar bone changes. *J Clinic Periodontol* 1990;17:14.

14. Benn DK: A review of the reliability of radiographic measurements in estimating alveolar bone changes. *J Clinic Periodontol* 1990;17:14.

15. Bennett TG, Paleway SA: Internal resorption, post pulpotomy type. *O Surg, O Med, O Path* 1964;17:228.

16. Bernick J: Central giant cell tumor of the jaws. *J Oral Surg*: 1948;6:324.

17. Berry HH, Ladwerlen JR: Cigarette smoker's lip lesion in psychiatric patients. *JADA*: 1973;86: 657.

18. Bhaskar SN: Periapical lesions; type, incidence and clinical features. *O Surg, O Med, O Path* 1966;21:657.

19. Bhaskar SN, Cutright DE: Multiple exostosis report of 16 cases. *J Oral Surg* 1968;26:321.

20. Blakemore JR, Eller DJ, Tomaro AJ: Maxillary exostosis. *O Surg, O Med, O Path* 1979;48:187.

21. Bragger U: Radiographic parameter: Biologic significance and clinical use. *Periodontol* 2000: 39, 73, 2005.

22. Browne, RM and Rivas, PH: Chondromyxoid fibroma of the Mandible: A case report. *Br J Oral Surg*: 1977;15:19.

23. Bruce KW, Royer RQ: Lipoma of the oral cavity. *Oral Surg*. 1954;7:930.

24. Bell WH, Callender RM, Pugh BR, Wood GD: The abrasion and cleaning properties of dentifrices. *B Dent J* : 1968;125;331.

25. Cabrini RL, Barros RE, Albano H.: Cysts of the jaws : A statistical analysis. *J Oral Surg*: 1970;28: 485.

26. Cameron CE: Cracked tooth syndrome. *JADA* 1964;68:405.

27. Cash CD, Royer RQ, Dahlin DC: Metastatic tumors of the jaws. *Oral Surg*. 1961;14:897.

28. Cavanha AO. Enamel pearls. *O Surg, O Med, O Path*: 1965;19:373, .

29. Cawson RA: Chronic oral candidiasis and Leukoplakia. *Oral Surg* 1966;22:582.

30. Chen SY, Miller AS: Neurofibroma and schwannoma of the oral cavity. *Oral Surg*. 1979;47:522.

31. Chew CL, Tan PH: Torus palatinus : A clinical study. *Aust Dent J*: 1984;29:245.

32. Clark WH Jr, Bernardino EA, Mihm MC.: The histogenesis and biologic behaviour of primary human malignant melanomas of the skin. *Cancer Res*. 1969;29:705.

33. Cohen S, Burns RC.: *Pathways of the pulp*, 3rd edition. C.V. Mosby Co., St. Louis, 1984.

34. Coley BL, Higginbotham NL, Groesbeck HP: Primary reticulum cell carcinoma of bone. *Radiology* 1950;55:641.

35. Corio RL, Lewis DM: Intra oral rhabdomyomas. *Oral Surg* 1979;48:525.

36. Crowley RE: Neurofibroma. *NY. Dent J*: 1951;17:457.

37. Dahl EC, Wolfson SH, Hangen JC: Central odontogenic fibroma : review of literature and report of cases. *J Oral Surg*. 1981;39:120.

38. Dahlin DC, Ivins JC: Benign chondroblastoma. A study of 125 cases. *Cancer* 1972;30:401.

39. Damm DD, Neville BW: Oral leiomyomas. *Oral Surg* 1979;l47:343.

40. De Aranjo FB, Rosito DB, Toigo E, Dos Santos CK: Diagnosis of approximal caries:

16

radiographic versus clinical examination using tooth separation. *Am J Dent* 1992;5:245.

41. Devlin H, Karayimni K, Mitsea A, Jacob R, Lindh C, Marjanovic E, Horner K: Diagnosing osteoporosis by using dental panoramic radiograph: The osteodent project. *O Surg, O Med, O Path* 2007;104:821.

42. Dick H, Simpson W: Dental changes in osteoporosis. *O Surg, O Med, O Path* 1972;34,408.

43. Einhorn J, Wersall J: Incidence of oral carcinoma in patients with leukoplakia of the oral mucosa. *Cancer* 1972;20:2189.

44. Eliasson S, Halvarson C, Ljungheiimer C: Periapical condensing osteitis and endodontic treatment. *O Surg, O Med, O Path* 1984;57:195.

45. Ellis GL, Cario RL: Spindle cell carcinoma of the oral cavity. *Oral Surg* 1980;50:523.

46. Espelid I, And Tveit A: Clinical and radiographic assessment of approximal carious lesions. *Acta Odontol Scand1991* 1986;44:31.

47. Espelid I, And Tveit AB. : Diagnosis of secondary caries and crevices adjacent to amalgam. *Int Dent J* 1991;41:359.

48. Eversole LR: Central benign and malignant neural neoplasms of the jaws: *A review. J Oral Surg*: 1969;27:716.

49. Faweett KJ, Dahlin DC: Neurilemmoma of bone. *Am J Clin Pathol*: 1967;47: 759.

50. Fitzergerald RJ, Adams BO, Davis ME: A microbiological study if recurrent dentinal caries. *Caries Res* 1994;28:409.

51. Flamant R, Hayem M, Lazar P, Denoix P: Cancer of the tongue: A study of 904 cases. *Cancer.* 1964;17:377.

52. Gamez-Aranjo JJ, Toth BB, Luna MA: Central hemangioma of the mandible and maxilla: Review of a vascular lesion. *Oral Surg.* 1974;37:230.

53. Gardner DG: The central odontogenic fibroma: An attempt at clarification. *O Surg, O Med, O Path* : 1980;50:425.

54. Gardner DG: The mixed odontogenic tumor. *O Surg, O Med, O Path* 1984;58:166.

55. Gardner DG: The peripheral odontogenic fibroma : an attempt at clarification. *Oral Surg* : 1982;54:40.

56. Gartner AH, Mack T: Differential diagnosis of internal and external root resorption. *J Endo* : 1976;2:329.

57. Giansanti JS, Waldron CA: Peripheral giant cell granuloma : review of 720 cases. *J Oral Surg* 1969;27:787.

58. Goldman HM: Spontaneous intermittent resorption of teeth. *JADA* 1954;49:522.

59. Goldstein BH, Laskin DM: Giant cell tumor of the maxilla complicating paget's disease of bone. *J Oral Surg* 1974;32:209.

60. Gould AW: An investigation of the inheritance of torus palatinus and torus mandibularis. *JDR* 1964;4:159.

61. Greene GW, Natiella JR, Spring PN: Osteoid osteoma of the jaws. Report of a case. *Oral Surg* 1968;27:787.

62. Greer RO, Berman DN: Osteoblastoma of the jaws: Current concepts and differential diagnosis. *J Oral Surg*: 1978;36:304.

63. Grotepass FW, Farman AG, Nortje CJ: Chondromyxoid fibroma of the mandible. *J. Oral Surg* 1976;34:988.

64. Hardman FG. Keratocanthoma on the lips. *Br J Oral Surg* 1971;9:46.

65. Hatziotis JC, Asprides H: Neurilemomma (Schwannoma) of the oral cavity. *Oral Surg* 1967;24:510.

66. Hausmann E, Allen K: What alveolar crest level on a bite wing Radiograph represents bone loss. *JP* 1991;62:570.

67. Hildebolt CF, Vanner MW, Zerbolio DJ, Shrout MK, *et al*: Radiometric based classification of alveolar bone health. *JDR* 1992;71:1594.

68. Hildebolt CF, Vannier MW, Shrout MK. Periodontal disease morbidity quantification II: Validation of alveolar bone loss measurements and vertical defect diagnosis from digital bite wing images. *Journal of Periodontol* : 1990;61:623.

69. Hollister DW, Klein SH, Dejager HJ, Lachman RS, Rimoin DL: Lacrimo-auriculo-dento-digital syndrome. *J Pediatr*: 1973;83:438.

70. Holst JJ, Lange F. Perimylolysis: Contribution towards the genesis of tooth washing from non-mechanical causes. *Acta Odont Scand* 1939;1: 39.

71. Horner K, Devlin H, Harvey L: Detecting patients with low skeletal bone mass. *J Dent* 2002;30:171.

72. Hurlburt CE, Wuerhman AH: Comparison of interproximal carious lesions detection in panoramic and standard intraoral radiography. *JADA*: 1976;93:1154.

16

73. Jacobsen JH, Hansen B, Wenzel A, Hintze H: Relationship between histological and radiographic caries lesion depths measured in images from four digital radiography systems. *Caries Res* 2004;38:34.

74. Kaffe I, Bouchner A.: Radiographic features of central odontogenic fibroma. *O Surg, O med, O Path*: 1994;78:811.

75. Kaffe Tamse A, Littmer MM: Radiographic manifestation of idiopathic external and internal root resorption. *Quint Int* 1982;13:339.

76. Kalathingal SM, Tyndall DA, Caplan DJ: *In vitro* assessment of cone beam local computed tomography for proximal caries detection. *O Surg, O Med, O Path* , 2007;104:699.

77. Kenr J.: Radiographic screening of edentulous patients. Sense or Non-sense. *O Surg, O Med, O Path*: 1986;62:463.

78. Kjaerheim A, Stokke T: Juvenile Xantho-granuloma of the oral cavity. *Oral Surg* 1974;38:414.

79. Kondell P, Wiberg J. Odontogenic Keratocysts. *Swed Dent J* 1998;12:57.

80. Kramer IRH. Cacinoma in situ of the oral mucosa. *Int Dent J*: 1973;23:94.

81. Krolls SO, Jacoway JR, Alexander WN: Osseous choristomas (osteomas) of intra oral soft tissues. *Oral Surg* 1971;32:588.

82. Larebke RG: Vertical crown root fracture in posterior teeth. *Dent Cl North Am* 1984;28:883.

83. Leider AS, Garbarino E: Generalized hypercementosis. *O Surg, O Med, O Path* 1987;63:375.

84. Levitas TC: Germination, fusion, twinning and concrescence. *J Dent Child* 1965;32:93.

85. Lin LM, Langeland K, Vertical foot fracture. *J Endo* 1982;8:558.

86. Mallow RD, Spatz SS, Zubrow HJ: Odontogenic fibroma with calcification. *O Surg, O Med, O Path*: 1966;22:564.

87. Massler M, Perreault JG: Root resorption in the permanent teeth of young adults. *J Dent Child* 1954;21:158.

88. Matalon S, Feuerstein O, Calderon S, Mittleman A, Kaffe I: Detection of cavitated carious lesions in approximal tooth surfaces by ultrasonic caries detector. *O Surg, O Med, O Path* 2007;103: 109.

89. Mcdonald JDS, Yeung RWK, Li T, Lee KM: Computed tomography of odontogenic myxoma. *Clinic Radiol* 2004;59:281.

90. Mejare J, Grondahl HG, Carlstedt K, Grever AC, Ottoson E: Accuracy at radiography and probing for the diagnosis of proximal caries. Scand. *J Dent Res*: 1985;93:178.

91. Melrose RJ, Abrams AM: Juvenile fibromatosis affecting the jaws : Report of three cases. *Oral Surg* 1980;49:317.

92. Mena CA: Taurodontism. *O Surg, O Med, O Path*: 1971;32:812.

93. Misch KA, Yi ES, Sarment DP: Accuracy of cone beam computed tomography for periodontal defect measurements. *J Periodontol* 2006;77:1261.

94. Mora MA, Mol A, Tyndall DA, Rivera EM: In vitro assessment of local computer tomography for the detection of longitudinal tooth fractures. *O Surg, O Med, O Path* 2007;103: 825.

95. Moore C: Smoking and cancer of the mouth, pharynx and larynx. *JAMA*: 1965;191:283.

96. Murdoch CA, Miles DA: Clinical and radio-graphic features of the lacrimo-auriculodento-digital syndrome. *O Surg, O Med, O Path* 1996;81:727.

97. Nair MK, Tyndall DA, Ludlow JB, May K: Timed aperture computed tomography and detection of recurrent caries. *Caries Res*: 1998;32:23.

98. Natkin E, Oswald RJ, Carnes LI: The relationship of lesion size of diagnosis, incidence and treatment of periapical cysts and granulomas. *O Surg, O Med, O Path* 1984;57:82.

99. Noffke CEE, Ranbenheimer EJ, Chabikuli NJ: Odontogenic Myxoma : Review of the literature and report of 30 cases from South Africa. *O Surg, O Med, O Path* 2007;104:101.

100. O'Brien, JE, Stout AP: Malignant fibrous xanthomas. *Cancer* 1964;17:1445.

101. Paissat DK: Oral submucous fibrosis. *Int J Oral Surg* 1981;10:307.

102. Phillips JR: Apical root resorption under orthodontic therapy. *Angle Orthodont* 1955;20: 1.

103. Pindborg JJ, Reibel J, Roed Petersen B, Mehta, FS: Tobacco induced changed in oral leukoplakic epithelium. *Cancer* , 1980;45:2330.

104. Potdar GG: Ewing's tumors of the jaws. *Oral Surg* 1970;29:505.

105. Poyton HG, Davey KW: Thalassemia: Changes visible in radiographs used in dentistry. *O Surg, O Med, O Path* 1968;25:564.

106. Priebe WA: The value of roentgenographic film in the differential diagnosis of periapical lesions. *O Surg, O Med, O Path* 1954;7:979.

16

107. Rabinowitch BZ: Internal resorption. *O Surg, O Med, O Path* 1972;33:263.

108. Regezi JA, Batsakis JG, Courtney RM: Granular cell tumors of the head and neck. *J Oral Surg*: 1979;37:402.

109. Regezi JA, Kerr DA, Courtney RM: Odontogenic tumors: An analysis of 109 cases. *J Oral Surg*: 1978;36:771.

110. Robinson M, Slavkin HC: Dental amputation neuromas. *JADA* 1965;70:662.

111. Rudolphy G, Loveren C, Van Amerongen, JP: Validity of radiographs for diagnosis of secondary caries in teeth with class II Amalgam restoration in vitro. *Caries Res* 1997;31:34.

112. Rudolphy MP, Van Amerongen JP, Tencate, JM: Grey discoloration and marginal fracture for the diagnosis of secondary caries in molars with occlusal amalgam restorations. An in vitro study. *Caries Res* 1995;24:371.

113. Sapone J, Hensen L: Traumatic bone cysts of the jaws, diagnosis treatment and prognosis. *O Surg, O Med, O Path*: 1974;38:127.

114. Schwartz S, and Shklar G: Reaction of alveolar bone to invasion of oral carcinomas. *O Surg, O Med, O Path*: 1967;24:33.

115. Selzer S, Bender IB, Smith J: Endodontic failures: An analysis based on clinical, roentgenographic and histologic findings. *O Surg, O Med, O Path*: 1967;23:500.

116. Sepheriadou-Mavpoulou T, Patrikiou A, Sotiriadou S: Central odontogenic fibroma. *Int J Oral Surg* 1985;14:550.

117. Shafer WG: Oral carcinoma in situ. *Oral Surg* 1975;39:227.

118. Sharp GS: Cancer of the oral cavity. *Oral Surg* 1948;1:614.

119. Shear M: Erythroplakia of the mouth. *IDJ* 1972;22:460.

120. Shklar G, Meyer I: Giant cell tumors of the mandible and maxilla. *Oral Surg* 1961;14:809.

121. Shootweg PJ, Muller H: Differential diagnosis of fibro-osseous jaw lesions: A histological investigation on 30 cases. *J Craniomaxillofac Surg* 1990;18:210.

122. Shrout KM, Hildebolt EC: Differentiation of periapical and radicular cysts by digital radiometric analysis. *O Surg, O Med, O Path*: 1993;76:356.

123. Sikri Vimal and Sikri, Poonam: Clinical and radiological examination of root surface caries: An in vitro study. *IJDR*: 1, Jan.-June, 1991.

124. Silverman S, Ware W, Gillody C: Dental aspects of hyperparathyroidism. *O Surg, O Med, O Path*: 1968;26:184.

125. Simon ENM, Merkx MAW, Vuhahula E, Ngassapa D, Stoelinga PJW: Odontogenic myxoma : a clinicopathological study of 33 cases. *Int J Maxillofac Surg* 2004;33:333.

126. Simon JHS: Incidence of periapical cysts in relation to the root canals. *J Endo* 1980;6:845.

127. Simpson HE: Internal resorption. *J Can Dent Assoc* 1964;30:355.

128. Smith JB: Cancer of the floor of the mouth. *J Oral Surg*. 1948;6:106.

129. Spouge, J.D. : Odontogenic tumors, a Unitarian concept. *Oral Surg* : 1967;24:392.

130. Stafne EC, Gibilisco JA: Oral Roentgenographic Diagnosis, Philadelphia, W.B. Saunders, 1975;149.

131. Stiff R, Lally R: Cliedocranial dysostosis. *O Surg, O Med, O Path*: 1969;27:202.

132. Stroncek GG, Acervedo A, Hiza LH: A typical odontogenic adenomatoid tumor, review of literature. *J Oral Med* 1981;36:102.

133. Struthers P, Shear M: Root resorption by ameloblastoma and cysts of the jaws. *Int J Oral Surg* 1976;5:128.

134. Summers CJ: Prevalence of tori. *J Oral Surg* 1968;26:718.

135. Syriopoulos K, Sanderink GC, Velders XL, Vanderstelt PF: Radiographic detection of approximal caries: A comparison of dental films and digital imaging systems. *Dentomaxillofacial Radiol* 2000;29:312.

136. Syrjanen S, Tammisalo E, Lilija R, Syrjanen K. Radiological interpretation of the periapical cysts and granulomas. *Dentomaxillofac. Radiol* 1968;11:89.

137. Takeda Y, Kudo K: Adenomatoid odontogenic tumor associated with calcifying epithelial odontogenic tumor. *Int J Oral Max Surg*: 1986;15: 469.

138. Tamse A, Littner MM, Kaffe I: Roentgenographic features of external root resorption in the permanent dentition. *Quint Int*: 1984;13:51.

139. Tsiklakis K, Syriopoulos K, Stamatakis HC: Radiogrpahic examination of the temporo-mandibular joint using cone-beam computed tomography. *Dentomaxillofac Radiol* 2004;33:196.

140. Van Daatselaar AN, Tyndall DA, Vandor Stelt PF: Detection of caries with local CT. *Dentomaxillofac Radiol* 2003;32:235.

16

141. Vandenberghe B, Jacob R, Yang J: Diagnostic validity (acuity) of 2D CCD versus 3D CBCT images for assessing periodontal breakdown. *O Surg, O Med, O Path* 2007;104, 395.

142. Walton RE, Michelich RJ, Smith GN: The histopathogenesis of vertical root fracture. *J Endo* 1984;10:48.

143. Weathers DR, Callihan, MD: Giant cell fibroma. *Oral Surg* 1974;37:374.

144. Welbury RR: Congenital epulis of the newborn. *Br J Oral Surg* 1980;18:238.

145. Wenzel A: Digital imaging for dental caries. *Dental Cl North America* 2000;44:319.

146. Wenzel A, Fejerskov O: Validity of diagnosis of questionable carious lesions in occlusal surfaces of extracted third molars. *Caries Res* 1992;26:188.

147. Wenzel A, Haiter N: Influence of spatial resolution and bit depth on detection of small caries lesions with digital receptors. *O Surg, O Med, O Path*: 2007;103:418.

148. Wenzel A, Larsen Hintze H, Mikkelsen L, Mouyen F: Radiographic detection of occlusal caries in non-cavitated teeth. A comparison of conventional film radiographs, digitized film radiographs and Radiovisiography. *O Surg, O Med, O Path* 1991;72:621.

149. Wenzel A, Larsen MJ, Fejerskov O: Detection of occlusal caries without cavitation by visual inspection, film radiographs, xeroradiographs and digitized radiographs. *Caries Res* 1991;25:365.

150. West RK: Differential diagnosis of abnormal dental radio-opacities. *JADA* 1956;54:271.

151. White SC: Computer aided differential diagnosis of oral radiographic lesion. *Dentomaxillofacial Radiol* 1989;18:53.

152. White SC, Yoon DC: Comparative performance of digital and conventional images for detecting proximal surface caries. *Dentomaxillofacial Radiol* 1997;26:32.

153. Wilcox IR, Walton RE: A case of mistaken identity : Periapical cemental dysplasia in endodontically treated teeth. *Endo Dent Trauma.* 1989;5:298.

154. Witkop RE, Michelich RJ, Smith GN: The histopathogenesis of vertical root fracture. *J Endo* 1984;10:48.

155. Wood NK, Goaz PW: Differential diagnosis of oral lesions. 45th ed. St. Louis: Mosby Year Book, 1991;393.

156. Young AH: Ameloblastic fibroma in an infant. *J Oral Max Surg*: 1985;43:289.

157. Zachariades N, Papanicolaous S, Xypolyta A: Cherubism. *Int J Oral Surg* 1985;14:138.

158. Zamir J, Fisher D, Sharav Y: A longitudinal radiographic study of the rate of spread of human approximal caries. *Arch Oral Bio* 1976;21: 523.

159. Zegarelli DJ, Zegarelli-Schmidt EC, Zegarelli EV: Verruciform xanthoma. *Oral Surg* 1974;38: 725.

16

G

Glossary

Abscess: A localised pus formation often accompanied by swelling and pain. In dentistry, a periapical abscess is usually located near the apex of the root of the infected tooth and may be chronic or acute. Appears radiolucent when large enough to be visible on a radiograph.

Absorption: The process through which radiation imparts some or all of its energy to any material through which it passes.

Absorbed dose: It is the energy imparted to matter by ionising particles per unit of the mass of irradiated matter at the place of interest. Unit of absorbed dose is RAD (Radiation Absorbed Dose).

Acidifier: A chemical (acetic acid) in the fixer solution that neutralizes the alkali in the developer solution and stops further action of the developer.

Acoustic meatus: The opening at the centre of the ear. It is a part of the temporal bone and appears on extra oral radiograph as a small radiolucent circle.

Activator: A chemical in the developer (usually Na_2CO_3) solution that cause the emulsion on the radiograph film to swell and initiates the reducing action of the developing agents. It makes the developer alkaline.

Acute: Having a rapid onset, short severe course and pronounced symptoms.

Acute radiation syndrome: Symptoms of short term radiation effect, after a massive dose of ionising radiation.

Adamantinoma: (Ameloblastoma) It is a tumor of the jaw especially the mandible, arising from enamel forming cells. May be partly cystic, partly solid and may reach a large size.

It is usually benign or may be low grade malignant. It may be unilocular or multilocular. If multilocular, may give honeycomb or soap bubble appearance.

Ala: The wing of the nose. In dental radiography, the depression at which the nostrils connects the cheek.

Ala-tragus line: An imaginary line or plane from the ala of the nose to the tragus of the ear (the cartilagenous projection in front of the acoustic meatus of the ear).

The plane is important in determining the correct position of the patient's head while using the bisecting technique.

Alpha particles: A form of particulate radiation. It contains two protons and two neutrons and is positively charged. Symbol (α).

Alternating current: A current in which there is a flow of electrons in one direction followed by a flow in the opposite direction alternatively.

Alveolar bone: That portion of maxillary and mandibular bone that surrounds and supports the roots of dentition.

G

Alveolar process: That portion of maxillae/mandible that immediately surrounds and supports the roots of the teeth and appears radiopaque in a radiograph.

Ammeter: An instrument calibrated in amperes that measures the electric current.

Ampere: Unit of intensity of electric current which is produced by one volt acting through a resistance of one Ohm.

Angstrom unit: A unit of measurement that describes the wave lengths of certain high frequency radiations.

One angstrom unit measures 10^{-10} of a meter.

Angulation: The direction in which the central rays and the Position Indicating Device of the X-ray machine are directed in relation to the plane of object and the film.

Anode: The positive electrode in a X-ray tube.

Anodontia: Congenital absence of teeth. Any tooth in dental arch may fail to develop. The most probable conditions are the absence of the third molars, the premolars and the maxillary lateral incisors.

Anterior nasal spine: The most anterior point on the floor of the nasal cavity. The point is located in the midsagittal plane.

Artefact: Any structure or feature produced by the technique used, not occurring naturally, presenting itself on the radiograph as an abnormal condition.

Atom: The smallest particle of an element that has the properties of that element. Atoms are extremely minute and are made up of a number of a subatomic particles (protons, electrons, neutrons).

Atomic number: Number of protons in the nucleus of an atom. It determines the number of electrons, their management and the physical and chemical properties of the substance (element).

Atomic weight: The relative weight of an atom as compared with the standard carbon atom isotope with a mass of 12. Therefore, carbon has an atomic weight of 12.

Oxygen - 16, hydrogen - 1.008, nitrogen - 14.008.

Autotransformer: A voltage compensator that corrects minor fluctuations in alternating current flowing through the X-ray machine. It consists of a wire wound around the soft iron core. Having primary and secondary coil for input and output currents respectively.

Background radiations: Ionising radiations that are always present. It consists of cosmic rays from outer space, naturally occurring radiation from the earth and materials around us. It excludes radiations from X-ray generator or any other radiation generating device. Also called natural radiations.

Beta radiations: A form of particulate radiations consisting of high speed negative electrons. Symbol - β.

Binding energy: The internal energy within an atom that holds its components together. It is equal to the energy required to dissociate various components, i.e. protons and neutrons.

Bisecting technique: An exposure technique in which the central beam of radiations is directed perpendicularly towards an imaginary line which bisects the angle formed by the recording plane of the film and the long axis of the tooth.

Bisector: The imaginary line that bisects the angle formed by the film and tooth (see bisecting technique).

Bite block: A small device usually made of plastic, styrofoam or wood that can be inserted between the teeth and held in place by biting pressure. It functions to hold the X-ray film in position while it is being exposed.

Bitewing radiograph: A radiograph that shows the crowns of both the upper and lower teeth on the same film. The wing of the film is clenched in the teeth such that the film is in the occlusal plane.

Buccal object rule: (see Clark's rule).

Cancellous bone: It is a bone having a reticular or latticework structure as the spongy tissue of the bone.

Cassette: A rigid film holder consisting of a light tight case with a hinged lid at the back side. The front side is kept facing the source of radiation.

Cassette holder: The part of a panoramic type of X-ray machine that holds the cassette steady while exposure.

G

Cathode: The negative electrode terminal in the X-ray tube. The cathode consists of a tungsten filament wire that is set in a molybdenum focusing cup that directs the cathode stream on the target on the anode.

Cathode streams: The streams of thermionically emitted electrons travelling from the heated filament of the cathode towards the target on the anode in the X-ray tube.

Cephalometer: A device used to orient or position the head of the patient for radiographic examination.

Cephalostat: A head-holder or precision instrument used to stabilize the patient's head during exposure. It holds the head parallel to the film and at right angles to the radiation beam (Gnathostat - used for jaws).

Central beam: The central portion of primary beam of radiation which is parallel to the long axis of the tube, also known as central ray.

Cephalometric radiographs: Lateral and postero anterior extra oral head films. More often used in orthodontic treatment.

Cervical burn out: A radiolucency often observed on the mesial and distal root surfaces near the cementoenamel junction. The radiolucent appearance is caused by the concave shape of the root at the cervical line and is frequently mistaken for caries when diagnostic radiographs are analyzed.

Charge couple device: It is a digital image receptor for intraoral imaging composed of light or X-ray sensitive array of semiconductors on a silicon chip.

Clark's rule: A rule for the orientation of structures portrayed in two or more radiographs exposed at different angles. Accordingly the object nearer to the source of radiation moves in an opposite direction to the direction in which the source is shifted.

Collimation: The restriction of the useful beam to an appropriate size and shape (generally to a diameter of 2-3/4 inch (7 cm) at the skin surface in round collimators).

Collimator: The diaphragm or tubular device of an X-ray machine usually made of lead, designed to restrict the dimensions of the useful beam.

Cone: A cone or cylindrical position indicating device (PID) is used to indicate the direction of the central beam of radiation. The length of the cone helps to establish the desired target source distance.

Cone beam computed tomography: It is a device with a two-dimensional director, which generates a scan of the entire region of interest as compared to conventional CT scanners whose multiple 'slices' must be stacked to obtain a complete image.

Contrast: The visual differences between shades ranging from black to white in adjacent areas of radiographic film. Generally, the use of increased kilovoltage results in the production of a radiograph with long gray scale contrast.

Control panel: The portion of X-ray machine which houses the major controls allowing the operator to stand away from the machine.

Corpuscular radiation: These are radiations constituted of minute subatomic particles such as protons, electrons and neutrons also α and β particles. These particles occupy space, have mass and weight and with exception of neutrons also have an electrical charge.

Cross-sectional technique: A technique used in occlusal radiography in which central ray is directed towards the area of interest and parallel to the long axis of the teeth and adjacent areas.

Cyst: A closed sac or pouch with a definite lining, that contains fluid or semifluid material lined by epithelium.

If filled with fluid or fibrous material, a cyst appears radiolucent on a radiograph when present in the bone.

Density: In radiography, it is the film blackening (it is the amount of light transmitted through a film). The simplest way to increase or decrease the density of a radiograph is to increase or decrease the milliamperage or exposure time.

Developer: The chemical solution used in film processing that makes the latent image visible by reducing the silver ions to silver atoms.

Developing agent: Substances like elon and hydroquinone that reduce the halides in the film emulsion to metallic silver. Elon brings out the details and hydroquinone brings out the contrast in the film.

G

Diagnosis: The art of differentiating or determining the nature of a problem or disease. Dental radiographs are an important factor in evaluating the dental condition of the patient and help in finalizing the diagnosis by being an adjunct to it.

Diaphragm: In radiology, a plate usually of lead with a central aperture so placed as to define the useful beam in terms of shape and also to reduce the scattered radiation.

Digital radiography: It is electronic dental imaging or filmless radiography. It produces a dynamic image in which visual characteristic of density and contrast can be manipulated for specific diagnostic and treatment requirements.

Digital subtraction radiograph: It is an image enhancement method that removes the structure noise from the images.

Direct current: Electric current that flows continuously in one direction.

Dosage: The radiation delivered to a specified area of the body measured in rads(R).

Dose: The amount of absorbed radiation in rads at any given point.

Dose rate: The radiation dose received per unit of time.

Dosimeter: A small device, usually the size of a fountain pen used to measure radiation. This device contains a small ionizing chamber and an electrometer that can be read by the person wearing the dosimeter.

Duplicating film: A photographic film that appears similar to X-ray film and is used to duplicate X-ray films in a contact printer type X-ray duplicating unit.

Edentulous survey: Radiographic examination of a patient without teeth for assessing the patient for dentures.

Electrical potential: In radiography and electricity, the difference in relative voltage or amount of electric charge between the negative and positive electrodes.

Electrode: Either of two terminals of an electric current, in the X-ray tube, either the anode or the cathode.

Electromagnetic radiation: Form of energy propelled by wave motion as photons of energy.

This is a combination of electric and magnetic energy.

Electromagnetic spectrum: Types of electromagnetic energies arranged in diagrammatic form as a continuous range. These include radio and television waves, infrared waves, visible light, ultraviolet waves, roentgen rays, gamma rays and cosmic radiations.

Electromotive force: The difference in potential between cathode and the anode in the X-ray tube which accounts for the speed of flow of electrons.

Electron: A small negatively charged particle of the atom continuously revolving around the positively charged nucleus.

Element: A substance that cannot be decomposed by chemical means and that is made up of atoms that are alike in their peripheral electronic configuration but may differ in their nuclei, atomic weight or radioactive properties.

Elongation: A term used in radiography to refer to a distortion of the image in which the object appears longer than the anatomical size (usually when the radiation are directed acutely to the long axis of the object).

Emulsion: The coating on radiographic film of a gelatinous solution containing silver halides.

Energy: The ability to do work and overcome resistance. In radiography the force that propels the electrons and enables them to penetrate the materials in their path.

Enhancement: Intensification of detail, making a radiograph easier to interpret.

Exposure: A measure of ionisation produced in air by gamma or α-radiations.

Exposure rate: The exposure of an object by radiations per unit time.

Filament: The spiral tungsten coil in the focusing cup of the cathode of the X-ray tube.

Film badge: A device containing a special type of film, worn by persons frequently exposed to radiations. When developed and interpreted, it gives an accurate measurement of the exposure to harmful radiation during the time the badge was worn.

Film holder: A mechanical device used to hold and stabilize dental X-ray in the mouth. It is usually made of plastic. Mason film holder is made of wooden block.

Film packets: The intraoral film that is wrapped and enclosed for dental use by the manufacturer. It contains one or two films with a dark protective paper on either side of the film and a thin sheet of foil on the back with a semimoisture proof outer wrapping.

Film placement: The act of positioning the film packet in the patient's mouth.

Filter: Absorbing material, usually aluminium, placed in the path of the beam of radiation to remove less penetrable X-rays.

Filtration: The use of radiation absorbing materials for selectively attenuating or screening out the low energy X-ray from the primary beam of X-radiations.

Fixer: In radiography or photography a solution of chemicals that stops the action of the developer and makes the image permanently visible.

Fixing agent: Sodium thiosulfate, also known as 'Hypo'. It is one of the several chemical ingredients of the fixer whose function is to remove all the unexposed and/or undeveloped silver bromide grains from the solution.

Fluorescence: The emission of a glowing light by certain mineral salts when they are struck by radiation of particular wavelengths. In radiography, calcium tungstate present in the emulsion of the intensifying screen of cassettes glows and gives off a bluish green light when the crystals are struck by the X-ray photons.

Focal spot: A small area on the target of the anode towards which the electrons from the focusing cup of the cathode are directed in the X-ray tube. X-radiations originate at the focal spot.

Focal trough: A term describing that area of the dental anatomy that is reproduced distinctly on a panoramic radiograph.

Focusing cup: A cup shaped depression in the face of the cathode that contains the tungsten filament. This is designed to project the free electrons towards the tungsten target of the anode.

Fog: A cloudy appearance of the finished radiograph caused by any of several factors such as, old or contaminated processing solution, exposure to chemical fumes, faulty safelighting or scattered radiations.

Fore shortening: A term used in radiography to refer to a distortion of the image in which the object appears shorter than their actual anatomic size. This is most often caused by excessive vertical angulation of the central X-ray beam.

Frankfurt's plane (Auriculo-orbital plane): A term used in cephalometric radiography to designate the horizontal plane between porion (lowest point on the margin of the orbit) and the orbitale (highest point on the margin of the auditory meatus).

Frequency: The number of crests of a wavelength passing a given point per second. The higher the frequency, shorter is the wavelength.

Gamma rays: A form of electromagnetic radiation with properties similar to X-rays. Usually produced spontaneously in the form of emission from radioactive substances. It consists of high energy photons having mass or charge.

Gene mutation: The alteration produced in genes which renders the cells to function permanently in a manner different from that prior to the alteration.

Genes: The fundamental units of inheritance arranged on the chromosomes which carry the individual traits of the organism.

Gene mutant: An altered gene that functions permanently in a manner different from that prior to the alteration.

Grid: A device made of parallel lead pieces used to screen scattered radiation while taking radiographs.

Half life: The period required for the disintegration of half of the atoms in a sample of any specific radioactive substance is called the half life of that substance.

Half value layer: The thickness of a specified substance that when introduced into the path of a given beam of radiation, reduces the exposure rate by half.

Hardening agent: Potassium alum, one of the chemicals of the fixing solution. It functions to shrink and harden the wet emulsion.

Hanging drop appearance: A radiographic feature seen in case of fractures of the floor of the orbit

G

when the tissues in the eye socket bulge into the maxillary sinus giving an illusion of a hanging drop.

Hard radiations: Rays of high energy and extremely short wavelengths. Essential for dental radiography.

Horizontal angulation: The direction of the central beam in a horizontal plane. Faulty horizontal angulation is the main cause of overlapping of the proximal structure during exposure.

Image: In radiography, the appearance of outline form of the structure exposed to radiation. A latent (invisible) image forms on the film when it is exposed. This latent image becomes visible after developing and final processing of the film.

Impulse: In radiography a measure of exposure time.

Incandescence: In radiography the stage in which the tungsten filament in the cathode becomes red hot and begins to glow, thus liberating free electrons that swarm around the glowing wire to form the electron cloud.

Intensifying screen: A card or plastic sheet coated with calcium tungstate or similar fluorescent crystals and positioned in the cassette so that it intimately contacts the film. When exposed to radiation, the fluorescent crystals glow, giving off a blue or green light that along with the radiations causes the latent image to form faster than is possible when radiations alone are used and hence reduce the exposure time by 10–40 times.

Interpretation: In radiography the ability to read what is revealed by the radiograph is called interpretation.

Intraoral radiograph: A radiograph produced when the film is placed within the mouth and exposed. It is of three types - Periapical, bite-wing and occlusal.

Inverse square law: A rule stating that the intensity of radiations is inversely proportional to the square of the distance between the source of the radiation and the point of measurement.

Ion: An electrically charged particle from an atom or a molecule which is formed due to the loss or gain of electrons or protons.

Ionization: The change that takes place within an atom when electrons or protons are gained or

lost from the atom. The atom loses its neutrality and becomes either positively or negatively charged.

Ionizing radiations: Radiation that is capable of producing ions when passed through a material by the process of ionization.

Irradiation: The exposure of an object or a person to radiation.

Isotope: An alternate form of an element having the same number of protons but different number of neutrons inside the nucleus. Thereby, having a difference in the atomic weight and the properties.

Kilovolt: A unit of electromotive force equal to 1000 volts, that drives the electric current through the circuit. High voltage is necessary for the production of X-rays by the resultant increase in the speed of electrons being emitted thermionically. Kilovoltage affects the quality of the X-rays.

Kilovolt peak: The crest value in kilovolts of the potential difference of a pulsating potential generator (kVp).

Lamina dura: A thin, hard layer of cortical bone (bundle bone) that lines the dental alveolus. It appears as a thin radiopaque line around the roots of the teeth on a dental radiograph.

Landmarks: In dental radiography this term refers to specific positions or points located on the hard or soft tissues of the head, face or oral cavity. The landmarks help in the projection of X-rays and also in the interpretation of radiographs.

Latent image: The invisible image produced when the film is exposed to X-rays. The image remains invisible until the film is processed.

Latent period: The time between exposure of a living being to radiation and the first clinically observable symptoms in the subject.

Latent radiograph: Extraoral film placed against either side of head and parallel to it. Used extensively in cephalometric radiography.

Lead protective apron: Apron made of lead or equivalent materials. It covers the patient's body to protect them from radiations, specially the gonadal areas.

Leakage radiation: The X-rays that escape out of the tube head at places other than the aperture.

These radiations should be checked because the operator is at a risk of overexposure due to these X-rays.

Lethal dose: The amount of radiation that will be or could be sufficient to cause the death of an organism.

Light fog: Clouding or darkening of radiographic film through accidental exposure to bright light or prolonged exposure to a safelight.

Maximum permissible dose: The maximum dose that a person or specified parts are allowed to receive in a stated period of time.

Mandibular plane: The term used in cephalometric radiography designating the line joining the gonion to the menton along the inferior border of the mandible.

Menton: A term used in cephalometric radiography to describe the lowest point on the contour of the mandibular symphysis.

Macromolecules: A very large molecule constructed from many smaller organic building blocks of molecules linked together by repetitive formation of covalent bonds and constructed into polymeric chain structures.

Magnetic resonance imaging (MRI): When certain atomic nuclei with an odd number of protons or neutrons or both are subjected to a strong magnetic field, they absorb and re-emit electromagnetic radiations. The analysis of the net magnetization vector's deflection provides the image information when radiofrequency pulses are provided.

Magnifications: Specific techniques used to purposefully magnify the radiographic image so as to make accurate assessment or measurements. It is of special use in implantology and caries assessment.

Markers: These are metallic pieces placed in the splint which is placed in the mouth before taking the radiograph. These act as guides for selecting the sites for cross-sectional tomographs.

Mach band: Shadow frequently apparent on the images of unaffected teeth below or above the occlusal enamel. It is an optical illusion liable to be confused with incipient caries.

Manual processing: Conventional method of developing the radiograph in which the exposed film is passed through various procedures of developing and fixing by the radiographer himself.

Mean active bone marrow dose: It is that dose of radiation averaged over the entire bone marrow related to a particular stochastic effect (Leukemia).

Milliampere: Unit of measurement of current flowing through a circuit. It is one thousandth of an ampere (mA).

MilliSievert: It is a unit of equivalent dose which is a measure of biologic effect of different radiations to a tissue or organ.

Monitoring devices: In radiation, the use of any of several devices to determine whether an area is within safe radiation limits or whether a person's exposure is within permissible limits.

Mounting: It is procedure of clipping the exposed films on to the hangers during the process of developing. The film positions are labelled with patients name to avoid any further confusion. Also it is a procedure of storage of exposed film in a film mount which helps in proper preservation, maintenance and handling of radiographs in a most satisfactory manner.

Monochromatic beam: Beam of radiations pertaining to or located within a single wavelength in a spectrum.

Mottled: A radiographic feature showing scattered regions of radiolucency or radioopacity characteristic of certain diseases or a term describing the appearance of poorly defined aggregates of small spicules of bone distributed throughout a radiolucent area.

Mutation: A change in the hereditary pattern due to permanent change in genetic material, usually restricted to change in a single gene but sometimes is used for any structural chromosomal exchange. It includes a loss or gain or exchange of genetic material.

Multilocular: Term describing a lesion that appears to be formed of multiple adjacent compartments within the bone.

G

Nasion: In cephalometric radiography, the most anterior point of the frontonasal suture in the midsagittal plane.

Negative: A photographic or radiographic film wherein light and dark areas of the subject are shown in reverse.

Negative angulation: Angulation achieved by pointing the tip or end of the tube upward from a horizontal plane. In the bisecting technique, negative angulation is used to make all mandibular exposures.

Negative ion: An ion that has a negative electric charge after gaining a surplus electron.

Neutron: One form of corpuscular radiation or subatomic particle. A neutron has no electric charge and has about the same mass as a proton. It is a constituent of the nucleus of an atom.

Nuclear medicine: It is method of assessing the metabolic status of the tissue of the body by induction of radionuclide labelled compounds or elements (traces). The basis is that the body is immune to detect the radioactive nature of material which aggregates at sites proportional to their metabolic activities. Subsequent radiographs reveal the site of aggregation.

Object: In radiography whatever tissue is being radiographed is object

Object film distance: It is the distance between the tissues to be radiographed and the film.

Occipitomental skull projection: see waters projection

Onion skin appearance (e.g. proliferative periosteitis): Formation of periosteal new bone in layers. When the growth of a lesion is slow, the body's response manifests itself in the form of bony layers.

Opacity: The state or quality of being impenetrable to X-rays.

Orange peel appearance: Radiographic pattern produced by many closely arranged, fine trabaculae. Also called 'ground glass', 'orange peel', or 'salt pepper' appearance. Used to describe the radiographic appearance of fibrous dysplasia, hyperparathyroidism and other diseases affecting the bone.

Orbitale: In cephalometric radiography the lowest point on the rim of the bony orbit.

Overexposure: When the exposure time is more than optimum for a specific film, it results in a dim radiograph and the film is said to be overexposed.

Overlapping: A term used in radiography to refer to a distortion of the tooth image in which the structures of one tooth are superimposed on the structures of the adjacent tooth. This is most often caused by faulty horizontal angulation of the central beam. It can also be seen in cases of overcrowding of the teeth.

Overdevelopment: Reduction of unexposed crystals by the developing solution due to prolonged immersion of the film in the developing solution leading to production of chemical fog on the film is known as overdevelopment.

Oxidation: In radiography the process during which the chemicals of the developing or fixing solutions combine with oxygen and lose their strength.

Oxidising agent: Any substance that produces oxidation in another substance.

Pantomography: A method of tomography for visualization of curved surfaces at any depth. In dentistry it may be used for radiography of the maxillary and mandibular dental arches and their associated structures (panoramic radiography).

Proton: A positively charged fundamental particle of the atom which has a mass approx. equal to that of the nucleus of a hydrogen atom (1.7×19^{-27} kg), about 140 times of an electron, and positive charge of 1.6×10^{-19} coulomb. It is constituent of all nuclei.

Photon: A unit of quantum of electromagnetic energy which has no mass or electric charge but has an effective momentum.

Pogonion: A craniometric landmark denoting the most anterior point in the contour of chin in a sagittal plane.

Panorax: Trademark for a radiographic system that uses two axes of rotation to obtain a panoramic radiograph of dental arches and their associated structures.

Parallax: An apparent displacement of an object as seen from two differential points.

Phlebolith: A calculus or concretion in a vein. It is a type of ectopic calcification.

G

Photostimulable phosphor (PSP): It is a digital image receptor for intraoral imaging made up of luminous substance (e.g. phosphor). On exposure to X-rays, energy from storage phosphor is released and the information pattern is converted into digital form.

Penumbra: Marginal sharpness or blurring, surrounding the true shadow of a radiographic image due to slight difference in the angles of X-rays that are projected on the object and the film from various points on the target.

Polychromatic radiation: Radiation exhibiting many colours or different wavelengths of radiations. Greater is the variation, lower is the quality of the radiograph.

Posteroanterior projection: It is so called because the X-rays pass in a posteroanterior direction from the skull. It is used to examine the skull for the presence of disease, trauma or any other developmental anomaly. It provides good visualization of facial structures including frontal and ethmoid sinuses, nasal fossae and orbits. Cassette is placed vertically in a holding device and the head is centered in front of the cassette with the canthomeatal line parallel to the floor.

Paralleling technique: When long axis of the film lies parallel to the long axis of the object upon tooth and the rays are directed perpendicular to either of the two, the image produced is of the same size as the object.

Panoramic radiography: It is a radiographic procedure that produces a single image of the facial structure including both maxillary and mandibular arches and their supporting structures.

Palatal shift: It is the outcome of parallax technique in which an object present palatally shifts along the direction of movement of source of radiation during two subsequent successive exposures. This technique is used to ascertain the palatofacial positioning of the two overlapping images.

Peripheral burnout: It is a result of physical phenomenon of diffraction as a result of which the peripheral region of a radiopaque object appears as a radiolucent region. In teeth it is often confused with caries.

Quantum: It is an elemental unit of energy according to the Quantum theory. The theory states that energy absorption and radiation is a discontinuous process in small amounts or units called quantum.

Quality control: A term used to describe series of tests to assume that the radiographic system is functioning properly and the radiographs produced are of an acceptable level of quality.

Quality assurance: It may be defined as any systematic action to assure that a dental office will produce consistantly high quality image with minimum exposure to patients and personnel.

RAD (Radiation Absorbed Dose): A unit of measurement of the absorbed dose of ionising radiations. It is equal to transfer of 100 grams of energy per gram of absorbing material.

Radiodontics: Dental radiology is also called radiodontics.

Radiotherapy: Treatment of a disease by ionising radiation. X-radiations are projected on diseases parts and in calculated dose.

Radiolucent: Pertaining to substances and materials that permit the passage of radiant energy such as X-rays. Radiolucent substances are adipose tissue, gas, air, etc. These appear dark on an exposed film.

Radiopaque: It pertains to the substance or material that resists or obstructs the passage of radiant energy such as X-rays, e.g. Bones, calcium containing tissues. These appear white on an exposed film.

Radiation caries: Patients who have received therapeutic radiation to the head and neck and consequently suffer the loss of salivary gland functions will demonstrate rampant destruction of teeth called rampant caries or radiation caries.

Radiolysis: A series of chemical changes that occur after exposure to ionising radiations is called radiolysis.

Rinsing: After developing a film, the emulsion gets swelled up and saturated with the developing chemicals. At this time film should be rinsed in water for 10–20 sec. before they are placed in the fixer. The rinse dilutes the developer and removes the alkali activator thus preventing the neutralization of the acid fixer.

G

Resolution: It is a measure of the visualisation of images of relatively small objects that are close together.

Restrainer: It is a component added to developing solution usually potassium bromide. Dissociation of potassium bromide results in the liberation of bromine ions which restrict the reduction of silver halide crystals because of a common ion effect thus acting as an antifogging agent.

Sequestrum: A piece of bone that has become separated during the process of necrosis from the surrounding healthy bone. Due to the absence of blood supply it easily gets infected and is a foci of pus formation.

Scattered radiations: The diffusion or deviation of X-rays produced by the medium through which it passes.

Shielding: Any protective structure used for preventing or reducing the passage of particle or radiation so as to avoid the harmful effects of radiations, e.g. lead protective apron.

Sialography: X-ray examination of salivary glands and ducts after injection of a radiopaque medium into the gland substance via the duct opening.

Sialolith: A calcareous concentration or calculus in salivary glands or its ducts involving most commonly the submandibular gland and seldom the minor salivary glands. It usually presents as a white yellowish stone composed mainly of calcium phosphate, carbonates, iron oxide, sodium chloride, Thiocyanide and magnesium compounds.

Shape distortion: It is a result of unequal magnification of different parts of the same object. It arises where two parts of an object are at a different distance from the focal point.

SLOB rule: It is an acronym often remembered conveniently for object localisation. If the object moves in the direction of the rotation of the X-ray tube, the object is located lingually. If the object moves distally on moving the tube mesially, then the object is on the buccal side. Then it is remembered as SLOB. Same lingual, opposite buccal. Also see Clarke's rule.

Submentovertex projection: It is used to demonstrate the base of the skull. It also reveals the position and orientation of condyles, sphenoid sinus, curvature of mandible, lateral wall of maxillary arch, the medial and the lateral pterygoid plates and foramina at the base of the skull. This projection is taken by placing the film cassette vertically in a holding device with the patient's head extended well forward so that the chin is in the centre of the cassette. The mid sagittal plane is kept perpendicular to the floor.

Supercoated films: An additional layer of gelatin is added as a supercoating on the film emulsion. This coating helps to protect the film from damage by scratching, contamination and pressure from the rollers when it is being processed in an automatic processor.

Sharpness: Sharpness is defined as the extent of clarity to which a radiograph will define a boundary between areas of different densities.

Snooke's hydrogen tube: It is exactly same as Crooke's tube but only difference is that in place of a mixture of gases only hydrogen is used. With increased hydrogen content the tube is called a hard tube and with decreased hydrogen content the tube is called a soft tube.

Soap bubble appearance: It is a radiographic appearance in which the compartments in the bone are separated by distinct septa that reach into the radiolucent area giving the appearance of a multilocular region/soap bubble appearance, e.g. Ameloblastoma, central giant cell granuloma.

Stochastic effects: Those effects which are dependent only on the dose for their occurrence and not dependent on the severity, e.g. radiation induced cancer.

Sun ray appearance: It is a production of sun ray image which is a result of a fast expanding lesion which resorbs the bone and carries along with it small pieces of bone arranged along the path of expansion of the lesion. It is typically seen in a sarcoma.

Step ladder appearance: It is a result of formation of coarse trabecular pattern resulting in large spaces. In between teeth only horizontal trabeculae are present thereby giving an illusion of a step ladder, e.g. sickle cell anemia.

Speed of film: It depends upon (i) duration of heating and temperature and (ii) grain size -

larger the grain the more sensitive the film. The speed of the film is designated by the alphabets ranging from A to F (slow to higher speed).

With an increase in the speed of film, exposure time is relatively decreased.

Tube shift technique: It is used to identify the spatial position of an object is called as the tube shift technique. The rationale of this procedure is demonstrated by the manner in which the relative position of radiographic images of two separate objects changes when the projection angles at which the images are made are changed (see SLOB).

Transformer: It is an electrical device used to increase or decrease the voltage. It is used to supply power to X-ray unit.

Target: It is a small block of tungsten embedded in the face of the anode which is bombarded by the electrons streaming towards it from the cathode.

Tube film distance: It is the distance from the target to the X-ray film or object. It greatly affects the intensity of the radiation and the subsequent quality of the radiograph.

Threshold dose: It is defined as the amount of radiations to the body above which the change begins to appear in the body to produce a detectable degree of any given effect.

Threshold erythema dose: That dose of radiation on the body which causes erythema on the skin.

Thermionic emission: When the tungsten filament becomes hot, it emits electrons which are separated from the outer orbit of tungsten atom at a rate proportional to its temperature by the process of thermionic emission.

Thermoluminescent dosimeter: Some materials have the property of emitting visible light when exposed to radiations. The emitted light is proportional to exposure to radiations. These are used for personal monitoring.

Transcranial view: It is done for the evaluation of TMJ problems. It depicts the changes in the articular surfaces of the TMJ in a lateral aspect. Closed mouth transcranial view is used for the evaluation of the position of the condyle in the mandibular fossa. Cassette and films are placed perpendicular to the floor. Head is positioned

in such a way that the ears, cheek and the temporal region touch the cassette.

Underdeveloped: It is a type of defect caused due to insufficient developing time, depleted developer or excessive fixation.

Underexposure: It is a type of defect produced due to improper exposure of the film to X-radiations. The defect manifests itself as insufficient contrast.

Ultraviolet radiation: These are a type of electromagnetic radiation having a wavelength of 400–420 nm and photon energy of 3.1–124eV.

Ultrasound: Diagnostic ultrasound examination uses a very high frequency (1.5–10 MHz) pulsed ultrasound beam which is directed to the body from a transducer placed in contact with the skin.

As it travels through the body some of it is reflected back by tissue interfaces to produce echoes which are picked up by the same transducer and then converted to an electrical signal. The electric signal is further converted into a visual echo picture image.

Ultra speed film: Speed E and F films are called the ultra speed films. With an increase in the speed of the film, the exposure time is decreased.

Vacuum: Space which contains neither air nor gas.

Voltage: A measure of electric charge (in volts) when moving between two points, e.g. voltage measured across cell membrane is approx. 90 millivolts.

Voltmeter: It is an instrument used to measure the electromotive force in volts.

Wavelength: The distance between one crest to the other is known as a wavelength. It is abbreviated with the Greek letter *lambda*.

Waters' projection/occipitomental projection: It is used for evaluation of the paranasal sinuses, orbit, frontozygomatic suture and the nasal cavity. It also demonstrates the position of coronoid processes of the mandible between the maxilla and the zygomatic arch. The projection is taken with the raised chin held against a vertical film such that canthomeatal line is elevated 37º above the horizontal.

Whole body radiations: When whole body of a mammal is exposed to low or moderate doses of radiations, it results in typical changes called as acute radiation syndrome.

Washing of film: After fixing, the film is washed with a sufficient amount of water for an adequate period of time to assure the removal of all processing chemicals that might affect the appearance and stability of the film.

Xeroradiography: A method which uses conventional X-ray equipments and positioning techniques but the film is replaced by an electrostatically charged selenium plate in a special cassette.

Zeugmatography: Also known as 'Nuclear Magnetic Resonance'. It is newer system in scan radiology with maximum potential for diagnosing tumors. It is still under budding stage of development.

Zonography: A type of tomography accomplished through narrow angle (less than 10°) and multidirectional movement of X-rays tubes. It is used for examination of structures that are at least several centimetres in thickness.

Index

I

Reader's Notes

Reader's Notes

Other Outstanding CBS Books in Dental Sciences

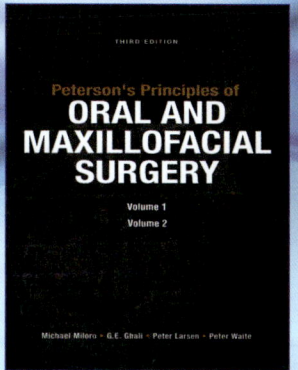

THIRD EDITION

Peterson's Principles of
ORAL AND MAXILLOFACIAL SURGERY

Volume 1
Volume 2

Michael Miloro • G.E. Ghali • Peter Larsen • Peter Waite

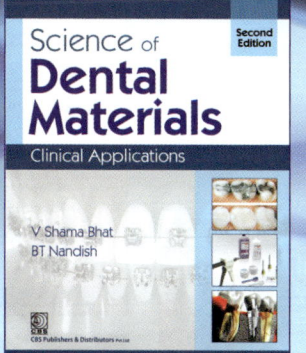

Science of
Dental Materials

Second Edition

Clinical Applications

V Shama Bhat
BT Nandish

CBS Publishers & Distributors Pvt Ltd

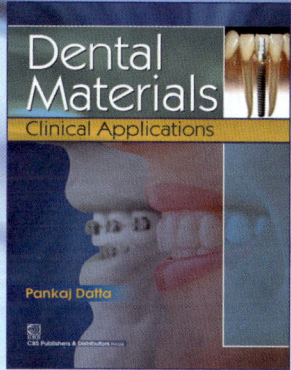

Dental Materials
Clinical Applications

Pankaj Datta

CBS Publishers & Distributors Pvt Ltd

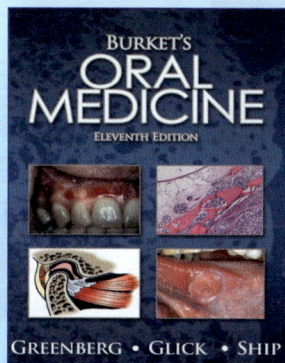

BURKET'S
ORAL MEDICINE

ELEVENTH EDITION

GREENBERG • GLICK • SHIP

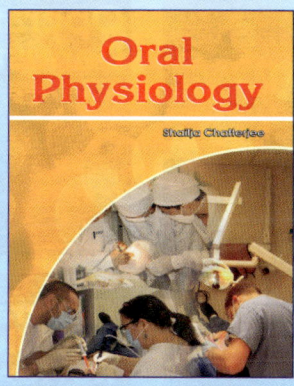

Oral Physiology

Shailja Chatterjee

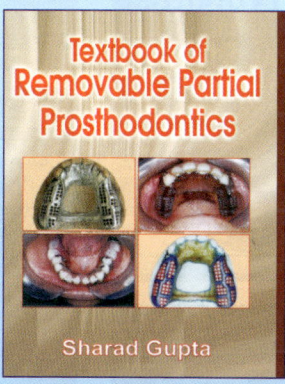

Textbook of Removable Partial Prosthodontics

Sharad Gupta

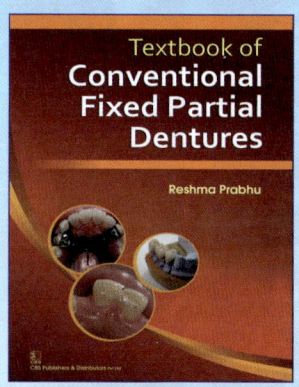

Textbook of
Conventional Fixed Partial Dentures

Reshma Prabhu

CBS Publishers & Distributors Pvt Ltd

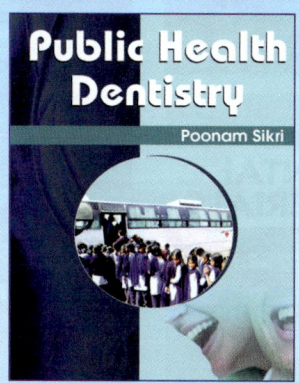

Public Health Dentistry

Poonam Sikri

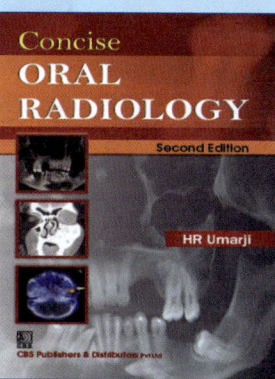

Concise
ORAL RADIOLOGY

Second Edition

HR Umarji

CBS Publishers & Distributors Pvt Ltd

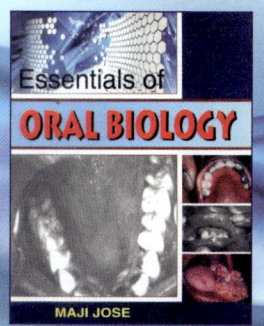

Essentials of
ORAL BIOLOGY

MAJI JOSE

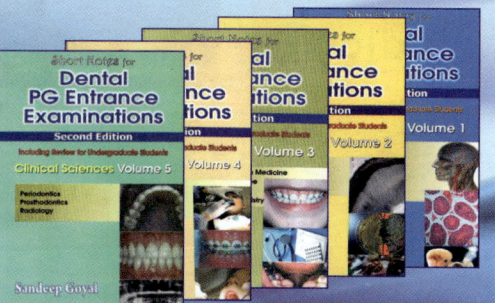

Short Notes for
Dental PG Entrance Examinations
Second Edition

Including Review for Undergraduate Students

Clinical Sciences Volume 5

Periodontics
Prosthodontics
Radiology

Volume 4

Volume 3

Volume 2

Volume 1

Sandeep Goyal

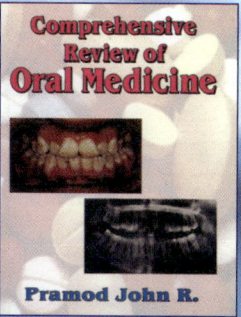

Comprehensive Review of Oral Medicine

Pramod John R.

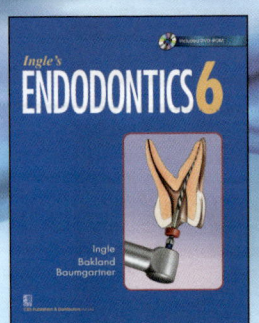

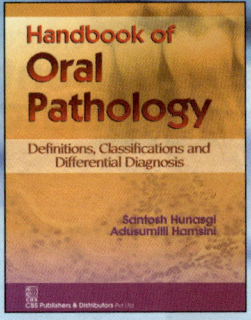

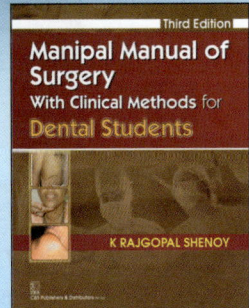

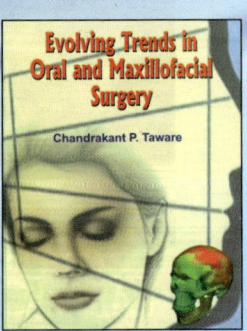

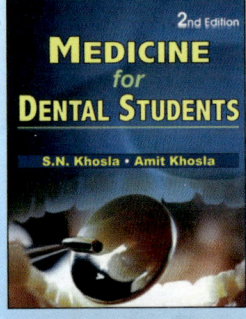

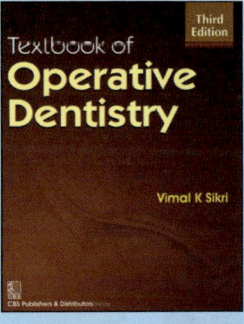

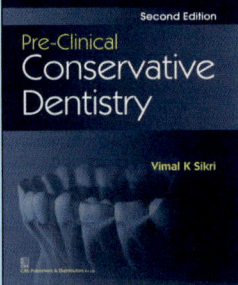

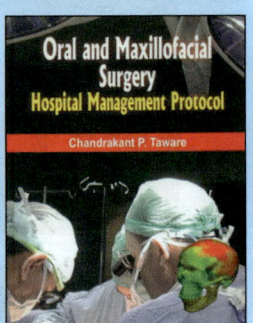

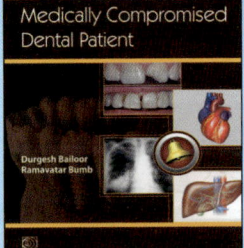

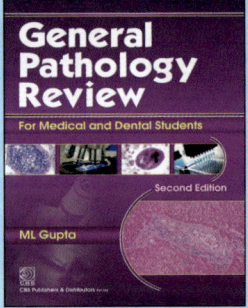

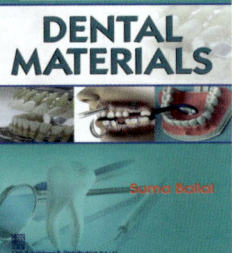

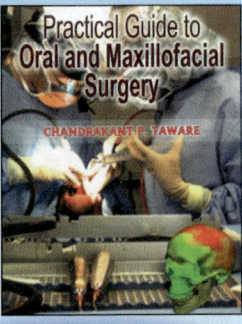

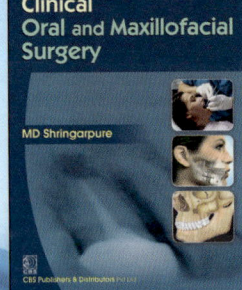

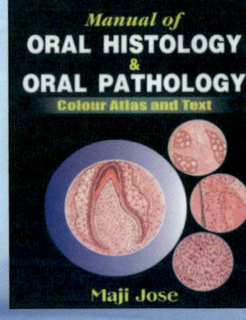

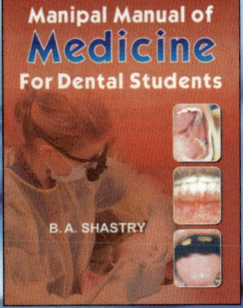

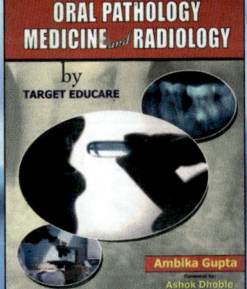